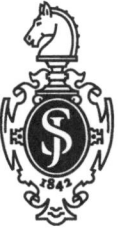

Springer-Verlag France S.A.R.L

Nathalie Bricout

Forewords by John Bostwick and Jean-Pierre Lalardrie

Breast surgery

With 610 drawings and photographs in black and white
and in color

Illustrations: Yves Morel, Nathalie Bricout

Springer-Verlag France S.A.R.L

Nathalie Bricout, MD
Plastic Surgeon
157, rue de l'Université
75007 Paris
France

ISBN 978-2-8178-0928-1   ISBN 978-2-8178-0926-7 (eBook)
DOI 10.1007/978-2-8178-0926-7

Based on: Nathalie Bricout: *Chirurgie du Sein*
© Springer-Verlag France, Paris, 1992

Translation by Dr David LeVay

© Springer-Verlag France, Paris, 1996
Softcover reprint of the hardcover 1st edition 1996

2918 / 543210 – Printed on acid-free paper

Contents

Forewords

The past twenty years has seen a remarkable growth and development of the field of aesthetic and reconstructive breast surgery. During this time, the focus of the management of breast cancer has changed from primarily radical ablation to consideration of aesthetics and psychology of breasts with conservative surgery and breast reconstruction. Plastic and reconstructive breast surgeons have responded to the patient's requests with a wide range of techniques for breast enlargement, reduction, lifting and reconstruction. Recent considerations have been the minimizing of scars, breast reconstruction with autogenous tissue and management of problems after lumpectomy-radiation.

It is to this setting that Dr. Nathalie Bricout brings us *Chirurgie du sein*. It is particularly valuable for an artistic teacher, sensitive of plastic and reconstructive surgery, to put together a comprehensive book on the subject. The student can get more from the text when there is a common thread of philosophy, a high level of artistry and care, excellent illustrations, and an honest and straight forward presentation of the results and discussion of complications.

The first chapter sets the tone for the book by bringing together the artistry and essentials of the normal breast with a detailed discussion of the vascular anatomy of the breast while including the history and appropriate citations in art history which reinforce the importance of the subject to artists throughout history. Dr. Bricout's experience with conservative surgery and radiation therapy is particularly valuable for plastic surgeons in countries where the technique is not yet popular. She presents guidelines for the excisions, and describes breast reconstruction after aesthetic and oncologic failures... usually with the need for autogenous tissue.

Her presentation of breast reduction is very comprehensive and is an excellent illustration of her versatility in several techniques. Of particular interest to me is her presentation of the techniques to minimize the scar to vertical, short horizontal as well as the periareolar pursestring mastopexy.

The chapters on breast reconstruction clearly present the highest level of artistry and aesthetic sensitivity. Surgeons interested in achieving excellent results with implants, tissue expanders, the latissimus dorsi flap and the T.R.A.M. flap should study these chapters. She presents the essential vascular anatomy and demonstrates the essential points for safe and aesthetically attractive breast reconstructions. Dr.Bricout has produced a benchmark text on surgery of the breast with a variety and range of techniques for excellent results in plastic and reconstructive breast surgery.

John Bostwick, M.D

Professor of Surgery and Chief of the Division of Plastic and Reconstructive
Surgery, Emory University School of Medicine, Atlanta, Ga.

To write today a book on the surgery of the breast that differs from the others, when so many works on this subject have recently been published, may seem to attempt the impossible.

These pages are evidence that it was necessary to do so, for they are manifestly the outcome of deep reflection and the fruit of long experience. In language accessible to both specialists and non-specialists, simple, clear and didactic, and thanks to illustrations which perfectly complement the text, all the problems posed by excisional surgery of the breast and its plastic and reconstructive surgery are analysed and dissected before forming the object of a synthetic view which is the only guarantee of intelligent surgical procedure.

The references to the past are limited to those necessary to the understanding of present-day ideas, supplemented by the informative account of a personal pilgrimage.

One is bound to be struck by the considerable space devoted to reconstruction of the breast. This is as it should be, since the different stages of such reconstruction embrace the entire plastic surgery of the breast. It is here that all the difficulties are displayed and every shade of meaning discussed.

These long compact chapters, every page of which is so authentic, must promote the awareness that the plastic surgery of the breast, especially its reconstructive surgery, is not a matter for improvisation. To obtain good results in this field, one must, with the modesty of the author, have studied greatly, considered greatly and worked greatly.

I would say in conclusion that my sole point of disagreement relates to the note in the foreword. It is my personal conviction that one can enjoy doing a disservice to the reader. The most recent texts and congresses are full of false notions on the surgery of the breast, full of erroneous assertions on the plastic surgery of the breast, which point readers or participants in directions that are to the ultimate detriment of the patients.

But here, all is sound, temperate and moderate. This book is a fine and a sound achievement.

Jean-Pierre Lalardrie, MD
Associate Professor of the Collège de Médecine des Hôpitaux de Paris,
Paris, France

Dedication
and acknowledgments

When I decided to write this book, the greatest difficulty was not that of starting it but of ever conceiving it as finished. A word-processor screen is less paralysing that the writer's famous blank sheet of paper, since it is much easier to use the keyboard than the pen to revise and change the order of a phrase and a paragraph, or to jot down some passing ideas at the foot of the page, jottings that will vanish with the printing. But to set a term to one's work, to accept that one has reached its conclusion and at last to entrust the manuscript to the printer will always remain an agonising episode in the production of a book.

I have had to live through the experience of producing this book, aiming at the best possible outcome, but constantly aware that some weeks or months later an indication might have been better defined, more carefully expressed, that a new technique might appear that would have deserved to be tried out, analysed and described. And hoping all the while – and hence an often frustrating caution in the writing – that another study would not arrive to invalidate the very points that had seemed so essential and on which so much stress had been laid.

But with too much insistence on perfection, nothing would have been achieved...

Every work of this type becomes obsolete in the fairly short term. Nevertheless, I hope, very egocentrically, that some of the ideas expressed here may consolidate the development of ideas in this field of plastic surgery. The dream is a permissible one.

There are those who may regard this book as incomplete, and it is. They will not find certain techniques that they are bound to hold dear; but, rather than an encyclopedic compilation, I prefer to report only that which I know from personal experience.

The information and the know-how conveyed here are certainly limited since they derive from one individual, from a single surgeon at a particular moment of her practice. The advantage for the reader takes the shape of a uniformity of surgical practice which does not promote enthusiasm for one particular idea or technique rather than another by a style of writing, or of illustration or presentation, that varies markedly from one chapter to another.

Note. This text is a summary of the mental state of every creator faced with the irresistible need to dosomething, while accepting that this 'monument' of frustration can, at best, be only a small grain of sand on the shores of achievement. And if nothing justifies suffering, to please onself, and possibly also to please others, can do no great harm.

To Didier,
To my children, Benjamin and Virginie,
To my mother,
> for their advice and their very great patience. I have promised them not to
> write another book for a long time.

To the memory of my father.

I sincerely thank Jean-Pierre Lalardrie, with whom I had the pleasure in 1987 of organising the course of annual congress of the Société Française de Chirurgie Plastique, Réparatrice et Esthétique on 'Mammary scars and plasties'. Although I was not strictly speaking his pupil, he has always over the years and during various congresses provided me with his stringent and well-meant criticisms.

I warmly thank Yves Morel for his superb drawings, the originality of which provides this book, at least so I hope, with an esthetic appeal unusual for a medical textbook.

The normal breast

Embryology

Although the breast is of double origin, ectodermal and mesodermal, the mammary gland may in fact be considered, strictly speaking, as a skin appendage, since the mesoderm provides only the vessels and the supporting connecting tissue.

It has even been argued, though we may find this somewhat pejorative, that the embryologic origin of the breast allows the assertion that it is no more than a specialised sweat-gland !

At the fifth week of embryonic development there appear the mammary strips, composed of two to four layers of ectodermal cells, which extend on the lateral wall of the chest and abdomen.

Between 6 and 7 weeks these strips thicken to form the primitive mammary ridges, extending symmetrically from the axillary region to the inguinal region.

There subsequently appear in pairs the primitive mammary buds (fig. 1), which normally in the human species regress completely except in the thoracic region at the level of the 4th pair.

From the 13th week onward, the cellular proliferation of ectodermal origin continues in depth in the underlying mesenchyme; 15 to 25 dense epithelial cords become embedded in the mesenchyme: these are the future lactiferous ducts and their deep extremities are the future acini.

At the 5th month there begins a phase of active growth. The main lactiferous ducts, composed of a double cell layer (glandular and myoepithelial), become hol-

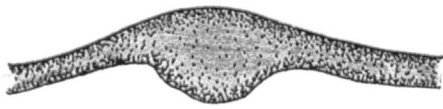

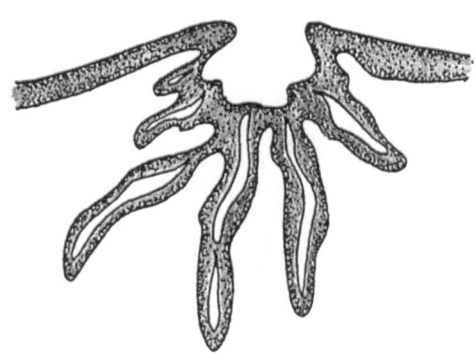

Fig. 1. Development of the breast:
- the primitive mammary bud (above)
- the development of the lactiferous ducts (around the 8th month)

lowed out with a lumen (20-25 weeks) and distal outgrowths forms the second-order lactifers. The nipple region forms a more marked prominence, with a peri-areolar sulcus, while the "primitive mammary field" is formed, the lower part of which is the future inframammary crease.

At the 8th month the lactiferous ducts open into the epithelial depression situated at the center of the rudimentary nipple (fig. 1) and in depth there develop the glandular acini, separated by connective tissue septa. Each lactiferous duct is thus at the origin of a separate primary glandular unit.

The nipple is formed during the perinatal period by proliferation of the subjacent mesenchyme. At birth, there is transient secretory and hyperemic activity as part of the genital activity of the new-born, but after two weeks everything settles down and the gland remains inactive until puberty.

Anomalies of development

The presence of supernumerary nipples, spread out along the nipple line (polythelia) is due to persistence of the primitive mammary buds. These accessory nipples are always situated on a line starting at the axillary fossa and ending at the pubis (fig. 2), corresponding to the course of the former mammary ridge (fig. 3). If this anomaly is accompanied by the development of an authentic accessory mammary gland (which may become functional in periods of lactation and is sometimes

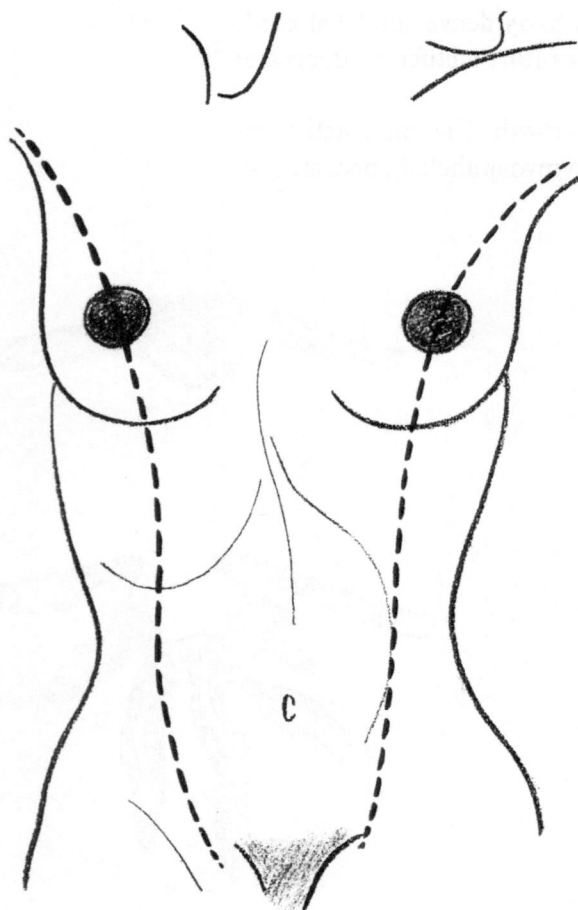

Fig. 2. Siting of accessory mammary glands and nipples along the mammary ridge

only identified at this time by the appearance of a milky secretion), it may be termed polymastia (fig. 4).

Amazia is a total absence of the breast, both gland and nipple-areolar plaque. It is usually unilateral and may well be accompanied by malformations of the upper limb. It should be noted that no gland, even if hypoplastic, can exist without a nipple-areolar plaque. In mammary aplasia there is a nipple-areolar plaque, often very small, without an underlying gland.

Mammary aplasias and hypoplasias (inadequate development of the gland) are generally revealed at puberty, except is cases with associated anomalies evident at birth such as a thoracic malformation or, in the case of Poland's syndrome, as a result of associated anomalies of the pectoralis major, or even malformations of the upper limb (phalangeal agenesia or dystrophy, syndactyly).

The mechanisms of malformation of the mammary gland are still little understood, and one must resort to hypotheses. The embedding of the mammary bud in the mesenchyme occurs under the influence of testosterone and the development of the secondary buds is dependent on estrogens.

There is not currently any satisfactory explanation for all of these anomalies. It is easy enough to conceive that the presence of accessory glands or nipples is due

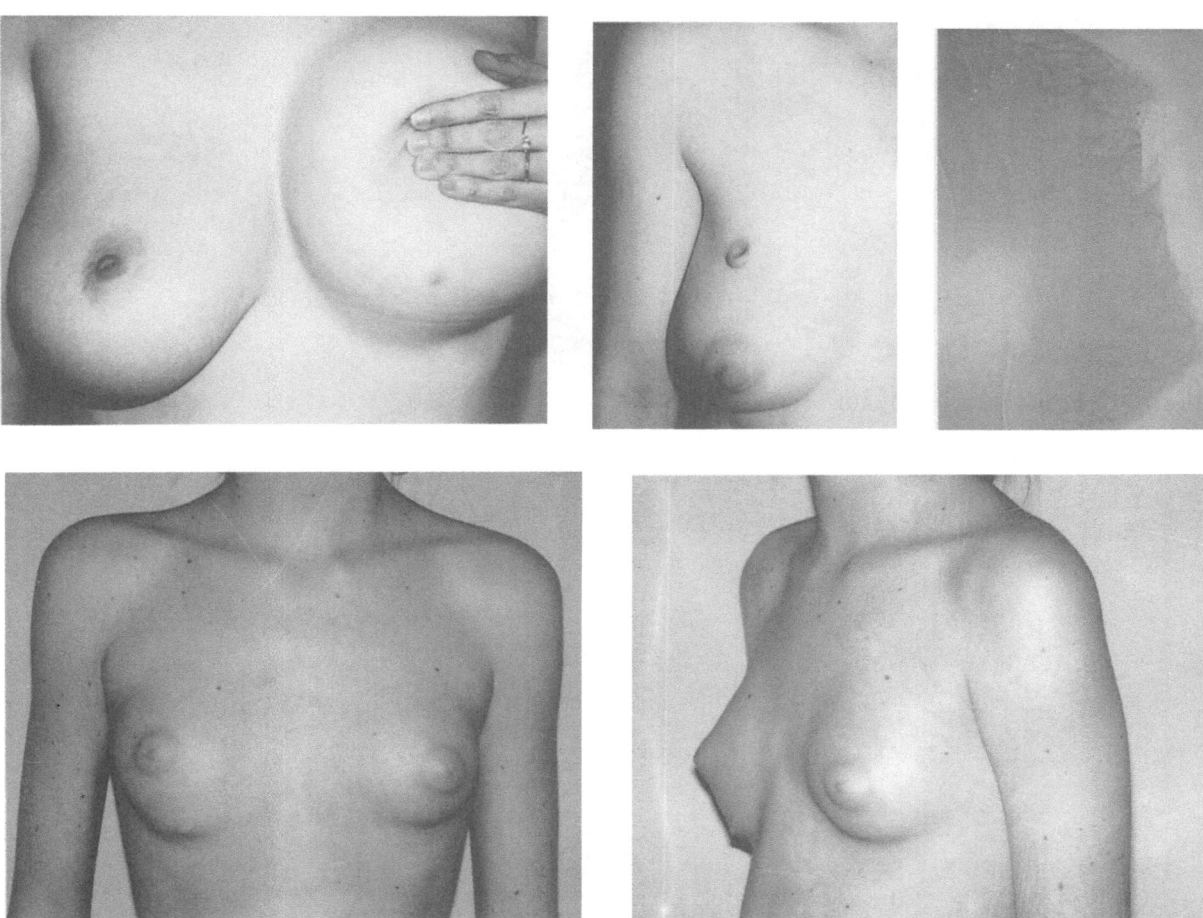

Fig. 3. Accessory nipple

Fig. 4 a-d. Polymastia. **a, b** Accessory gland and nipple on the upper part of the mammary ridge, clinical and xerographic appearances; **c, d** accessory gland and nipple in the inframammary fold

to the persistence (abnormal in women but quite normal in other mammals) (fig. 5) of primitive mammary buds other than those of the fourth pair, but the mechanisms of such defects must remain hypothetical: absence of development or complete regression of the mammary ridge, teratogenic factors coming into play at the precise moment of development in cases of associated malformations of the upper limb or thorax.

The ectodermal origin of the gland must always be borne in mind, as this accounts for the close relations between the gland and the skin; hence their essential unity and their interdependence at the vascular level because of the penetration of the ectodermal buds into the ensheathing mesenchyme.

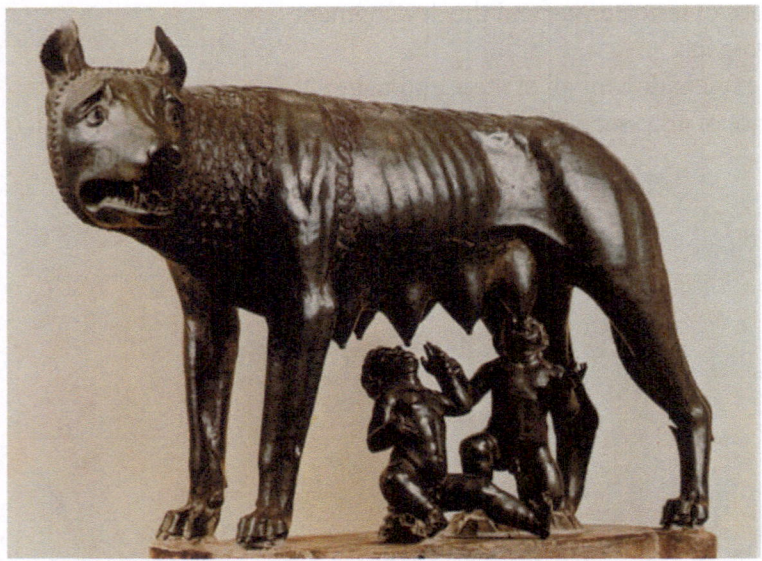

Fig.5. The Capitoline wolf (6th century AD)

Anatomy and morphology of the breast

While the descriptive anatomy of this variably sized organ has been well known for decades, so that recent reviews have been unnecessary, this does not apply to factors relevant to the vascular and morphologic anatomy discovered in recent years.

In fact, progress and developments in plastic surgery of the breast and rapid improvement in the treatment of breast cancer have refined our knowledge of the vascularisation of the breast and its lymphatic drainage, justifying — if there were any need — the confirmation of our empirical notions derived from clinical experience by anatomic studies directed beyond a simple description of the classical pedicles towards a better understanding of the different vascular plexuses. The concepts so defined have in their turn affected clinical practice, allowing technical variations excluding any further risk of vascular impairment.

At the same time the morphologic anatomy has become more demanding, a number of definitions corresponding to precise concepts — the term residual mammary volume, to cite only one example — having made their appearance within the last twenty years.

These concepts are really essential to correct analysis of our results, allowing a better evaluation of what constitutes the harmony of an operated breast, and certainly a better and more constructive understanding of defects and inadequacies.

Descriptive anatomy

Structure

The mammary gland, ie everything contained within the cutaneous envelope of the breast, consists, in proportions varying from one woman to another and at the different stages of reproductive life, of glandular tissue proper, connective tissue and adipose tissue.

Glandular tissue

Histologically, the glandular tissue is composed of acini grouped in clusters, constituting the basic units or lobules, surrounding alveolar ducts into which they empty. The alveolar ducts drain into an intralobular duct, the assembly of lobules grouped around the same intralobular duct forming a mammary lobe. The excretory ducts of the lobes, or lactiferous ducts — one per lobe — converge towards the nipple after exhibiting just beneath this a dilatation called the lactiferous sinus. The lactifers open to the exterior by the lactiferous orifices.

This structure of the breast results in the glandular elements predominating at the periphery, while the excretory structures and the connective tissue are predominant in the central portion of the gland. The glandular tissue itself is not distributed uniformly in the four quadrants; it is denser in the superolateral quadrant and the axillary tail, which may account for the greater frequency of malignant lesions in this region.

Although the lobules, and also the lobes, are separated by fibrous septa which are thicker around the lobes than the lobules, it is not possible to define a mammary lobe so as to allow segmental surgery of the breast. The gland is divided into quadrants for topographic purposes only.

Adipose tissue

Its ectodermal embryologic origin implies that the glandular tissue is intermingled with the subcutaneous adipose tissue. The adipose lobules are present in variable amount amidst the glandular tissue, the proportion varying with the degree of general obesity, age, pregnancy and lactation.

In fact, we have observed in young girls operated in the post-pubertal period two very different types of mammary hypertrophy. If the relation between height and weight has remained normal during this period, the hypertrophic breast is most often firm, elastic and rather white on section, and histologic study of the operative specimen shows a preponderance of glandular tissue. If puberty has been associated with excessive weight gain, and whether or not the patient has subsequently lost weight, the breast is of softer consistence, independent of the degree of skin distension, and markedly yellower on section, while the glandular tissue is proportionately reduced and sometimes present mainly in the retro-areolar region, histologic study confirming the predominance of adipose tissue.

Although every pubertal weight increase is not associated with mammary hypertrophy, a period of rapid weight gain at the time of puberty is harmful, apart from its other affects, as it may lead to the development of hypertrophy of a predominantly fatty nature. This stresses the importance of monitoring the weight in this sometimes tricky period of reproductive life.

The adipose tissue is also present at the periphery of the gland, forming an anterior layer constituting the subcutaneous adipose sheet, and a thinner posterior retroglandular layer.

The thickness of the subcutaneous fatty layer varies with the general degree of adiposity, and decreases from the periphery towards the areolar region, where the gland is now separated from the coverings of the areola and nipple only by a little connective tissue and the areolar muscle.

Posteriorly, the adipose tissue is less thick. In any case, it remains intermingled with the glandular tissue and is situated in front of the superficial fascia.

Connective tissue

Contrary to some assertions, the mammary gland does not possess a capsule properly so-called. The lobes and lobules are separated by thin fibrous septa identifiable in the histologic sections, but not on naked-eye inspection.

At the anterior aspect of the gland the connective tissue bundles extend into the subcutaneous adipose layer at right angles to the skin surface, and terminate in the dermis. These are the ligaments of Cooper, responsible for the fibroglandular ridges of Duret (fig. 6).

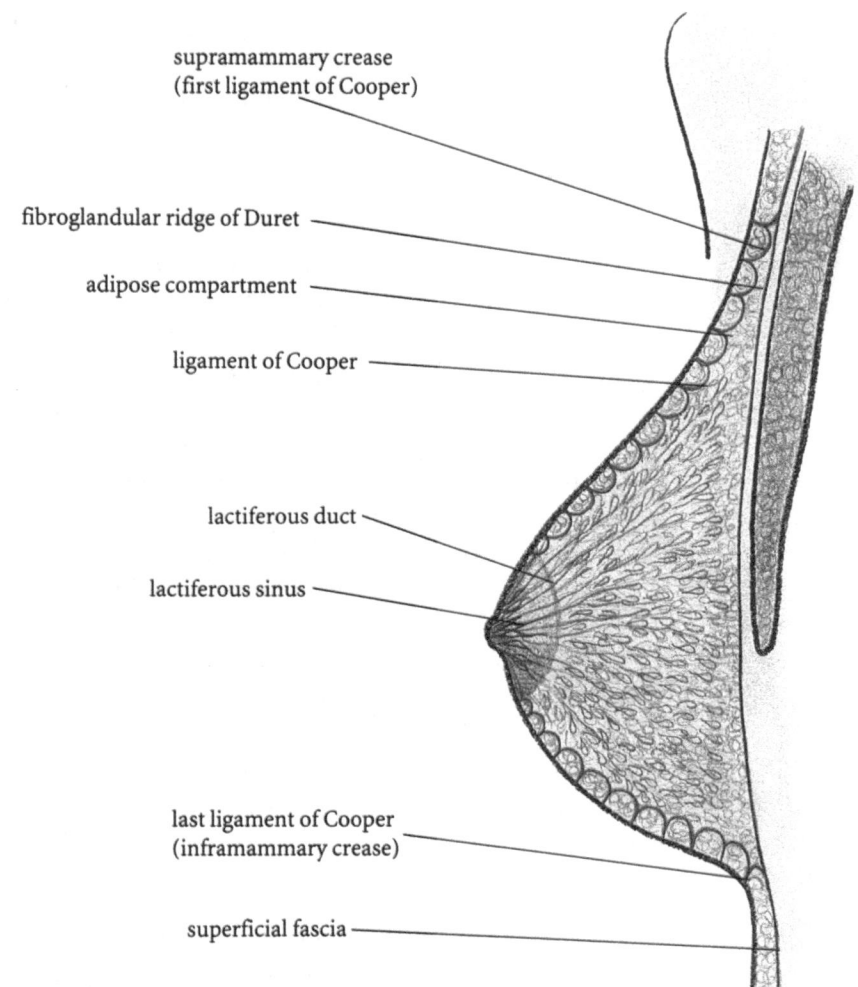

supramammary crease
(first ligament of Cooper)

fibroglandular ridge of Duret

adipose compartment

ligament of Cooper

lactiferous duct

lactiferous sinus

last ligament of Cooper
(inframammary crease)

superficial fascia

Fig. 6. Structure of the breast

The tethering and invasion of the ligaments of Cooper by the development of an underlying neoplastic process accounts for the 'orange peel' phenomenon, justifying sacrifice of the skin over the lesion.

The absence of an anterior fibrous septum is one of the reasons why subcutaneous mastectomy is so much decried. When the patient is slender, and glandular tissue is predominant in the midst of the gland, it is relatively easy to find a plane of cleavage between the subcutaneous fatty layer as such and the glandular tissue.

This artificial plane is more difficult to find in an obese woman and when the breast exhibits some degree of fatty involution.

It is true that the ligaments of Cooper are preserved, and probably the extremities of the crests of Duret. This is why subcutaneous mastectomy is so much criticised in terms of carcinology. But when one considers the changes in skin sacrifice in the indications for mastectomy, often reduced to an ellipse opposite the initial tumor and the areola, there remains as much of the crests of Duret and therefore of residual glandular tissue under the remaining skin envelope as in a correctly performed subcutaneous mastectomy.

At the posterior aspect of the gland, the supporting connective tissue forms a more marked layer, allowing easy separation from the aponeurosis of the pectoralis major muscle. This is actually the superficial fascia.

Superficial fascia

The majority of authors are agreed that the superficial fascia passes entirely behind the mammary gland, which is explained once again by its ectodermal origin. Others describe a division of the superficial fascia at the level of the breast into two layers, one anterior and preglandular, the other posterior and retroglandular, separating the deep aspect of the gland from the muscle plane. But even these recognise that the preglandular component of the superficial fascia cannot be identified separately as soon as the peripheral limit of the gland is reached, because of the presence of the crests of Duret prolonged by the ligaments of Cooper. We therefore retain the concept that the superficial fascia passes entirely behind the mammary gland, which is logical in terms of its embryonic development and corresponds to the following surgical realities:

The fixity of the inframammary crease in relation to the skin, the facility of surgical cleavage behind the gland and in front of the pectoralis major muscle (without necessarily supporting Chassaignac's hypothesis of a serous bursa), the difficulty of surgical cleavage between skin and gland in the case of subcutaneous mastectomy, where the surgeon must always hesitate between leaving glandular tissue or damaging the preglandular vascular plexus and inflicting skin damage.

Skin

The cutaneous envelope of the breast does not have the same characteristics everywhere. The skin is thicker at the periphery of the gland than near the areola, and thicker also near its lower limit (inframammary crease) than at the upper pole, which may be the effect of gravity.

This must be borne in mind during procedures of skin stripping, which must be done more cautiously and superficially as one approaches the areola and when the skin seems thinned, exhibits striae and is distended by excessive weight, so as to safeguard the subdermal vascularisation.

Opposite the areola, where the skin is thinner, it is closely attached to the gland by fibrous tracts without the interposition of fatty tissue, and also lined by a subcutaneous muscle, the mammillary muscle, composed predominantly of circular fibers and to a lesser extent of radial fibers. The quality of the skin also varies from one woman to another, independent of age. Some have a 'tonic' skin with a thick dermis, others a much finer skin with a thin dermal layer.

This also has an effect on the stability of the outcome of a plastic surgical procedure, particularly as regards the correction of hypertrophy and ptosis. If the skin is thick, and generally of good elastic quality, a good structural result will be easier to obtain, with relatively shorter scars, in cases of reduction of the skin envelope, but the scars may well be hypertrophic.

If the skin is fine, with a thinned dermis, the structural stability of the result is less certain, with a greater risk of recurrence of the ptosis. If care is not taken to safeguard a short vertical subareolar distance (not exceeding 4 to 4.5 cm) at the end of the procedure, even by attaching the inferior pole of the breast to the chest wall at the level of the crease, secondary glandular ptosis may develop with slipping of the inferior pole of the gland under the horizontal scar, even if it was initially correctly sited in the crease. It may be postulated that such skin, with a thin dermis, is associated with ligaments of Cooper which are also thin and stretched, so that they no longer fulfil their function of supporting the breast in relation to the skin. On the other hand, the scars will very likely be finer.

Nipple-areolar plaque

The areola, which is approximately circular in shape, with an average diameter of 35 to 50 mm for a breast of normal size, is pigmented and its color varies greatly in different women and also changes with the stages of reproductive life. The peripheral limit of the pigmentation is very ill-defined. Its surface is irregular, and studded with the tubercles of Morgagni, which are actually sebaceous glands.

The ill-defined peripheral border of the areola, associated with a progressive change of color between the pigmented areolar zone and the rest of the skin of the breast, conduces to placing the incision in a curved areolar surgical approach very sligthly within what appears to be the visible margin. The scar, usually of excellent quality, will be less apparent than a scar placed exactly at the periphery, which risks making the boundary more obvious and definite than the rest of the areolar circumference. The numerous variations of color of the areola also evidence the importance of tattooing in areolar reconstruction, which offers more variants than the various donor sites of grafts and allows shading off of the pigment peripherally.

At the center of the areola is the nipple, itself variable in shape and size in relation to the former, variably prominent and variably spread out, cylindrical or conical. Its surface is rendered more irregular than that of the areola by depressions corresponding to the orifices of the 15 to 25 lactiferous ducts.

Permanent longstanding umbilication of the nipple is not detrimental (apart from any problems of lactation that it may cause) since it is associated with shortness of the lactiferous ducts, and its surgical treatment can be effective only if these are divided. On the other hand, recent and irreducible development of umbilication of the nipple should be a cause for suspicion, as it may indicate the development of an underlying disease process.

Fixation of the breast

Anatomists have exercised their ingenuity in describing the factors involved in suspension or fixation of the breast:

    – prolongation of the clavi-pectoro-axillary aponeurosis towards the axillary pole of the gland,

    – a "capsule" of the breast, which, as we have seen, does not exist,

    – thickening of the anterior layer of the superficial fascia (unidentifiable)

    – vascular pedicles (?)

In fact, the sole support system of the breast is represented by the skin, by reason of its close connexions with the gland via the ligaments of Cooper.

As clinical examination shows, the mammary gland is mobile on the chest-wall and the muscle plane, but not in relation to the skin. The nipple-areolar plaque represents the keystone of the system, since it is the point of convergence of all the intraglandular fibrous septa, and the place where adhesion between glandular tissue and skin is closest because of the absence of any subcutaneous fatty layer at this level.

The absence of other effective means of support explains why ptosis develops as soon as the skin can no longer tolerate exaggerated distension beyond the stretch limits of the elastic fibers, as may be provoked by the development of pubertal glandular hypertrophy, possibly exacerbated by overweight, or by the glandular enlargement of pregnancy.

Age changes

Under the influence of age, hormonal variations in the different stages of reproductive life and weight changes, the mammary gland undergoes fatty involution of varying degree, which is well shown radiologically.

But this adipose nature is deceptive in terms of plasticity. In fact, it is more difficult to remodel a gland during a breast reduction at the age of 50 than at 20. This fatty involution is associated with sclerosis of the connective tissue, both within the gland and at its connexions with the skin. It seems as if the normal unity of skin and gland, based on the ligaments of Cooper, increases to the extent of creating an inseparable and unmalleable fibrous block.

Vascular anatomy

Arterial vascularisation

While there is a certain number of arterial pedicles as the source of the vascularisation of the mammary gland, it should be stressed at the outset that the ectodermal origin of the gland accounts for the close interdependence of the cutaneous and glandular blood-supply in this region. Knowledge of these close connexions has allowed the development of modern techniques of mammoplasty; in particular, it largely validates the importance of avoiding cleavage between skin and gland, a safety factor in terms of vascularity.

Three plexuses play unequal parts in the blood-supply of the breast:
– a subdermal plexus,
– a preglandular plexus,
– a retroglandular plexus, connected with the above by an intraglandular anastomotic system.

Origin of the plexuses

These plexus are derived from:

– the thoracoacromial artery (fig. 7)
This arises from the axillary artery at the upper border of the pectoralis minor muscle, at the junction of the medial and middle thirds of the clavicle, perforates the clavipectoral aponeurosis and divides into two branches: acromial and thoracic.

The thoracic, medial, branch is the one of interest to us since it is distributed by very rapid division into two branches to the pectoral muscles and the mammary region. The deep muscular branch is retropectoral. This gives rise to the perforating rami, which emerge at the lower border of the pectoralis major muscle and at right angles to it, and enter the gland from its deep aspect. The superficial subcutaneous branch is shorter and terminates at the level of the 3rd intercostal space, where it anastomoses with the anterior cutaneous perforating branch;

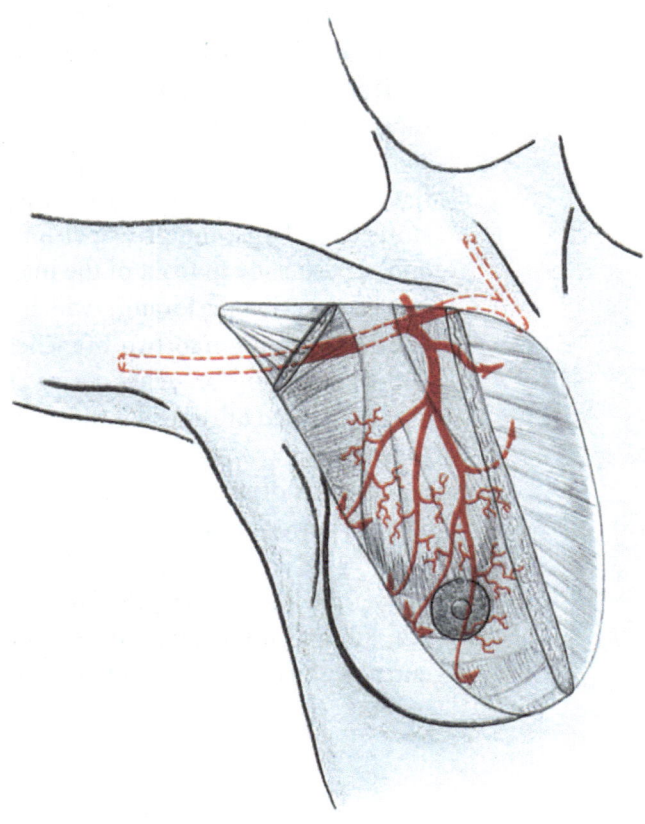

Fig.7. Thoracoacromial artery

– the lateral thoracic (external mammary) artery (fig. 8)

This arises from the axillary artery behind the pectoralis minor muscle, and travels downward, inward and forward following the lateral border of the pectoralis major. It ends by dividing into three branches:

• an anterior branch supplying the skin which anastomoses with an equivalent branch derived from the medial thoracic artery via the 3rd anterior thoracic perforant;

• a posterior muscular branch which anastomoses with the subscapular branches and gives off branches destined for the pectoral, serratus anterior and intercostal muscles;

• finally, its glandular branch (principal external artery) penetrates the gland at its axillary prolongation and divides into two branches which join in forming the periareolar circle by anastomosing with the homologous branches derived from the medial thoracic artery;

– the medial thoracic (internal mammary) artery (fig. 9)

This arises from the inferior aspect of the subclavian and travels downward and inward on the anterior slope of the dome of the pleura, behind the subclavian vein and the clavicle to enter the thorax. It passes behind the sternocostal shield as far as the 6th intercostal space, where it divides into its two terminal branches: one lateral, the musculophrenic a. and the other medial, the superior epigastric a. During its course it gives off posterior collateral branches destined to the mediastinum and thymus, internal branches for the sternal shield, anterior or anterior perforating thoracic vessels which traverse the intercostal spaces for distribution to the pectoralis major and mammary gland, and lateral or anterior intercostal branches which anastomose with the posterior intercostal or aortic vessels.

It shares in the supply of the mammary gland via the anterior perforating thoracic vessels, especially the 2nd, 3rd and 4th, and to a lesser degree the 5th and 6th.

The 3rd perforating thoracic vessel, which emerges at the medial end of the 2nd intercostal space, is the largest. (They are all called, as is that of the 3rd space when sufficiently large, the principal internal arteries.). It travels almost transversely and superficially in front of the mammary gland in the subcutaneous tissue, giving off anterior perforators which anastomose with the subdermal plexus and ends by dividing into two branches which anastomose at the periareolar circle with homologous branches derived from the main lateral thoracic artery.

The 5th and 6th anterior thoracic perforators emerge at a greater distance from the midlline (some 9 cm for the 5th and 13 cm for the 6th). They penetrate the gland on its deep aspect and play a much less important part in its blood-supply. The 5th perforator is also called the artery of the nipple;

– and, to a lesser degree, the infracostal arteries (fig. 10), collateral branches of the 7th, 8th and 9th aortic intercostal arteries, which give off perforating branches entering the inferolateral quadrant of the breast on its deep aspect.

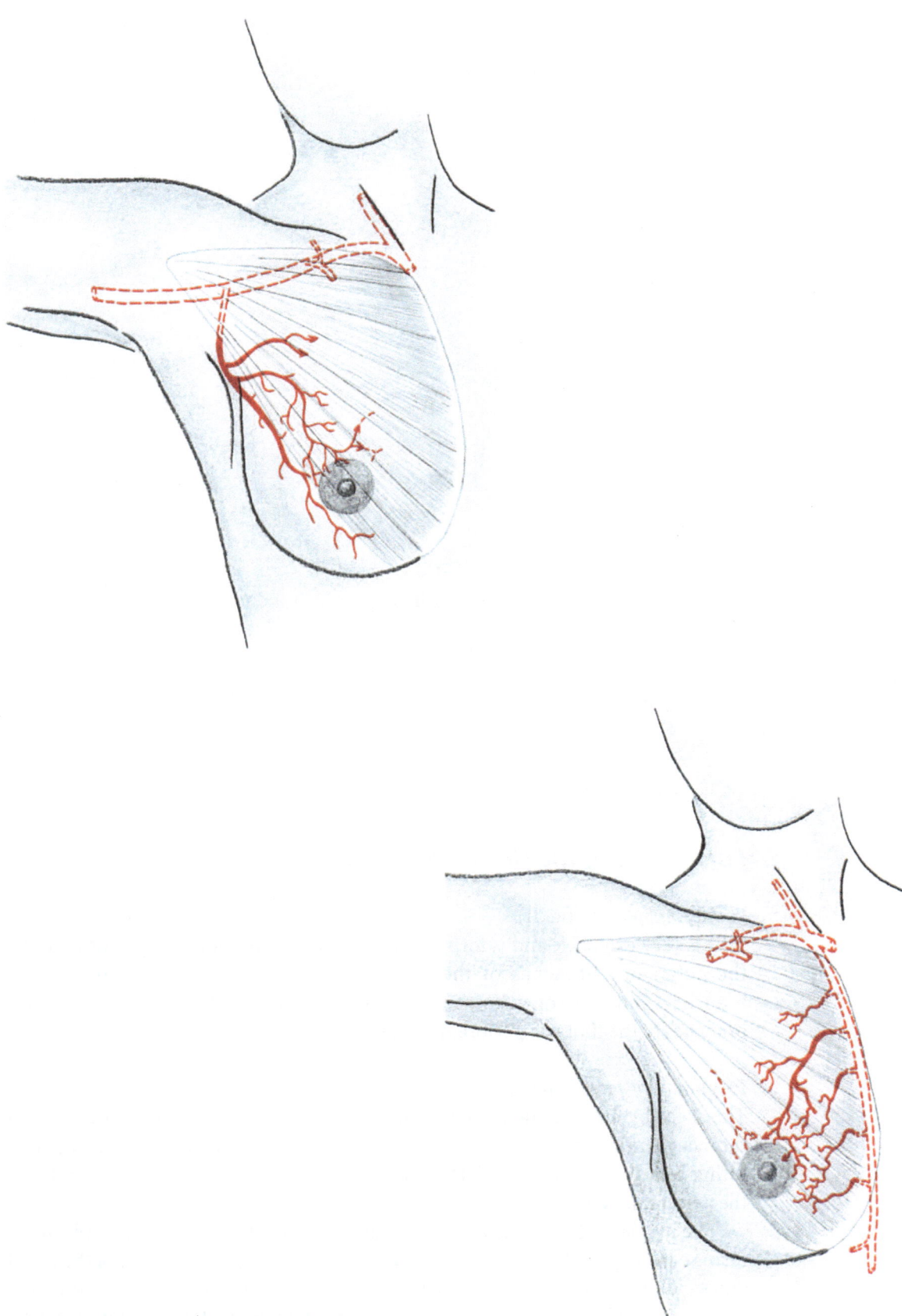

Fig.8. Lateral thoracic *(external mammary)* artery

Fig.9. Internal thoracic *(internal mammary)* artery

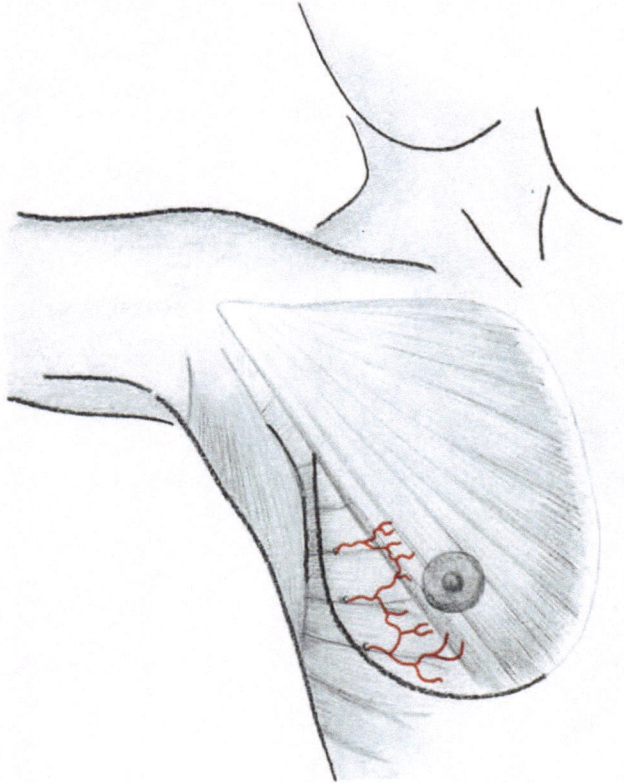

Fig.10. Infracostal arteries

Formation of the three plexuses

Subdermal plexus (fig. 11)

This is very extensive and is formed by an abundant anastomotic plexus between the cutaneous branches of the thoracoacromial a. (acromial and thoracic branches) and those of adjacent arteries, ie: subclavian, subscapular and anterior branches of the thoracic perforators derived from the medial thoracic a.

Preglandular plexus (fig. 12)

This is fed by the anterior and glandular branches of the lateral thoracic a., the 3rd thoracic perforator of the medial thoracic a., and the other anterior thoracic perforating vessels. The two main lateral and medial arteries anastomose to constitute the periareolar circle.

The preglandular plexus is widely anastomosed with the subdermal plexus. It forms a widely-meshed plexus which covers the entire anterior aspect of the gland and sends branches in depth, perpendicular to the surface. These travel within the interlobar and interlobular septa and surround the acini and the lactiferous ducts.

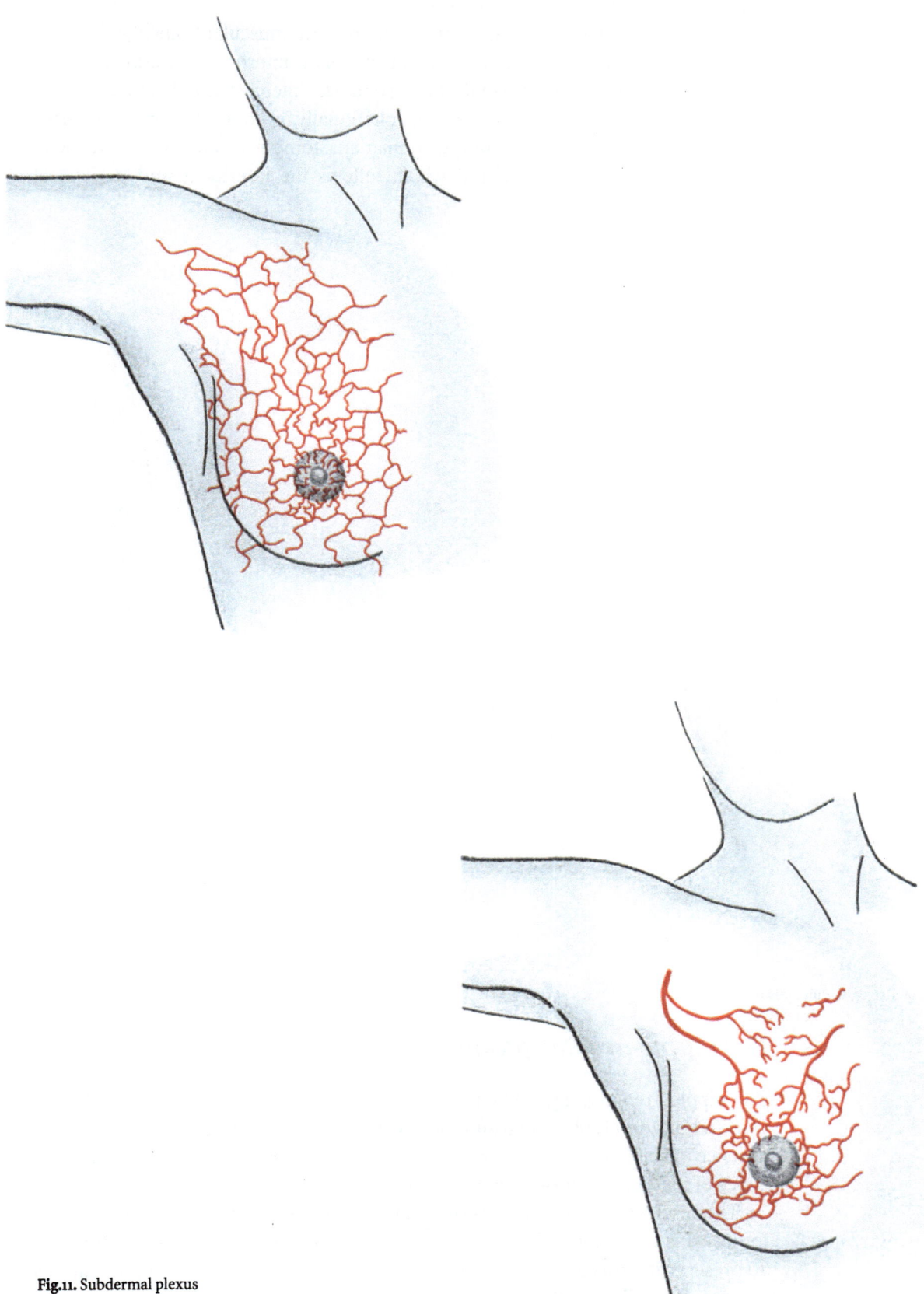

Fig. 11. Subdermal plexus

Fig. 12. Preglandular plexus

Retroglandular plexus (figs. 13 and 14)
This is formed by the perforating branches of the deep muscular branch of the thoracoacromial artery, the deep divisional branches of the internal perforating intercostals (2nd, 3rd, 4th and 5th) and of the lateral or aortic intercostals (7th, 8th, 9th).

This plexus, which is less important functionally, is connected to the anterior cutaneoglandular system by an intraglandular anastomotic plexus which is virtually perpendicular to the surface and which follows the interlobar and perilacteal connective tissue septa.

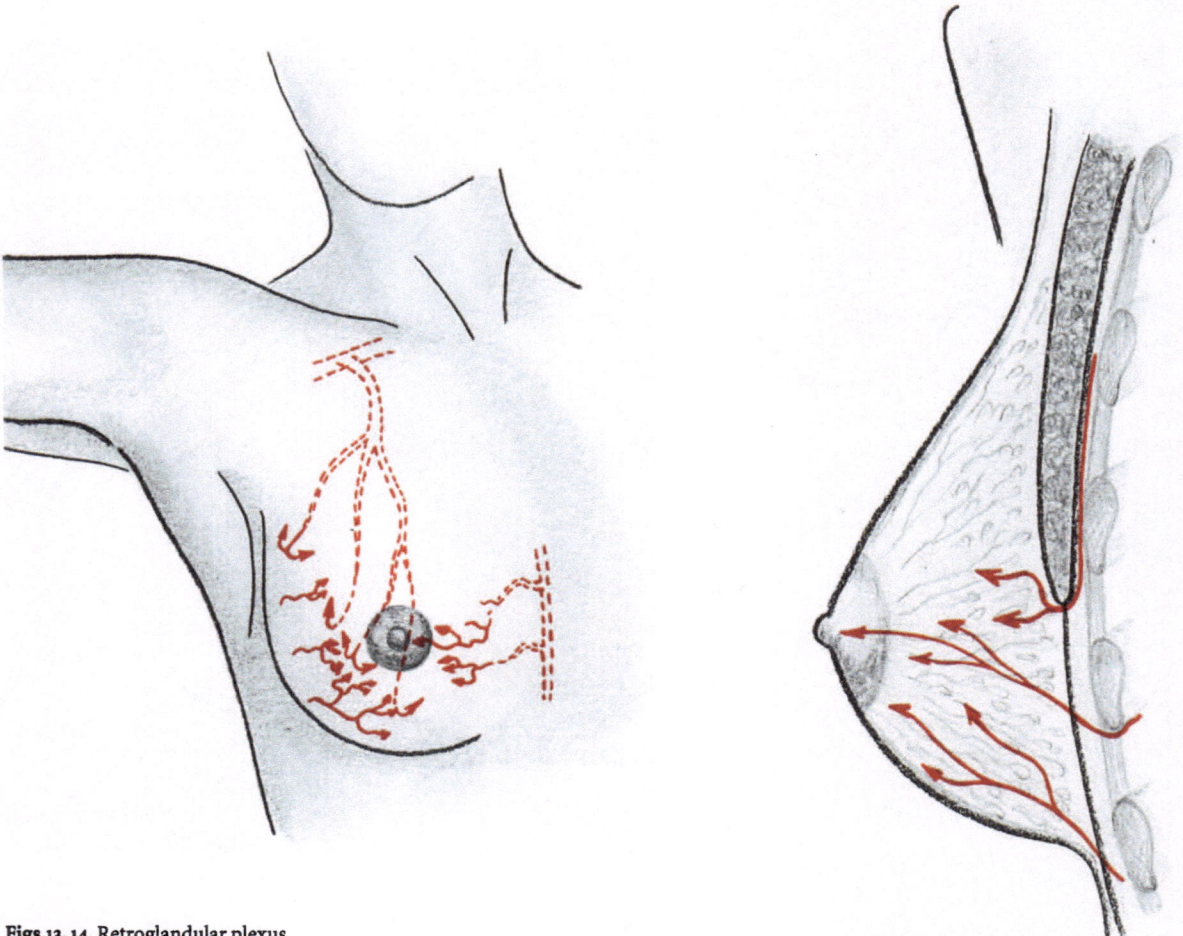

Figs.13, 14. Retroglandular plexus

The nipple-areolar plaque

The nipple-areolar plaque, like the gland as a whole, benefits from a double network, a horizontal subdermal and a vertical glandular plexus, characterised by the absence of a subcutaneous fatty layer between skin and gland and by the convergence of the lactiferous ducts at the nipple.

The subdermal areolar plexus (territory of the thoracoacromial a. and its anastomoses) is very superficial by reason of the fineness of the skin cover at this site. To preserve it, procedures involving skin stripping must therefore be very cautious and very superficial at this level.

Additionally, there is behind the nipple a plexus of perilactiferous capillaries perpendicular to the skin, whose origin is represented by the artery of the nipple, a medial perforating intercostal vessel derived from the 5th space (figs. 14 and 15). Finally, the periareolar arterial circle, formed mainly by the two branches of the internal and lateral thoracic aa., and situated beside and at the deep aspect of the areola, gives off recurrent deep arteries whose divisional branches anastomose with the subdermal and perilactiferous plexuses.

Surgical applications

What emerges from these anatomic concepts is that the arterial supply of the breast is marked by the existence of three plexuses, of which the most abundant are the subdermal and preglandular plexuses, anastomosing with each other, particularly in the periareolar region (fig. 16).

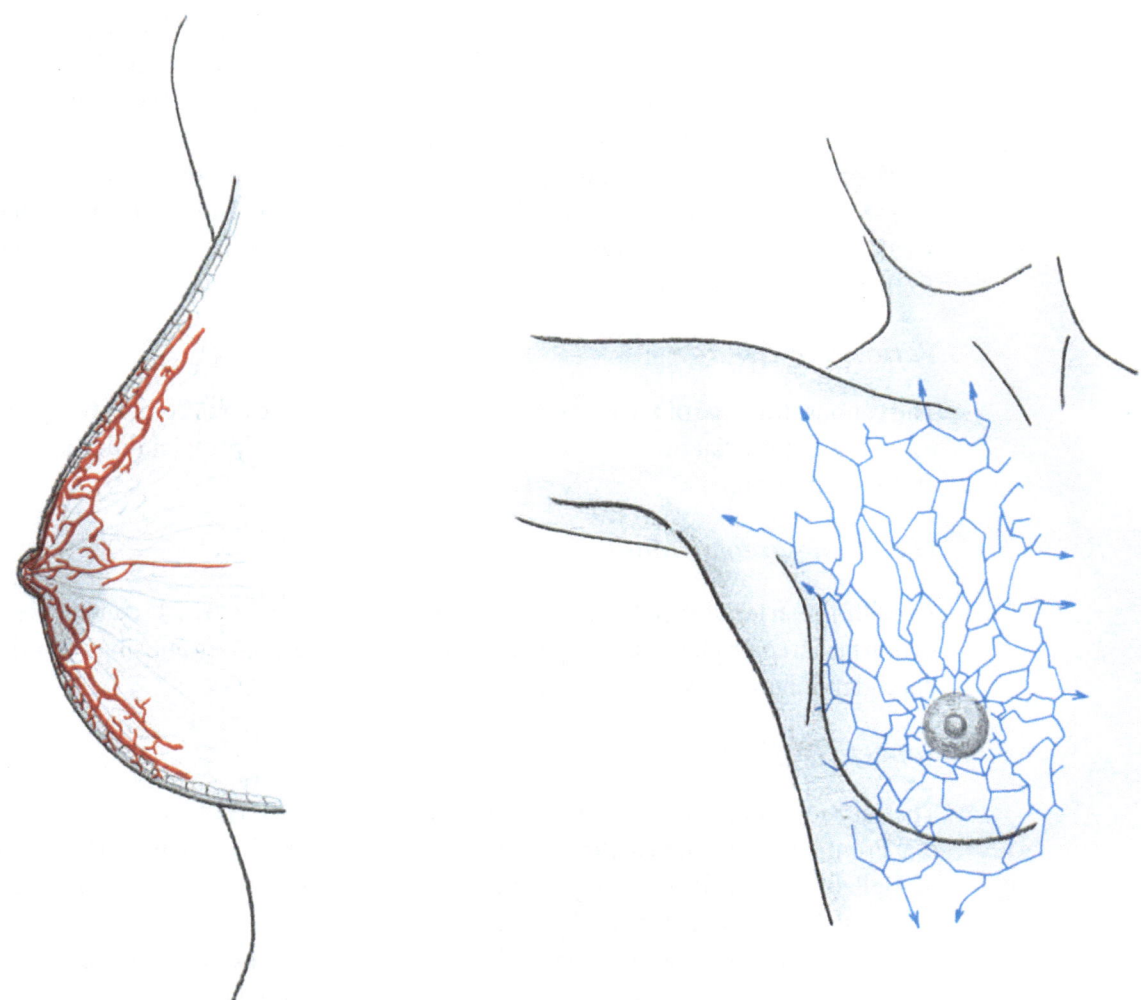

Fig. 15. Anastomoses between subdermal and preglandular plexuses

Fig. 16. Superficial venous drainage

This explains why numerous techniques of mammoplasty have been described, based on preservation of one or more pedicles.

However, certain techniques are more reliable than others as concerns survival of the skin, the nipple-areolar plaque and the gland.

As regards the nipple-areolar plaque, its survival may be ensured equally well by the subdermal or the glandular plexus; therefore, one of these two systems must be left in place and in particular the communication between both systems must be safeguarded. Hence the necessity, in techniques involving cleavage between skin and gland, of preserving a periareolar zone stripped of skin (Schwartzmann's maneuver). This problem does not arise in techniques without cutaneo-glandular cleavage since the de-epithelialised zone not only protects the areolar region but actually constitutes a nipple-bearing flap.

As for the risks of skin or glandular necrosis, although the posterior pedicle techniques have recently revived the idea of skin-gland cleavage, they are not devoid of risk when ptosis is marked (poor assessment of the site of penetration of the deep vessels into the gland, risk of glandular necrosis if these vessels are not fully respected, risk of skin necrosis at the angles of the inferior resection in an inverted T, which are at the extreme range of the skin plexus).

The most reliable techniques, permitting varied and unlimited resections, are those which respect the connexions between the skin, areola and gland, and which are therefore based on avoiding cutaneo-glandular cleavage and on the use of de-epithelialised nipple-bearing flaps.

Venous drainage

The venous drainage of the breast has no particular features. There exist two plexuses, one superficial and one deep, anastomosed via the intraglandular system and at their periphery.

The nipple-areolar plaque

As with the arterial supply, there exists a subdermal plexus which constitutes a major periareolar plexus and a plexus around the nipple, anastomosing with the deep glandular plexus around the lactiferous ducts.

Superficial flow

The very superficial subdermal veins constitute the circle of Haller around the areola. From here is formed a plexus with a very wide mesh, the subcutaneous plexus of Haller, very evident during pregnancy and lactation, which drains into the superficial veins of the region (fig. 16):

– above, into the superficial cervical plexus (anterior and external jugular veins);

– laterally, into the cephalic vein via the thoracroacromial vein ;

– below, into the superficial veins of the abdominal wall, notably the superficial thoraco-epigastric by communication with the plexus of the opposite breast.

Deep flow

The deep veins are satellites of the arterial branches; they travel in the connective tissue tracts and septa which separate the glandular lobes and drain into the two main currents:
  – laterally, into the lateral thoracic and then the axillary vein ;
  – medially, into the medial thoracic vein;
  – posteriorly, there is a less important flow towards the system of intercostal perforators.

Anastomoses between the two systems

The two systems communicate extensively with each other:
  – perpendicularly to the surface and superficially, by the perforating veins which travel in the ligaments of Cooper and by way of intraglandular anastomoses;
  – also at the borders of the gland, giving the impression that this has developed within a network whose meshes and aspects have diverged during the development of the gland (Ricbourg).
  The entire venous network of the breast is completely devoid of valves.

Surgical implications

As the superficial system predominates, it is necessary to preserve it, which is easy in procedures not involving cleavage between gland and skin but much less so in procedures that do involve such cleavage, where it is essential to avoid plication of the gland which might constitute an obstacle to the venous return, and possibly causes necrosis of the nipple-areolar plaque, or of the gland, or both.

Lymphatic drainage

The pattern of the lymphatic system of the breast can be superimposed on that of the arterial system. The abundance of anastomoses, so important as regards the arterial system and its surgical applications, becomes of prime importance with a malignant lesion; no sector of the breast has an exclusive drainage pathway.

Plexuses of origin

The well-developed superficial plexus, which drains the major part of the lymph, may be divided into an avalvular subepidermal plexus and a valvular subdermal plexus. These two plexuses become increasingly dense in approaching the areola, where they anastomose together to form the periareolar plexus.
  The deep plexus, also very developed, is formed of perilobular efferents which drain along the interlobar spaces, and of perilactiferous efferents. Both types of efferents drain mainly towards the periareolar plexus.

Lymph currents

From these two plexuses, superficial and deep, abundantly anastomosed in the periareolar region, the lymph current follows two main pathways towards the regional efferents:

– a lateral current, the most important, drains into the external mammary nodes and then the axillary nodes;

– a medial thoracic flow drains behind the sternum into the medial thoracic nodes;

– finally, an accessory and minor posterior flow reaches the infraclavicular nodes.

Lymph nodes (fig. 17)

Axillary nodes

Although these drain the greater part of the lymph, they do not correspond to any particular breast territory, and also drain the lymph of the upper limb and the thoraco-abdominal wall.

Classically, 5 groups may be distinguished:

1) the lateral thoracic (or pectoral axillary) group is divided into two groups, subpectoral and pectoral. It is situated along the lateral thoracic vessels, hidden behind the pectoralis major muscle, which covers it, and behind and below the pectoralis minor. It corresponds to the first two stages of Berg and includes 5 to 10 nodes;

2) the brachial (or lateral axillary) group is situated along and behind the axillary vessels, between the origin of the axillary vein and the inferior border of the pectoralis minor. It drains the upper limb and consists of 1 to 6 nodes. To prevent the development of lymphedema, it should be preserved during axillary nodal clearance by halting the dissection at the inferior border of the axillary vein;

3) the subscapular (or inferior scapular) group accompanies the subscapular pedicle and consists of up to 5 nodes; it may be stripped from the vessels and the nerve to the latissimus dorsi while preserving these. Although it drains the posterior part of the thorax, this group should be removed during axillary dissection for a lesion of the breast because of the anastomoses it forms with the lateral thoracic group;

4) the central axillary group, as its name indicates, occupies the center of the axillary fossa. Situated slightly below and behind the pectoralis minor, it consists of 2 to 6 nodes and drains the three preceding groups. It corresponds to the upper part of Berg's second stage;

5) the subclavicular (apical axillary) group is situated at the upper border of the pectoralis minor muscle at the apex of the axillary fossa and consists of up to 11 nodes. It represents Berg's third stage, and serves as a relay between all the preceding groups and the supraclavicular region, where the lymph flow rapidly empties via the subclavian trunk into the jugulo-subclavian venous confluence.

We should also note the presence of a direct accessory subclavian pathway, which emerges from the upper regions of the breast and reaches the subclavian group directly by traversing the pectoral muscles;

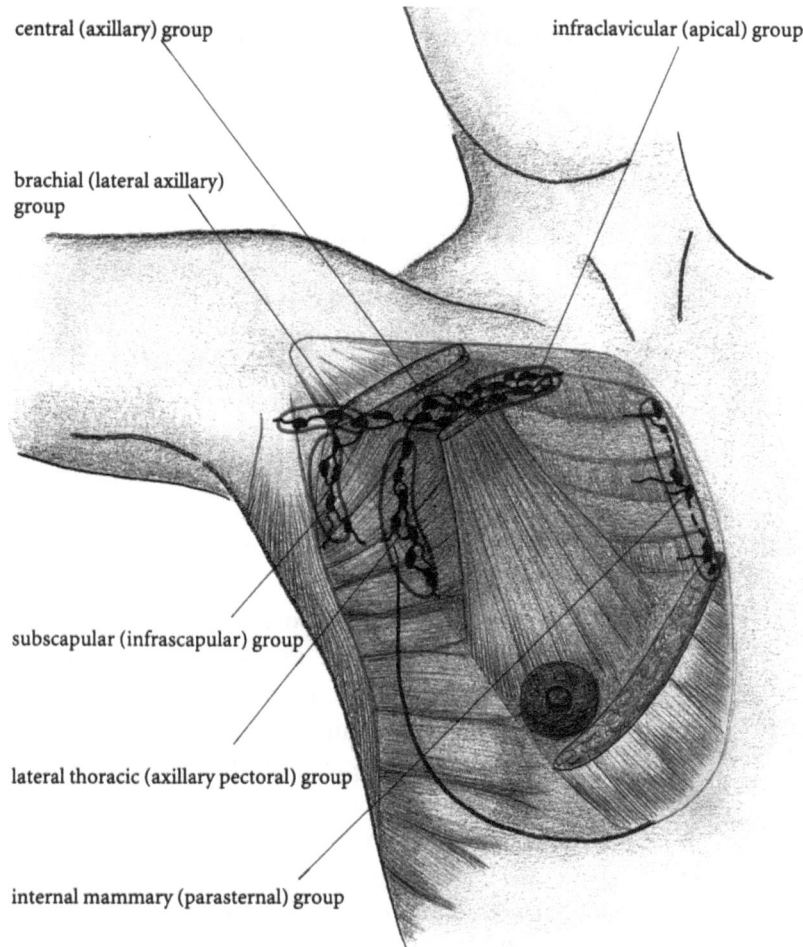

central (axillary) group

infraclavicular (apical) group

brachial (lateral axillary)
group

subscapular (infrascapular) group

lateral thoracic (axillary pectoral) group

Fig. 17. Lymph nodes

internal mammary (parasternal) group

The medial thoracic (parasternal) nodes
These are situated in contact with the internal thoracic vessels and extend the length of the first six intercostal spaces, especially the first three.

Surgical applications

These are of particular relevance to the modalities of axillary nodal clearance for cancer of the breast. Such a clearance must preserve the brachial group if the development of lymphedema of the upper limb is to be avoided, especially — but not solely — if associated radiotherapy is given.

It is also necessary to preserve, by careful dissection, the nerves and pedicles of the latissimus dorsi and serratus anterior muscles so as to maintain the possibilities of using a latissimus dorsi flap and to avoid the penalty of functional impairment due to a serratus palsy (slackening of the scapular attachment to the chest-wall).

Innervation

The innervation of the mammary gland and of its cutaneous envelope are intimately connected, a further reminder of the ectodermal origin of the gland.

Although certain nerves are entirely cutaneous, their role is minor compared with those to be considered as cutaneo-glandular, which all derive from the intercostal perforating nerves.

Cutaneous nerves

The strands of the supraclavicular branch of the superficial cervical plexus play only a minor role since they barely descend beyond the 2nd rib.

Cutaneo-glandular nerves

These are homologs of the arterial plexus and are derived from the perforating branches of the intercostal nerves to constitute two groups:

1) the anteromedial group comprises the anterior perforating branches of the 2nd, 3rd, 4th, 5th and 6th intercostal nerves; they travel in front of the gland and provide branches to the gland and the overlying skin.

The 5th intercostal nerve occupies a place apart since it passes directly to the nipple.

2) The lateral group is more important. It is formed by the external mammary branches of the 3rd, 4th, 5th and 6th lateral perforators of the intercostal nerves, which enter the gland on its deep aspect, near its outer border, after having perforated the chest-wall at the level of the mid-axillary line.

After having given off the cutaneous branches, their main trunks pass to the deep aspect of the gland, behind the superficial fascia, and regularly provide glandular branches with a postero-anterior course.

They also give off perforating branches around the areola which travel along the ligaments of Cooper and innervate the periareolar skin coverings.

Surgical implications

Despite its direct course to the nipple, the 5th perforating intercostal nerve does not play an exclusive part in sensation of the nipple. In fact, having always used techniques without cutaneo-glandular cleavage in the surgical treatment of hypertrophy, but with wide posterior stripping and glandular resection at the deep aspect of the gland, we have only rarely observed, and only in major glandular resections, any deterioration in the sensibility of the nipple-areolar plaque, which often already existed to a minor extent before the operation, due doubtless to the skin stretching. Moreover, this decrease of sensibility was as a rule temporary.

On the other hand, in two cases, and in one case in a definitive manner on one side, loss of sensation of the nipple was observed after having used a superior pedicle technique for moderate hypertrophy in both cases, where the sole error that can be recalled was to section the nipple-bearing flap laterally a little too high, at the margin of the outer periareolar circle, to facilitate its upward displacement. This would seem to confirm the important role of the branches of the lateral group of nerves.

It is commoner to observe loss of sensation after a formal subcutaneous mastectomy, which seems more logical since the plane of cleavage in this case passes flush with the crests of Duret, and therefore in front of the nerves, which travel just in front of the glandular plane in the case of those derived from the anteromedial group, and also in front of the laterally originating rami since these reach the surface via the depth of the gland.

Morphologic anatomy

The base of the breast (fig. 18)

This corresponds to the implantation of the breast on the thorax.

The area of projection of the base of the breast is more or less constant and extends, on average:

- from the 2nd intercostal space above,
- to the 6th intercostal space below,
- from the lateral border of the sternum medially,
- to the anterior axillary line laterally.

These limits are particularly well-defined below (inframammary crease) and medially (except in the very rare cases of synmastia). They are less definite above (supramammary crease) and laterally, and more difficult to assess when the patient is obese. They correspond to a patient examined in the standing position, since the inframammary crease in particular is fixed in relation to the skin plane, while the breast is relatively mobile as a whole in relation to the costo-muscular plane, to which it is only weakly adherent.

The orientation of the base of the breast depends on the shape of the thorax, the two bases forming an angle varying from around 30 to 50 °; hence the breasts are normally divergent, their lateral contours being normally longer and more convex than the medial.

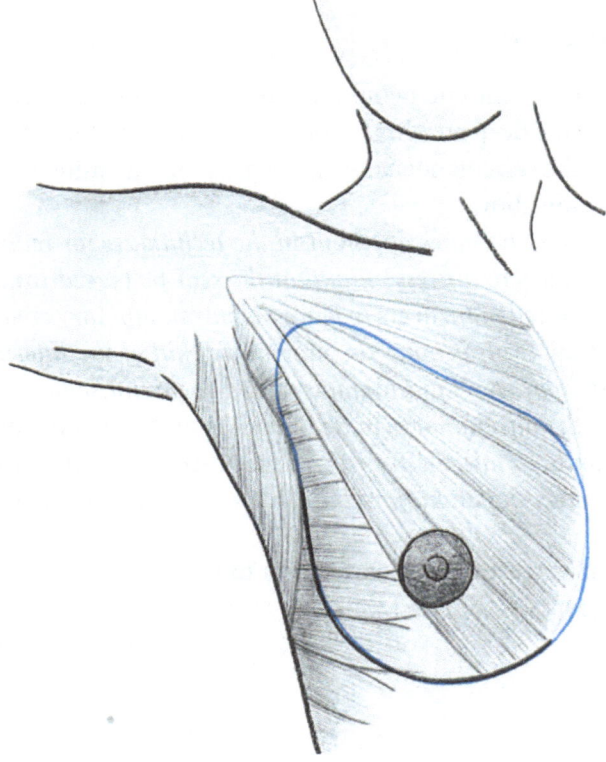

Fig. 18. The base of the breast

While study of this factor is only moderately important in the surgical treatment of breast hypertrophy (where the satisfactory techniques are those that deliberately control the reduction of the base of the breast, and this in proportion to its anterior projection so as not to encourage ptosis), it must be taken into more precise account on cosmetic grounds in the placement of implants and in breast reconstruction:
– in hypoplasias, the prosthetic implant must be centered on the existing areola, while being situated correctly in relation to the lateral border of the sternum. The necessary diameter of the implant will impose a certain size, as will be seen ;
– in reconstructions, the basal surface of an implant of the correct width and position will condition the ideal position of the areola, and therefore any plastic procedure on the opposite breast, since the whole must remain harmonious in relation to the patient's general and thoracic build.

Posteriorly, the base of the breast projects, but only partially, on the pectoralis major muscle, which is overlaid by the two superior quadrants and the greater part of the inferomedial quadrant. The inferolateral quadrant projects below and lateral to the pectoralis over the 4th, 5th, 6th and even 7th digitations of the serratus anterior, depending on the shape of the thorax and the extent of that muscle. But in no case does the serratus extend as far as the midline and there is a zone of varying size, depending on the shape of the thorax, at the junction of the inferior quadrants, where there is no longer any supple abundant muscle tissue like the fibers of the serratus and the pectoralis major. This zone consists only of the rigid aponeurosis of the intercostal muscles, and possibly of the rectus abdominis at its inner border.

This less fleshy region is of some importance during an immediate breast reconstruction or a subcutaneous mastectomy. The dissection must be very cautious here so as to preserve the retroglandular fascia, in order to ensure that the prosthetic implant has a continuous muscular and fascial covering to isolate it from the cutaneous layer.

The inframammary crease

This is a fixed element in relation to the cutaneous layer and is anatomically determined, since it corresponds to the deep attachment behind the gland of the superficial fascia, which here leaves the subcutaneous layer. It marks the transition from thoracic skin below to breast skin above.

The importance of this element becomes apparent in the techniques for reduction of the hypertrophic breast, where it is essential that the scar be placed transversely at this level. Any exaggerated maneuvers to place the inframammary crease higher up, in mammary skin, by transforming the mammary skin of the inferior part of breast segment III into thoracic skin (attempts aimed to minimise the scar defect) are doomed to failure, the inframammary crease returning to its original position after a few weeks or months, while the transverse scar ascends on the lower slope of the breast to become more apparent than if it had been placed correctly in the crease initially.

Though the inframammary crease is fixed in relation to the skin, it is mobile with the remainder of the breast over the chest wall.

This can be seen also after the surgical cure of hypertrophy, where the breast, relieved of its excessive weight and with its base reduced in extent, reascends with the crease on the chest wall because of the skin retraction associated with its elasticity.

The supramammary crease

This marks the upper limit of the breast, but is not evident in the standing position, or even spontaneously in the supine position. It can be demonstrated in the reclining patient by displacing the breast upward.

It is important to determine its limit as a landmark to be reached in separating gland from skin during a subcutaneous mastectomy, or in the Patey type of mastectomy.

The height of the breast

This corresponds to the distance between the supra- and inframammary creases and thus measures the vertical diameter of the base of the breast.

The quadrants of the breast

On topographic but not anatomic grounds, the breast seen from in front is divided into four quadrants: superomedial, superolateral, inferomedial and inferolateral, along two axes, vertical and horizontal, passing through the nipple.

The segments of the breast (fig. 19)

If the patient is examined standing, with the breast seen in profile, four segments can be defined on what is generally called the thoraco-mammary line, and study of these is useful in evaluating the position of the areola in relation to breast size and degree of ptosis:

- segment I, or infraclavicular thoracic segment, extends from the inferior border of the clavicle to the upper limit of the mammary gland, also known as the supramammary crease.

It varies in thickness with that of the subcutaneous fatty layer and of the pectoral muscles; apart from these two factors, it also varies in its obliquity downward and forward with the shape of the chest wall;

- segment II, or supra-areolar segment, extends from the supramammary crease, the point of attachment of the first ridge of Duret, to the upper limit of the nipple-areolar plaque. In a normal breast without ptosis, and in the standing position, it corresponds to two-thirds of the height of the breast base; ideally, it is slightly convex and faces forward and slightly upward. In fact, segment II very rapidly become slightly concave, at least in its upper part, this reversal of curvature being the first sign of developing ptosis;

- the nipple-areolar plaque, interposed between segments II and III, faces slightly upward and outward.

This orientation, which corresponds to the normal breast, is not that to be aimed for at the end of an operation to correct hypertrophy, where the areola should face forward, or even very slightly downward, and outward. In practice, the inevitable postoperative structural changes, which stabilise in around two months, are

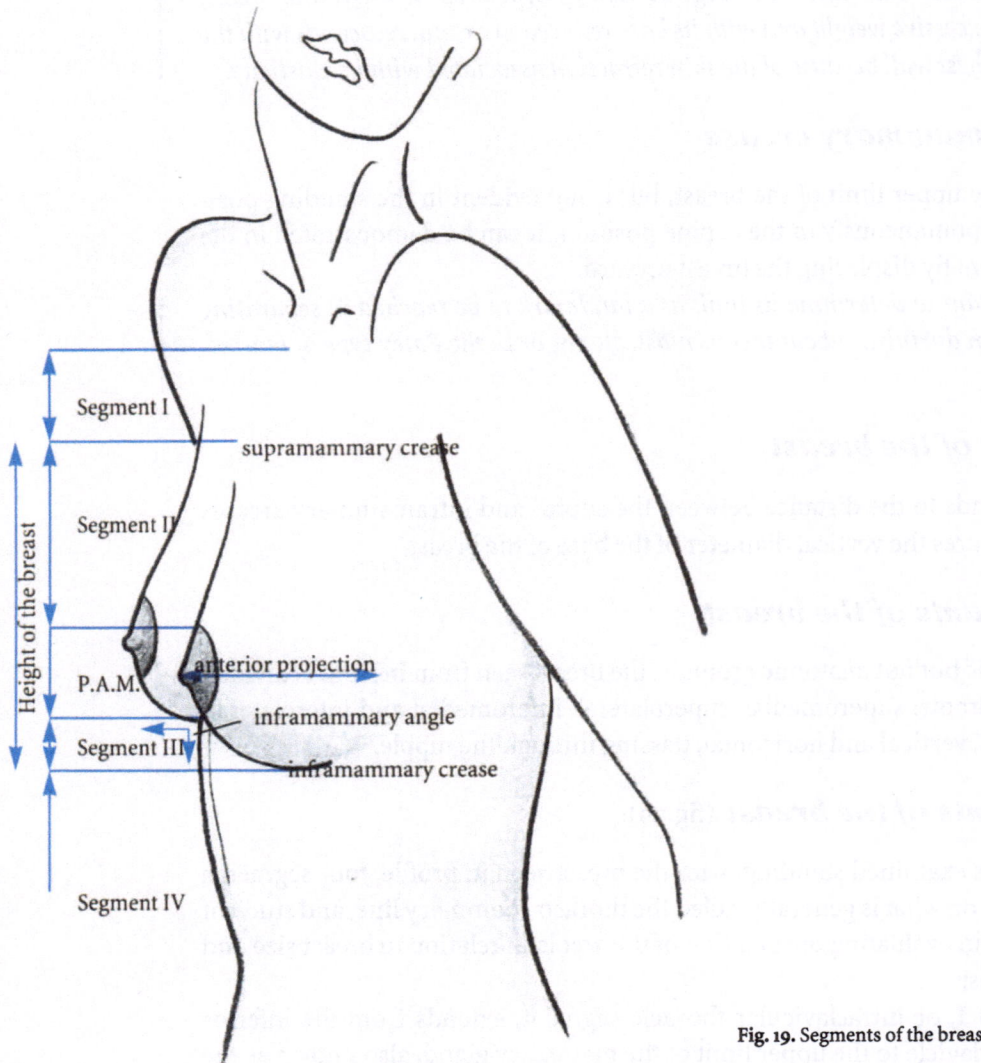

Fig. 19. Segments of the breast

evidenced by an inevitable relaxation of the skin envelope to an extent varying with its quality. To prevent ptosis, it is necessary that, at the end of the procedure, the reduction of the skin envelope should correspond to a moderate degree of overcorrection which achieves precisely this orientation of the areola, subject to other criteria to be considered;

– segment III, or subareolar segment, extends from the lower border of the nipple-areolar plaque to the inframammary crease. It corresponds to the inferior third of the extent of the base of the breast, and even in a breast without ptosis it is more convex than segment II;

– segment IV, or inframammary thoracic segment, extends the thoracic skin beyond the lower limit of the breast.

The anatomic separation between segments III and IV is very definite, since it corresponds to the inframammary crease, the lower limit of the last of Duret's ridges, and especially to the point where the superficial fascia of the subcutaneous plane passes into the retroglandular plane.

Anterior projection of the breast

This is measured from the midaxillary line behind to the tangent to the most anterior point of the breast volume in front. In a normal breast, without ptosis, it does not exceed a third of the basal diameter of breast implantation. It is an oblique line and cannot be an exact measurement of projection in the mathematical sense, since this would require the construction of a perpendicular on the chest wall passing through the breast meridian; and it becomes more inacccurate the more the breasts diverge.

Inframammary (or dihedral) angle

This is formed by the tangent taken from the inframammary crease at the lowest level of segment III and the vertical tangent to segment IV. It is one of the parameters used in assessing the degree of ptosis, which develops when it becomes less than 90°, another being the measurement of the distance between a horizontal plane passing through the lowest point of the inframmary crease and the horizontal plane passing through the most dependent point of the breast.

Breast size

It is quite difficult to define an ideal breast size in absolute terms since portrayal of the breast in different historical periods shows that the ideal breast has varied greatly in shape and size, according to the prevailing symbolic value attributed to it and the personal conceptions of the artist.

Starting with the abundant breast, confined to the gigantomasty of the Neanderthal Venus, a symbol of fecundity necessary to survival of the species, and with the polymazia of the Artemis of Ephesus (fig. 20), of similar significance, we pass to Egyptian, Greek and Roman statuary (fig. 21), where a more esthetic conception of the feminine image appears, together with a very marked decrease in the size of the ideal breast, which becomes rounded and whose base contracts, sometimes so much as almost to suggest the periprosthetic contracture so abhorred at the present day! The painters of the Middle Ages and of the Renaissance nearly always show us very small breasts (figs. 22 and 23), almost amounting to our current concept of hypoplasia. These breasts, unaffected by ptosis, regain their amplitude with the paintings of Rembrandt (fig. 24) and then of Rubens (fig. 25), a concept which persisted in representation of the female body up to the last century, ending in our own epoch with a breast of moderate size in harmony with the more linear silhouette of the modern woman and more compatible with the active life she so often leads.

Thus the notion of a normal breast size is very subjective, and varies with the period, fashion, ethnicity, and a number of socio-cultural factors which differ greatly in different countries (the breasts that we consider as bordering on hypertrophy in France being almost an indication for implant insertion in the United States!) and certainly with individual opinion.

It is therefore much more useful to seek to define an ideal breast size in terms of the general build of the patient and the shape of her thorax, and thus to reestablish harmony between the breasts and the figure generally. In these conditions, the correct breast volume will vary between 200 and 350 cm^3.

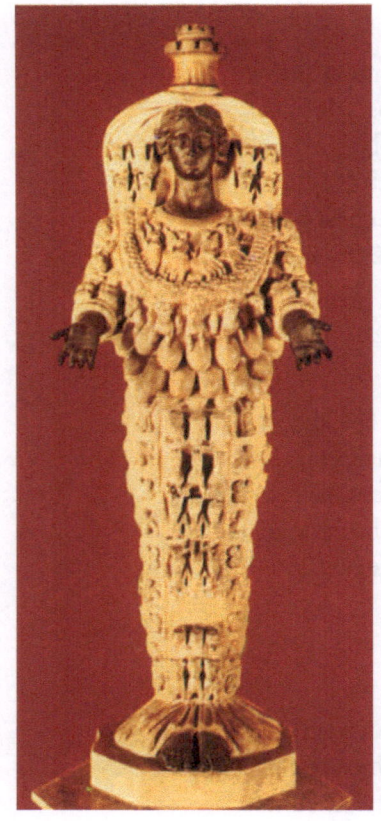
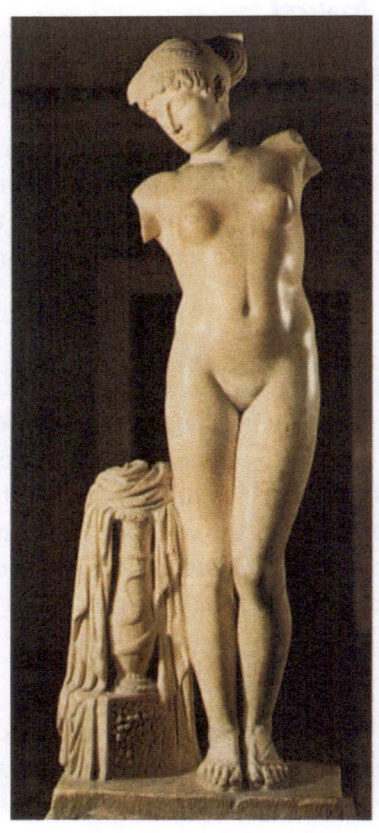
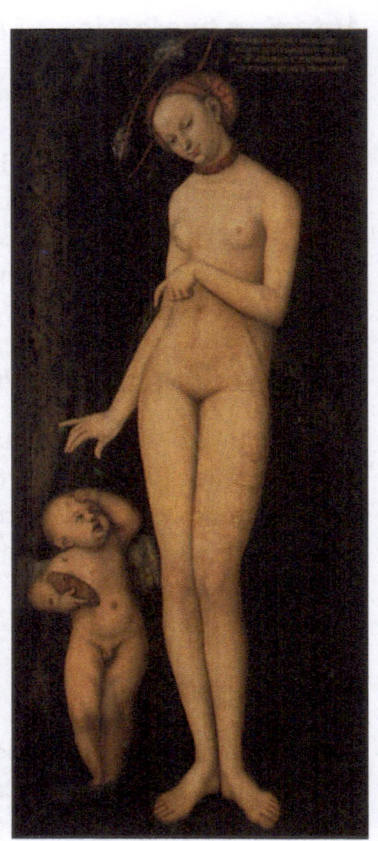

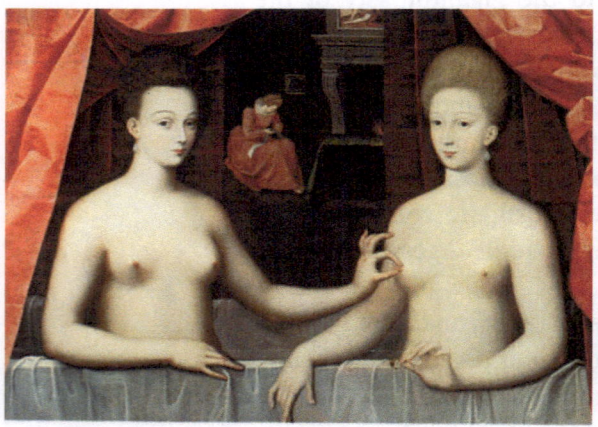
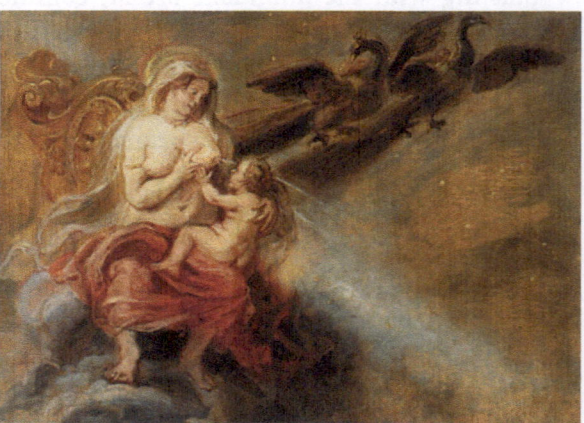

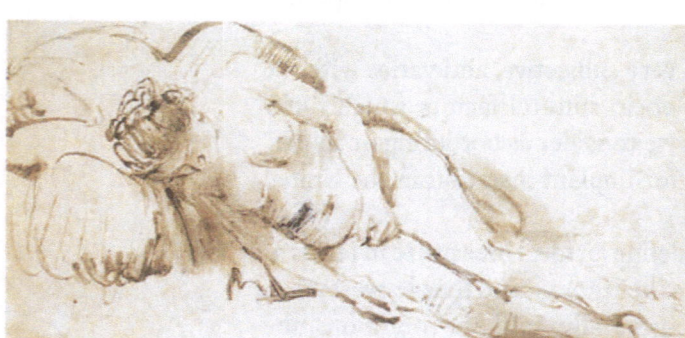

Fig. 20. Artemis of Ephesus (Rome, Capitoline Museums)

Fig. 21. Esquiline Venus, First Century BC (Rome, Capitoline Museums)

Fig. 22. Venus and Cupid, Lucas Cranach (1472-1553) (Belgian Royal Museum of Fine Arts, Brussels)

Fig. 23. Gabrielle d'Estrées and one of her sisters, School of Fontainebleau, late16th century (Paris, Louvre)

Fig.24. Juno suckling Hercules, Peter Paul Rubens (1577-1640) (Belgian Royal Museum of Fine Arts, Brussels)

Fig. 25. Nude woman on a pillow, Rembrandt Harmensz Van Rijn (1606-1669) (Amsterdam, Rijksmuseum).

Such concepts, already represented in the book by Lalardie and Jouglard, are not arrived at by measurement of breast volume, which is not easy to assess, but more simply by observation of the volumes used to fill the implants used in breast reconstruction.

Residual breast volume

In the surgery of breast reduction this is a much more important concept to define than simple breast size, for on it depends in great part the quality of the result.

The residual breast volume is that which remains after glandular resection. It is a function of the reduced base of implantation and of the anterior projection. If it is too small, the scar defect is much too obvious for the gain in shape. If too great, it carries the risk of short-term recurrence of the ptosis.

The object of a mammoplasty is not so much to resect a predetermined amount of tissue in terms of a certain initial size, as to obtain residual breast volumes, whatever the extent of the hypertrophy and the possible degree of asymmetry, which are equal, harmonious, related to the reduction of the breast base, and adapted to the general physique of the patient.

This is to stress the importance of techniques of breast reduction which allow reduction of breast size by any desired amount, and the adaptation of the breast base to this reduction, whatever the degree of the initial hypertrophy.

Conclusion

There certainly exists no single ideal type of breast, a concept false in absolute terms and one which must be integrated with the general conformation of the patient, independent of the taste of anyone else, whether painter, surgeon or even the patient requesting operation. Hence the importance, once again, of the preoperative assessment...

Though the ideal normal breast does not exist, the ideal operated breast will satisfy certain morphologic criteria, its dimensions being justified above all by the fact that this breast must have a harmonious shape which will protect it from ptosis, whether this be glandular or cutaneous.

It is in this light that it is conventional to respect certain measurements, though these distances should always be adapted to the shape of the chest wall and the patient's general build (fig. 26).

These criteria are as follows;

In a woman between 1.60 and 1.70 m in height:

– from the suprasternal notch to the areola: 17 to 19 cm;

– if this measurement is made on the axis of the breast based on a horizontal line passing through the suprasternal notch but 5 cm from the latter, this is shorter, since it corresponds roughly to the longer side of a right-angled triangle and not to its hypotenuse: 15.5 to 17 cm;

– from the midsternal line to the inner border of the areola: 8 to 9 cm;

– from the inferior border of the areola to the inframammary crease: 4.5 cm;

– for an areola of 4 to 4.5 cm diameter.

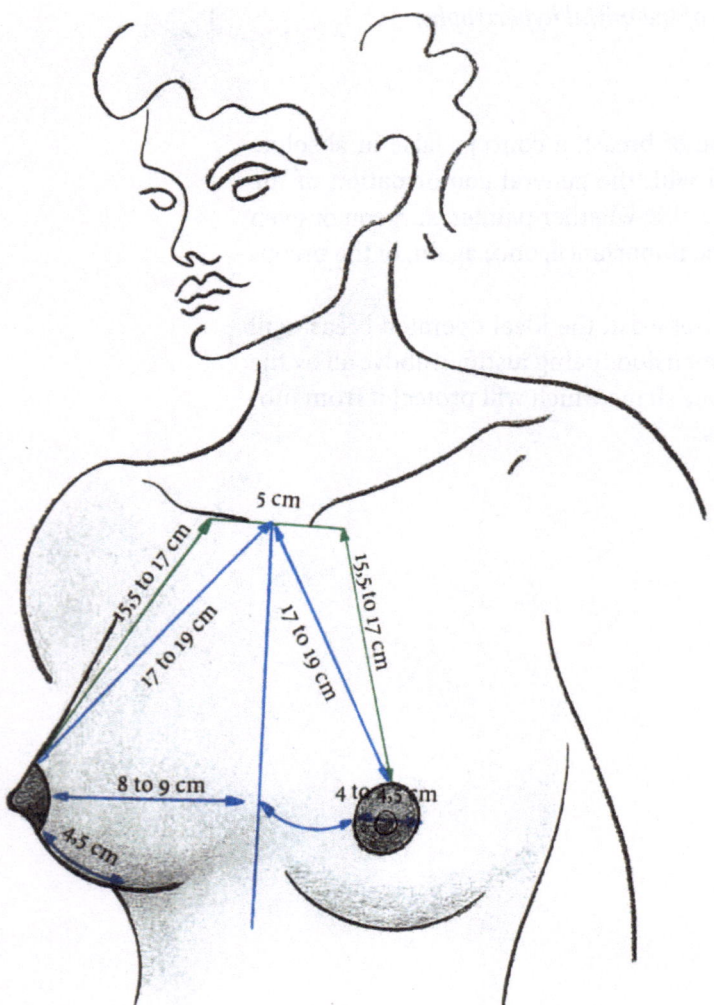

Fig. 26. Adequate dimensions of an operated breast

Photography

For the plastic surgeon the aims of photography are to provide a bank of illustrations easy to utilise, both for the personal analysis of results and for the purposes of audiovisual or written communication, or even for medicolegal purposes, by means of equipment that is relatively simple but of good quality, readily transportable and allowing work under simple conditions, either in the consulting room or in the operating room.

Equipment

Camera

Cameras of the type Reflex 24 x 36 are currently most used by amateurs like ourselves. It is convenient to have available a camera allowing TTL (through the lens) flash photography; the light intensity is measured through the lens by the camera cell, the flash (which does not have its own cell) being connected directly to it.

Since an additional light source is practically always necessary, given that the photography is made indoors, this measurement of exposure through the lens guarantees virtually constant correct exposure.

Professional photographers normally work with lighting arranged around the subject, or with multiple flashes allowing the conjunction of several light sources, and a manual exposure meter. While this type of photography may be of a more artistic nature, this is not the chief aim in our practice, since the necessary equipment is cumbersome and has to be installed on site in a precise location, which is hardly suited to our normal conditions of working.

Lighting

A single flash, fixed on a camera in frontal position, is usually satisfactory. Those which can be variably angled are preferable. Forward angulation is useful for close-up views, whereas in some cases it may be desirable to direct the light up to the ceiling and to photograph in reflected light.

The annular flash has important indications, especially in macrophotography, endobuccal photography and close-up views of the face. However, it is inadvisable for the shots that interest us in the surgery of the breast, since it tends to "flatten" the subject by eliminating the relief.

Some operative photographs are more striking when taken in transillumination, as for the demonstration of a vascular pedicle. This can be done by using a scialytic lamp as additional lighting opposite the lens and shining through the subject being photographed (fig. 27), with the flash physically separate trom the camera but connected to it by a flex, so as to ensure correct exposure (fig. 28).

Lenses

Two fixed-focus lenses suffice. It is better to use fixed-focus lenses rather than a zoom lens to standardise the shooting conditions and to provide comparable films.

The pre- and postoperative films are made with a small tele-lens of 105 mm, allowing for macrophotography. Although this focal length is not the same as that of the human eye, it does allow flash photography with satisfactory illumination, more easily with the subject at a reasonable distance (about 1.50 m for the thorax), without exaggerated shadows or appreciable image distortion.

This distance of 1.5 to 2 m is also that corresponding to human relations at the normal distance of observation between two persoms. A closer approach implies an idea of intimacy — or aggression — which is not suited to the doctor-patient relationship and may make the latter uneasy.

In the operating room we use a macro lens of 50 mm focal length, which corresponds to the human eye and allows for close-up views.

Films

Transparencies (reversible film) are the films of choice.

This type of film is immediately available for audiovisual presentations and easy to store (storage sheets). The reversible film allows direct printing on colored paper and even, without need for an inter-negative, on black and white paper thanks to small instantaneous developers (Vivitar, Polaroid) which provide films of quite satisfactory quality, allowing for the low-level enlargement used in publications. Our preference for some years has been for Kodachrome 64 ASA, and more recently Kodak Ektachrome Elite 100 ASA, whose average sensitivity is associated with a high resolving power and a warmer dominant than Ektachrome Standard. Moreover, Kodachrome film currently has the longest known shelf-life.

Choice of background

A constant background is essential for the correct evaluation of results.

It is no longer acceptable, in photographs intended to be of medical quality, to be able to distinguish a doorknob, the folds of a towel, the corner of an operating room, or reflections on a glossy wall.

We have resolved this problem by means ot two identical roller blinds whose matt material does not give rise to reflections, one installed in the consulting-room, the other at the hospital. The color is a medium blue-green, agreeable to the eye and flattering to the skin, which enhances a flesh tint by complementarity (fig. 29). Black backgrounds, because of contrast and compensation of exposure (unless one works with a manual light-meter), often give an unduly pallid tint to the skin, while over-exposure may conceal the details, particularly scars, whereas white backgrounds, on the contrary, give the skin a more sombre hue, with a tendency to under-exposure which exaggerates shadows.

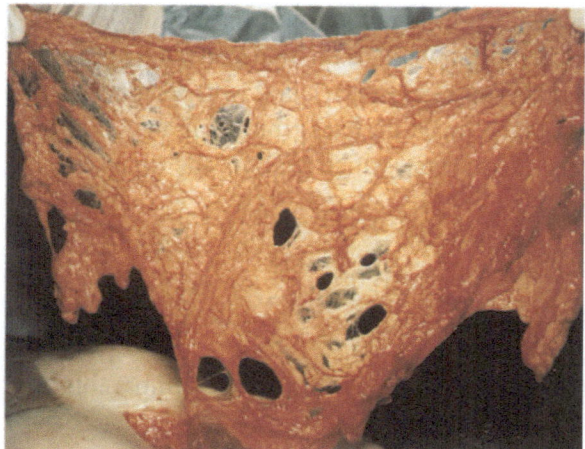 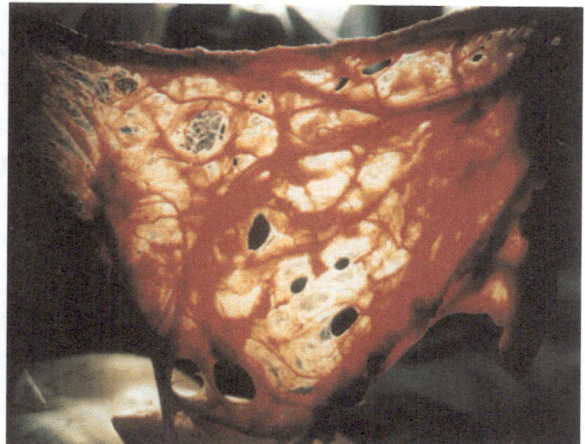

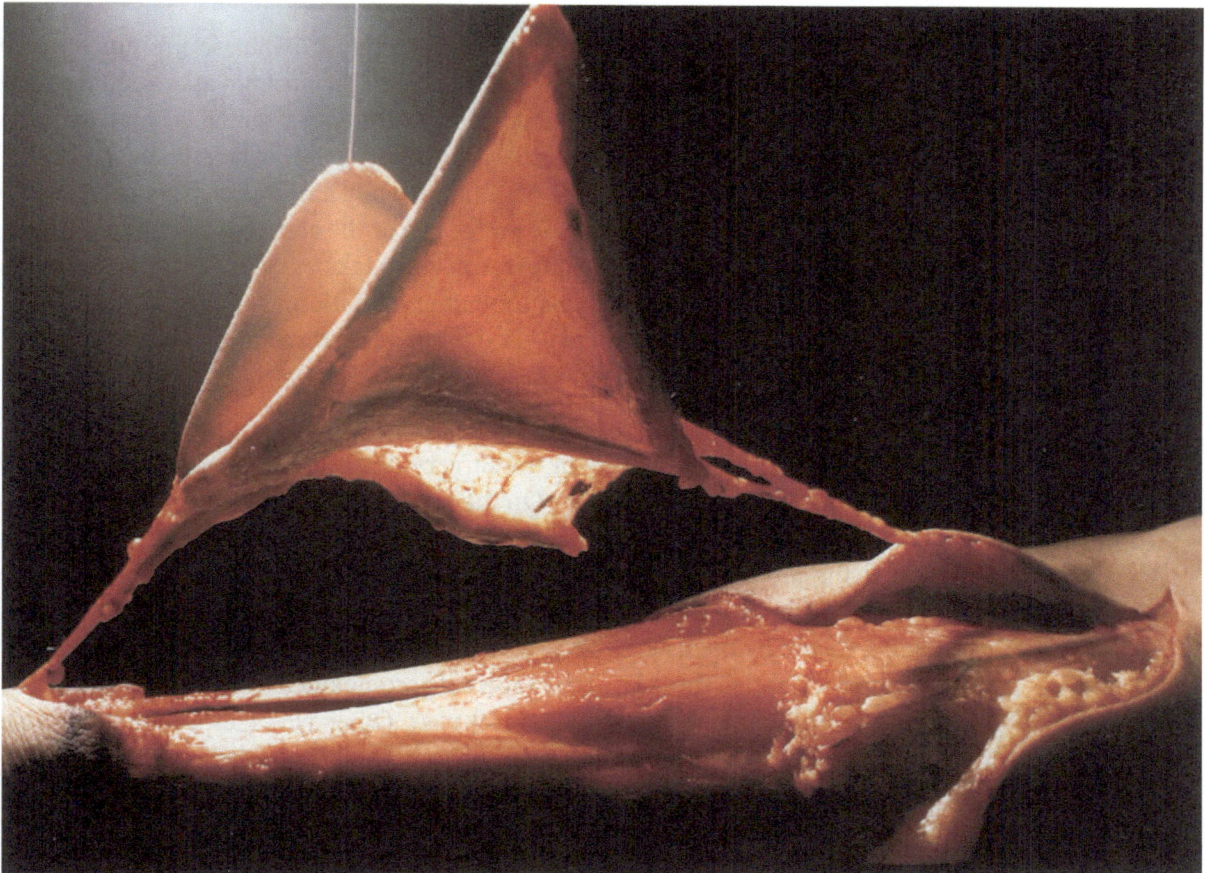

Fig. 27 a, b. Transillumination: omentoplasty. **a** The omentum is illuminated from in front and behind by two scialytic lamps, **b** only the lighting behind the omentum has been retained

Fig. 28. Transillumination: so-called "Chinese" forearm flap: the vascular plexus is clearly visualised. A single light source is used, with the flash connected to the camera by a flex, placed above and in front of the subject photographed, which is also useful in eliminating the background

The ideal would be to work with a neutral gray background (at 18%), but this hue is somewhat gloomy in our opinion, and a medium blue-green background is not only pleasing in projection but also appears in black and white prints as virtually neutral. The disadvantage of black or white backgrounds is that they give direct prints on paper with excessive contrast, which impairs the quality of the image.

Shooting

Views and setting must be absolutely standardised to provide comparable pre- and postoperative films.

Subject

While jewellery may possibly be retained, provided it is not so prominent as to attract excessive attention, garments and underclothes must not appear on the photograph as they tend to deprive the study of the neutrality essential to objectivity and to the medical anonymity of the film. Again, they are rarely of an esthetic nature.

The marks of too tight underclothes are equally a nuisance. This is rarely the case in the preoperative films made on the eve or the actual day of operation, but may be so sometimes during postoperative views taken in the consulting room. As these photographs are taken some time after operation, we advise the patient at the preceding consultation not to wear tight underclothes for the next visit.

Framing (fig. 29)

It is easy to respect anonymity in the surgery of the breast, since the face has no place in this type of photography. On the other hand, the view should not be too close-up, or it will give the eye a disagreeable impression of being situated too close to the subject.

Such close-up views, which do not provide an overall view of the operated region, do not by themselves allow objective analysis of the result. These films, or the films of a detail, should only be shown if accompanied by an overall view.

All the films are to be taken in axial view. Other views, especially low-angle shots in three-quarter views, risk being unrealistically flattering.

Views

A minimum of five basic views must be routinely taken pre- and postoperatively, supplemented as required by certain views specific to the procedure, apart from any peroperative views.

Frontal
This is the essential and indispensable view. As Vilain has pointed out, the outcome of a mammoplasty is judged from in front. Hence one should be wary of articles which shows a frontal view preoperatively and a three-quarter view for the result !

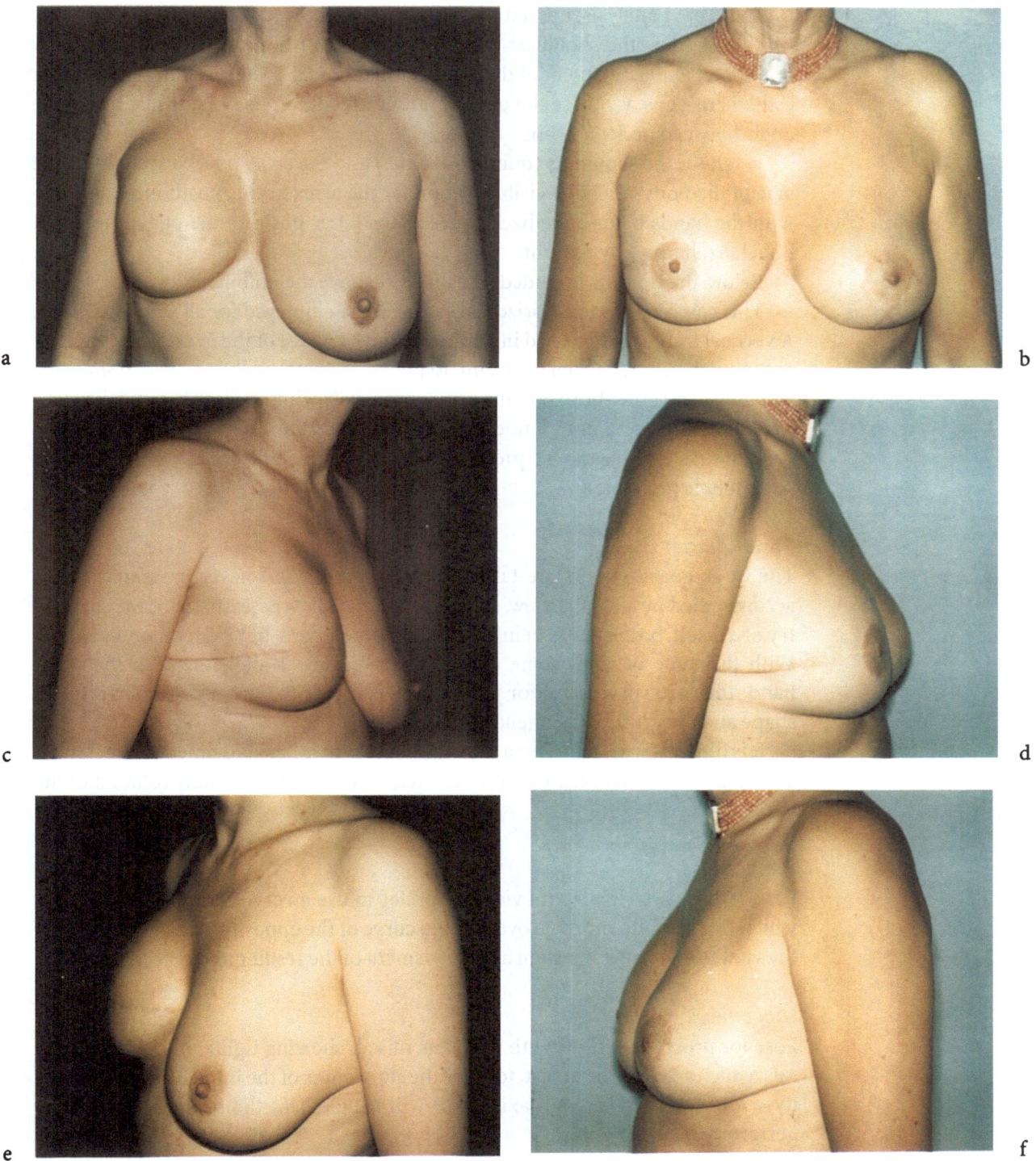

Fig. 29 a-f. Background and frame. a, b a black or very dark background is not very flattering, unlike a medium background. c, e three-quarter views are difficult to standardise, but are useful in assessing curvature. d, f skewed lateral views showing the curve of the other breast allow better assessment of any asymmetry and are more objective than the two false profiles shown (d seems to show symmetric curvatures but the asymmetry suggested by the frontal view is confirmed in f)

Breast reconstruction:

a, c, e: mastectomy — immediate reconstruction by expansile prosthesis, films taken at end of expansion b, d, f: after change to a definitive inflatable implant, reduction plasty of opposite breast, reconstruction of areola by tattooing and graft from opposite nipple

For proper analysis, the setting must respect certain conditions. The top of the film must show the shoulders entirely, allowing verification that they are really horizontal and assessment of the shape of the thorax. To ensure this, and also for esthetic reasons, we place the upper limit of the film in the viewer just below the angle between neck and chin.

Laterally, the shoulders (quite horizontal) and the arms (placed straight by the side of the body) must be visible. We prefer the arms in this position rather than with the hands behind the back, since in the latter position the patient may not hold herself properly upright.

Below, the frame is bounded by a line just above the umbilicus.

This corresponds to a horizontal setting to be employed for all standard views. A vertical frame may be used in addition to give an idea of the overall morphology of the subject, but, if taken from chin to pubis, it is not usually possible to show the shoulders and outer border of the arms completely without also showing the face. Retention of a horizontal frame for every view has the additional advantage of a harmonious and pleasanter presentation during an audiovisual communication with double projection.

Three-quarter

The three-quarter views are taken from both sides and never presented unless accompanied by a frontal view, since they do not allow assessment of the symmetry of a result, both breasts being viewed simultaneously but from different angles. With this type of view, some asymmetries disappear altogether. On the other hand, they are very useful for judging the curve of the breasts, particularly the shape and curvature of segments II and III.

It is difficult to standardise a 3/4 view without making guidelines on the floor at 45° for the position of the feet; it is also necessary to eliminate any rotation of the back.

Profiles

Rather than a strictly lateral view, we prefer to use a very slightly skewed profile which reveals, with minimal overlap, the curve of the opposite breast. The angle of the view is thus more constant and assessment of the result more objective.

Other views

Pose for prostheses: films with the arms raised, showing tightening of the pectorals, which squeeze the breast, to show the suppleness of the implant and its mobility with the breast. A high axial view will supplement the visualisation of any periprosthetic contracture.

Breast reconstruction:

– views centered on the reconstructed areola, frontal and lateral (to show the nipple outline),

– views from the back in cases with reconstruction using the latissimus dorsi, even with a brassière postoperatively, to show the position of the donor site scar. The entire trunk in frontal, lateral and possibly three-quarter views for reconstructions with a rectus abdominis flap. Views showing the design of the flap.

Timing of photography

Preoperatively: the five basic views and possibly other views appropriate to the operative procedure.

Postoperatively:

– films taken before 6 months are of little value, except when taken before a second-stage procedure, as the shape and scars are not yet stabilised;

– the postoperative films are valuable:

• after 6 months, where the essential shape is usually achieved,

• subsequently, films taken at 1 and 2 years, and later when possible.

Conclusion

It is relatively simple, and possible, for every surgeon to produce correct and objective photographs suitable for analysis and publication.

It should no longer be acceptable to see:

– poor frames, taken every which way, showing background features such as the corner of a toilet or a door, the shiny windows of an operating room, the anesthetic equipment, more or less well hidden by a drape creating folds and held across by the assistant, whose hands and even face are visible,

– films so dark as to be uninterpretable,

– more serious, films taken in conditions that verge on manifest intellectual dishonesty, because:

• routinely under-exposed preoperatively,

• and over-exposed postoperatively, which has the "advantage" of blurring the scars and, in facial surgery, of considerably improving the effects of a face-lift on the wrinkles,

• taken in high-angle preoperatively, and low-angle postoperatively, which is much more flattering for the curve of a breast, especially in three-quarter view.

The use for all views, apart from certain technical peroperative views, of the same background, and identical lighting conditions thanks to the same flash, placed in the same position on a TTL reflex camera, while taking care to retain the same frame, guarantees the best conditions for objectivity and therefore credibility.

References

Bostwick J (1990) Anatomy and physiology of the breast: Plastic and reconstructive breast surgery, Vol. 1, pp 57-97. Quality Medical Publishing Inc, Saint-Louis

Flageul G (1989) Analyse morphologique du sein, rapport du XXXIVème congrès de la Société Française de Chirurgie Plastique, Reconstructrice et Esthétique, pp 29-38, Paris

Guntz M (1975) Nomenclature anatomique illustrée. Masson, Paris

Lacotte B, De Mey A (1991) Anatomy and Physiology of the Breast, Vth European Course in Plastic Surgery, pp 2-7, Lejour M, Bruxelles, 16-21 Sept

Lalardrie JP, Jouglard JP (1974) Chirurgie Plastique du sein. Masson, Paris

Lalardrie JP, Jouglard JP (1974) La morphologie et l'anatomie du sein normal. Chirurgie Plastique du sein, pp 1-25. Masson, Paris

Langman J (1968) Embryologie médicale. Masson, Paris

Laurent B (1990) L'acte photographique en chirurgie plastique, reconstructive et esthétique, Thèse pour le doctorat en médecine, Tours

Ricbourg B, Hidden G (1989) Anatomie du sein. In: Hypertrophie mammaire, rapport du XXXIVème congrès de la Société Française de Chirurgie Plastique, Reconstructrice et Esthétique, Paris

Rouvière H. (1962) Anatomie humaine, tome 3. Masson, Paris

Rouvière H (1967) Appareil génital de la femme, Mamelles, Anatomie Humaine, descriptive et topographique, tome II, pp 528-531, 10ème édition. Masson, Paris,

Salmon M. (1988) Arteries of the skinr. Churchill Livingstone. New York

Tuchmann-Duplessis H, Haegel P (1970) Embryologie. Masson, Paris

Surgical approaches
to the breast

Despite all the progress in accessory investigations, and whether the lesion is palpable or revealed by imaging, the surgical approach often constitutes the sole and definitive means of obtaining a precise histologic diagnosis and of studying the glandular architecture, while at the same time constituting a therapeutic procedure.

The approach to a breast lesion must satisfy several requirements :
– it must be sufficiently extensive and properly sited so as to permit unhampered excision of the lesion;
– while minimising as far as possible the price paid in terms of scar defect and alteration in shape;
– and without hindering or compromising by its positioning a more extensive excision (eg, it should lie within the path of a possible future mastectomy) or a subsequent plastic procedure.

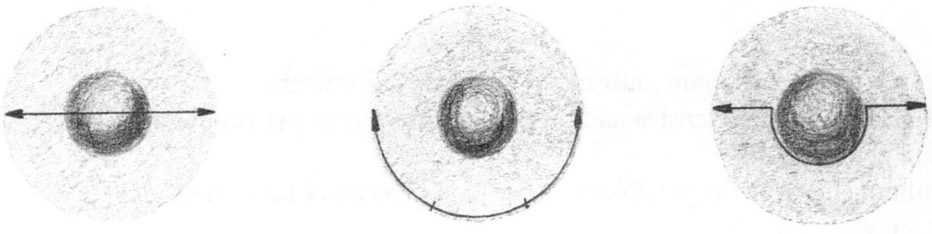

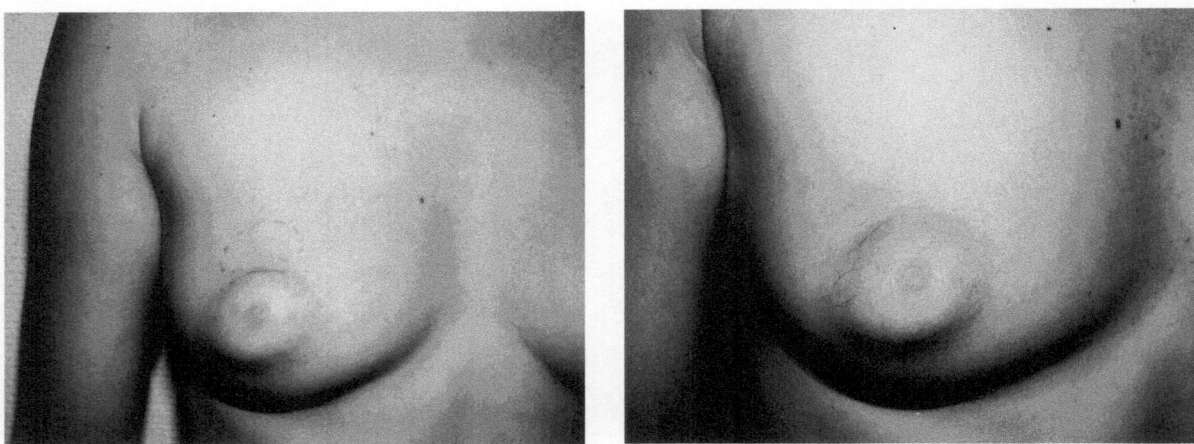

Fig. 30 a,b. a Areolar approaches. a Above, center : hemiareolar incision; two small nicks with the scalpel on this very slightly infra-areolar incision serve as landmarks for correct approximation at closure; above, left : transareolar and trans-nipple incision; above, right : transareolar incision around the base of the nipple. In these last two cases, it is helpful to approximate the nipple by a deep suture at its base to prevent retraction and deformation; **b** adenoma of superolateral quadrant : approach by superior intra-areolar route c appearance of scar at 6 months

The different approaches
to benign tumors

Intra-areolar approaches

These are the preferred routes of access to superficial lesions of the gland. A medium-sized nodule (3-5 cm in diameter) can be removed without difficulty up to at least 5 to 7 cm from the peripheral boundary of the areola.

Placement of the incision depends on the size of the areola and the topography of the lesion (fig. 30).

The incision may be horizontal transverse, splitting the nipple at its middle or skirting its base. In both cases, before closure of the superficial layers, it is important to appose the two parts of the base of the nipple by a deep suture so as not to produce any deformation or retraction.

A curved peripheral incision is the other alternative, especially when the areola is small, as it has the advantage of being relatively longer. It is best to place the incision very slightly within the periphery of the areola (1 mm), which is often not clearly defined, rather than to make the incision at or outside this boundary; the residual scar will be less evident.

When the lesion is accessible to palpation, its position is marked on the skin with ink.

For smaller or deeper lesions, help is provided by the use of ultrasound on the morning of operation and in the operative position; with the patient supine and the arm beside the trunk the radiologist makes a skin marking with a felt pen and indelible ink at the level of the lesion.

If the lesion, such as a focus of microcalcification, is not palpable, ultrasonic or stereotactic location with insertion of a transfixing harpoon is the best technique, followed by radiography of the excised specimen. The use of a harpoon is preferable to a simple needle, which may be displaced during the dissection.

While radiography of the operative specimen is essential to confirm excision of the relevant focus, it should be borne in mind that it is better not to request immediate histologic examination, which is difficult to interpret and is likely to give false-negative results. It is preferable to keep the entire specimen intact for histologic examination after embedding.

The path of the incision is drawn with a fine brush. For a semicircular incision, two small scratches made superficially with the scalpel at right angles to the incision will facilitate approximation of the skin margins at the end of the operation.

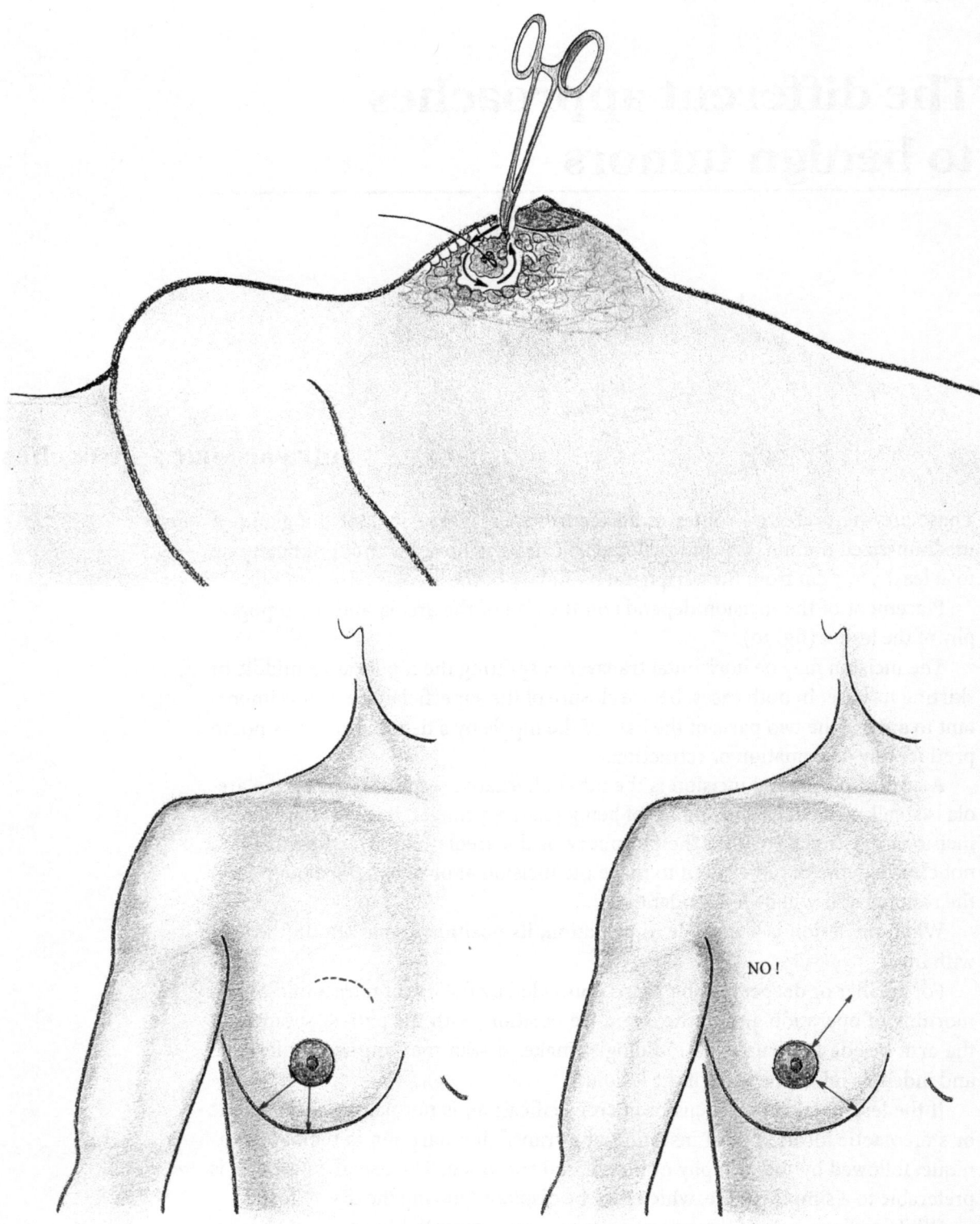

Fig. 31. Excision of lesion by transareolar route after location with harpoon

Fig. 32. Radial incisions give an acceptable scar defect when vertical or oblique/lateral. If a radial incision is necessary in the upper quadrants it is better curved

Fig. 33. Radial incisions should not be used in the medial quadrants

The incision of the superficial layers is made perpendicular to the skin with a 15 scalpel-blade and the margins are elevated with skin hooks.

The dissection is continued with Metzenbaum scissors, their concavity turned towards the gland, passing to the deep aspect of the subcutaneous tissue and dividing the ridges of Duret flush with the gland as far as the level of the lesion (fig. 31).

The lesion is then excised with scissors (Mayo's scissors are better then Metzenbaum's when the gland is firm) by plunging into the gland. A diathermy knife may also be used, provided the access is wide enough for good retraction of the margins of the incision so as to avoid damaging them.

Drainage is unnecessary in cases where the residual cavity is small, provided hemostasis is scrupulous and a moderately compressive dressing applied. If drainage is desired, it is best to use a superficial suture to approximate the gland and to place the drain beneath this, and to check before applying the dressing that the dead space does not create a depression which would risk perpetuating a skin dimple opposite the zone of excision; or the tissues may be left to fill in over a simple rubber dam rather than a suction drain.

In most cases closure can be done without suture of the gland at the level of the excision. However, suture of the deep glandular layer with a fine absorbable suture can be done opposite the incision, taking care to avoid any deformation of the areola.

Suture of the superficial layers is made at two levels : the deep dermal layer with interrupted inverting 4/0 absorbable sutures, the superficial dermal layer with a continuous intradermal suture of rapidly absorbable 4/0 material or monofilament 3/0 or 4/0 nylon which is removed around the 12th postoperative day.

The dressing is made with adhesive strapping to approximate the skin edges, gauze pads and adhesive elastic bandages. This dressing is retained for 24 to 48 hours, while the adhesive skin strips are left at least until removal of the sutures if the latter are not absorbable.

Radial approaches

These are indicated if the lesion is bulky, to extend a semicircular intra-areolar approach.

The incision may be vertical and subareolar or lateral and oblique (fig. 32).

Radial incisions in the inferolateral or superior quadrants are undesirable for cosmetic reasons (fig. 33). There is also a not inconsiderable risk of scar hypertrophy when the midline is approached.

Closure of such an incision is also made in two layers, placing the margins under slight tension by two hooks at both ends of the incision, so as to prevent slippage. The deep dermal layer is closed with inverting interrupted sutures of slowly-absorbed 3/0 or 4/0 gauge, the superficial intradermal plane with rapidly-absorbed fine material or monofilament nylon.

Axillary route

This allows easier access to a lesion situated in the axillary prolongation of the gland.

If the lesion is very low down, the incision is made behind and parallel to the palpable prominence of the inferolateral border of the pectoralis major (fig. 34).

If the lesion is situated higher up, at the lower part of the axillary fossa proper, a horizontal incision which is very slightly concave upward and situated in a natural flexion crease, at about 3 cm from thre apex if the axilla, is preferable. Its anterior end should not transgress on the prominence of the pectoralis major (fig. 34).

After stripping the skin, the lower border of the pectoralis can be freed and retracted, the muscle being best relaxed by placing the arm in 90° of abduction and anteflexion), but the muscle or its tendon must not be incised for fear of producing very ugly depression or adhesion at the scar.

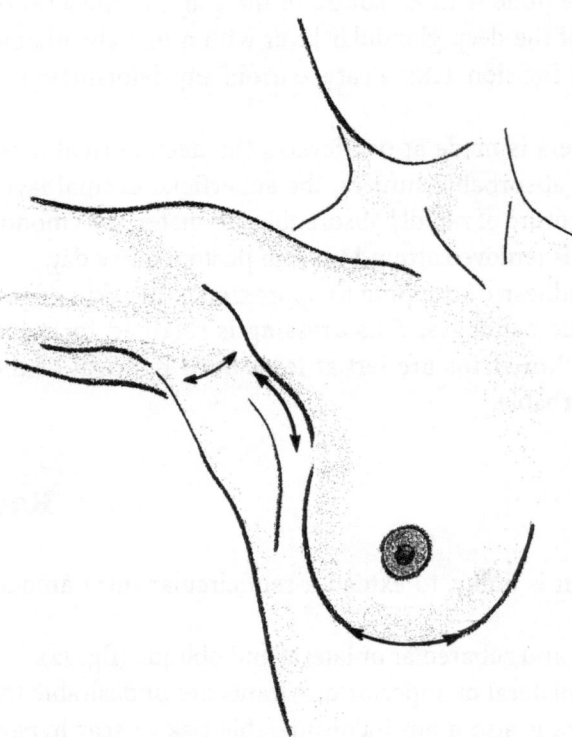

Fig. 34. Axillary and "inframammary" approaches; actually the latter incision should be placed strictly in the inframammary crease

Inframammary route

This is the route of choice for accessing bulky or deeply situated lesions, whatever their site, or lesions of the inferior quadrants, and for performing routine biopsies in all four quadrants or in the case of diffuse lesions, as it gives excellent exposure of the whole of the deep aspect of the gland.

The scar defect is altogether minor provided it is placed strictly in the inframammary crease (fig. 34). Therefore the crease is drawn with a skin pencil or a fine indelible felt pen in the standing or seated patient before operation, if this is to be carried out with the patient supine. Alternatively, and preferably, the operating table can be placed in the semi-seated position once the patient is anesthetised.

If the breast is deformed and stretched by a bulky lesion, such as a phylloidal tumor, correct placement of the crease may be difficult to locate as it will appear artifically lower. One must then be guided by symmetry with the inframammary crease of the opposite breast.

The incision (a few cm is usually adequate) is centered at the middle of the inframammary crease. If greater access is necessary, it can readily be extended laterally, still in the crease, but one should not approach the midline too closely for two reasons : the crease is less well defined medially than laterally, so that the scar may be more obvious; also, in approaching the midsternal region, the risk of a hypertrophic or even keloidal scar cannot be excluded.

After incision of the superficial layers, it is useful to retract the upper margin of the incision with hooks or a clawed retractor to remain at the level of the muscular plane. Care should be taken after the first stage of stripping to avoid involvement with the digitations of the serratus anterior musccle laterally and the intercostal muscles medially, or under the lower edge of the pectoralis major posteriorly.

Tissue adhesions require dissection with scissors or scalpel as far as the lower border of the pectoralis. This is where hemostasis becomes more important. Once the lower border of the pectoralis is crossed, stripping is much easier and can be done by blunt dissection, which is virtually bloodless. In the case of superior quadrant lesions, stripping can be taken as far as the upper pole of the gland without difficulty.

After confirming hemostasis, if need be with the help of a retractor, it is preferable to close over a suction drain. It is unnecessary to tether the lower pole of the gland to the parietal tissues (a procedure which may even be harmful by creating adhesions above the crease), because the inframammary crease is so well-marked anatomically.

Summary

The choice of incision depends on:
- the size of the areola,
- the topography of the lesion and its bulk.

Small superficial lesions situated close to the areola should be accessed by the areolar route, using either a horizontal transverse or a curved peripheral incision, involving a quarter or even half the areola.

It is certainly preferable to avoid curved incisions if they necessarily involve the whole of the upper half of the areola. They may, in fact, compromise survival of the areola when a mammoplasty is envisaged in the near future, using one of the techniques with a superior pedicle that form the basis of modern methods. This situation is not exceptional and may be encountered if biopsies are made on the opposite breast during the first stage of a breast reconstruction, or in the context of considerations that may result in possible subcutaneous mastectomy.

Bulkier lesions of the lower quadrants may be accessed by an inferior semicircular route extended by a radial incision, either vertical or oblique lateral, or by an inframammary route, depending on the distance between the lesion and the areola or the creased.

Lesions situated near the inframammary crease are accessed by the inframammary route, as are all bulky or deep lesions.

Lesions of the superolateral quadrant, at the axillary extremity of the gland, are accessed by the axillary route.

The problem of mammary discharge

Isolated mammary discharge

After having identified the lactiferous duct responsible (by expressing the gland in each quadrant), one may resort to galactography by injecting a dye, methylene blue, through a fine catheter, using very little of the medium so as to avoid staining of the operative field. It is often easier to insert a bristle into the orifice of the sinus as far as possible until arrested, so as to guide the excision and confine it to the ramification concerned.

A transverse areolar incision is made circumscribing the orifice identified, through which a pyramidectomy is done, step by step, from the surface to the depths, so as to extract the whole length of the lactiferous sinus involved by removing all the affected territory (fig. 35). This can be assisted by traction on a suture but this traction should not be excessive, so as not to damage the branching system.

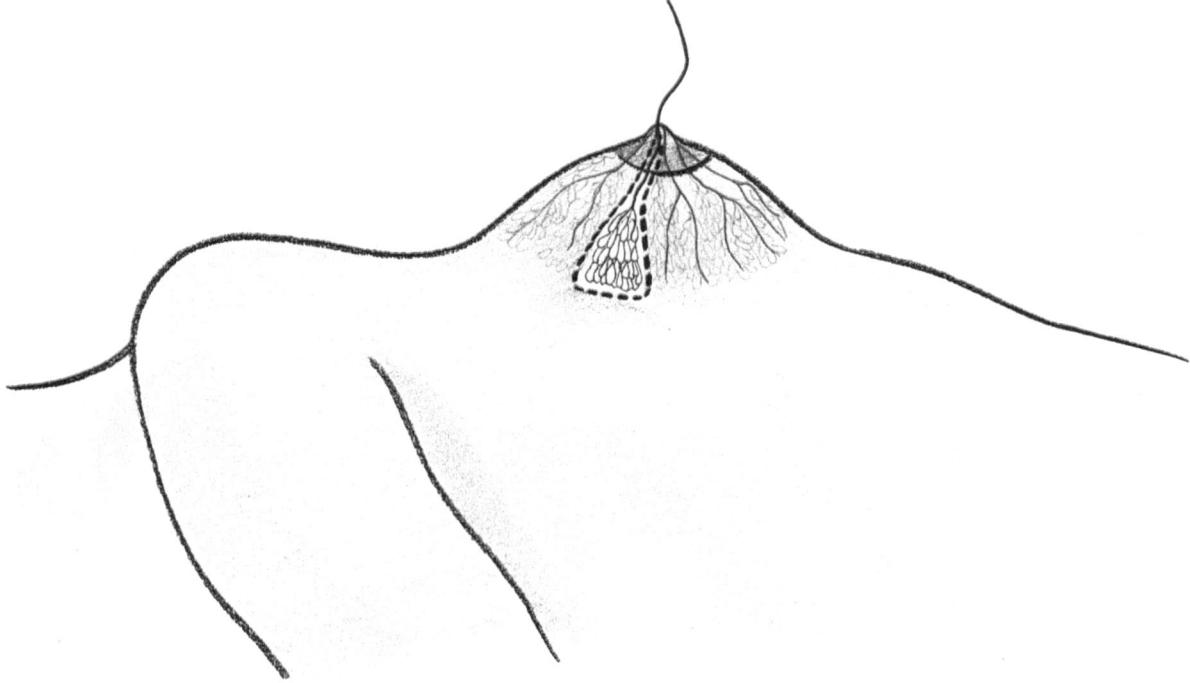

Fig. 35. Pyramidectomy

Discharge associated with a nodule

If the discharge is associated with a nodule or an abnormal radiologic image, the associated lesion must of course be removed as a priority, with a request for immediate histologic examination if there is the least clinical or radiologic suspicion.

Tumorectomy

Approach

Classically, it is indicated to use a direct approach over a suspect lesion because of the associated skin sacrifice. Actually, skin loss will be routine only if the lesion is superficial or if there are skin changes at this level. In practice, when the lesion is remote from the superficial layers and the breast is somewhat bulky or ptosed, the skin segment "over" the tumor is variable, depending on whether the patient is examined in the standing or lying position, and skin sacrifice is much less logical since it is more dificult to assess unless there is an associated plastic procedure.

Direct incision with initial skin sacrifice is therefore indicated only in superficial lesions of the gland with changes in the overlying skin and a very strong suspicion of malignancy. Otherwise, skin sacrifice, if it does prove necessary, can always be made after immediate verification of malignancy.

However, one must ensure that it remains within the bounds of a possible future mastectomy. If this is not the case, it is preferable to use a superior hemiareolar incision for tumors of the upper quadrants, and a radial incision for tumors of the lower quadrants. However, the inframammary incision remains the preferred route to perform an extensive tumorectomy (with a safety margin of at least 2 cm in all directions), once the lesion is found not to be superficial, since it allows easy access to the whole of the deep aspect of the gland by posterior stripping, with excellent exposure even of the upper quadrants.

Radial incisions in the upper quadrants are to be avoided because of the poor cosmetic results; if direct access is necessary here, it is better to use a curved incision.

Tumorectomy

After incision of the skin and subcutaneous layer, the tumor is located by palpation and a wide excision is performed with an adequate safety margin in all directions, well away from the boundaries of the tumor as palpated, so as to avoid disrupting the lesion with possible residual malignant potential.

The glandular incision may be made with a diathermy knife, starting at the plane of the pectoralis major and stripping the deep aspect of the gland with the finger widely, beyond the anticipated margins of the excision; this allows good identification of the margins of the lesion and simultaneous exploration of the adjacent regions.

The specimen is immediately identified by several metal wires or locators if immediate radiography of the tumor is desired, and is sent for histologic examination with a corresponding diagram. The margins of the excision are checked in a search for any abnormal induration which might indicate supplementary resection.

Depending on the size of the gap created by the tumorectomy in relation to the remainder of the gland, the deep layer may be brought together by a few sutures, or the tissues may be left to fill in the cavity gradually provided hemostasis has been scrupulous and drainage is by a suction drain, or by a rubber dam if it is feared that suction may give rise to deformity.

If an extensive tumorectomy is performed on a breast of small or moderate size, and if there is a risk of subsequent deformity, the question of filling in the gland by a plastic procedure arises. Should this be the case, it should be done by a simple maneuver, usually a rotation by posterior stripping of the margins at the level of the muscle plane (fig. 36). This type of plasty is one that least modifies the architecture of the gland. Where the margins are approximated, one or more metal locators are placed to facilitate subsequent mammographic surveillance and to serve as landmarks for any subsequent radiotherapy (fig. 37).

If radium therapy is foreseen, with the insertion of guide cannulas preoperatively, the radiotherapist, in collaboration with the surgeon, will place markers on the gland margins before these are approximated so as to precisely identify the margins of the excision.

The associated lymph node clearance is performed through a separate incision from the tumorectomy, to avoid scar contracture or retraction of the nipple. This axillary incision is placed behind and parallel to the pectoralis major tendon. It is only with tumors of the superolateral quadrant that the incision may become common to both procedures, but its direction should then be changed at midpoint to avoid secondary contracture.

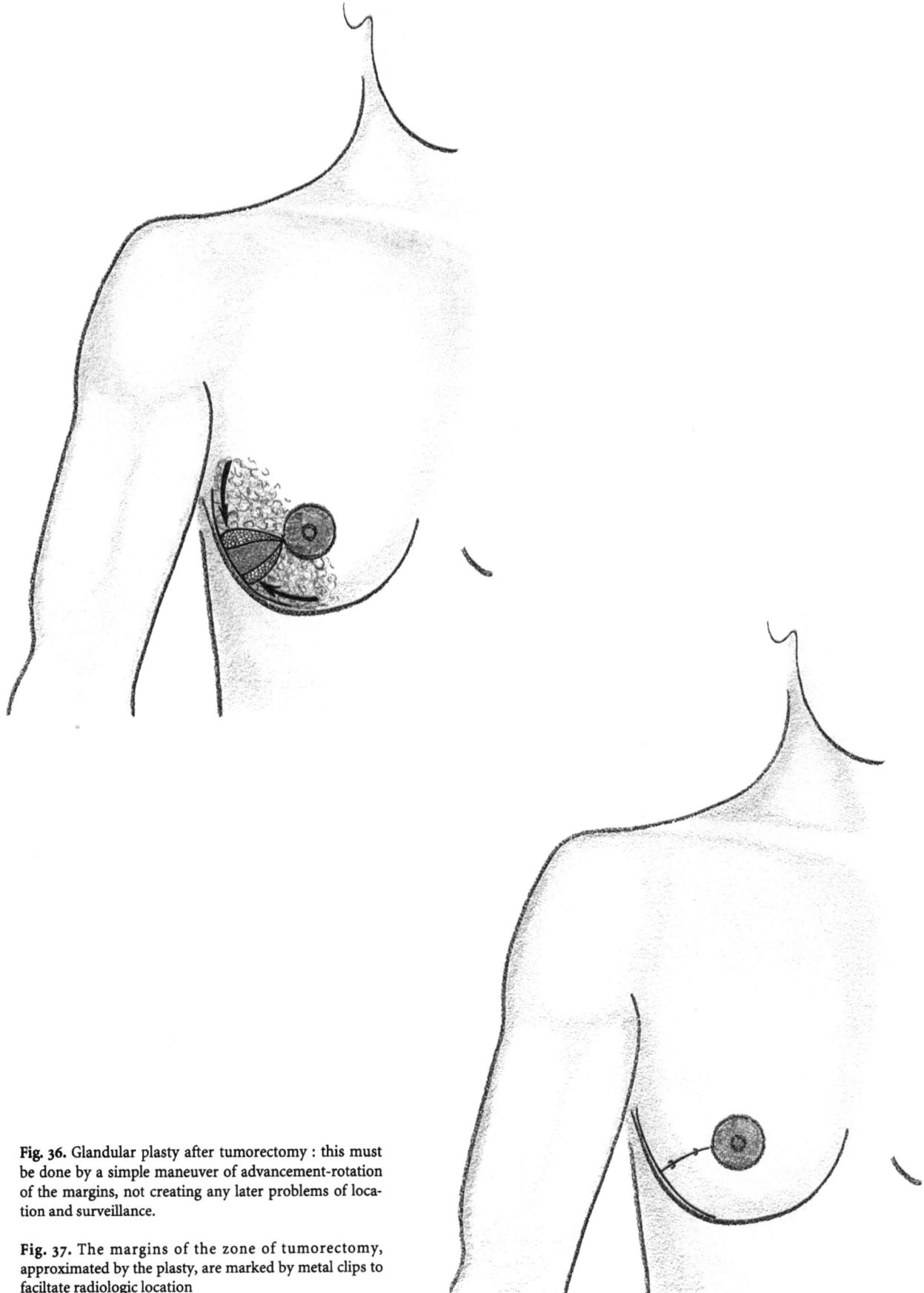

Fig. 36. Glandular plasty after tumorectomy : this must be done by a simple maneuver of advancement-rotation of the margins, not creating any later problems of location and surveillance.

Fig. 37. The margins of the zone of tumorectomy, approximated by the plasty, are marked by metal clips to faciltate radiologic location

Quadrantectomy

We need not say much about this. It is a procedure to be avoided if it amounts to a true quadrantectomy, especially of the medial quadrants, since it gives very poor cosmetic results and creates problems of plastic reconstruction that are much more difficult than those raised by a mastectomy, and often with disappointing results. When such an excision is necessary it may legitimately be asked whether a mastectomy would not be preferable, with immediate or subsequent reconstruction.

Mastectomy

Halsted's operation

Radical mastectomy was described by Halsted in 1890.

A very wide elliptical skin excision whose main vertical axis is slightly oblique downward and outward allows the performance of a block excision of the mammary gland and both pectoral muscles, associated with extensive nodal clearance of the axillary fossa; this clearance is taken up as far as the clavicle, laying bare the axillary vessels and in turn the subclavian vessels, taking care to respect such structures as the nerves and pedicles of the latissimus dorsi and serratus anterior.

In some cases a medial thoracic nodal clearance may be added, not without risk to the pleura.

Apart from the functional impairment associated with sacrifice of the pectorals, particularly its effect on the function and position of the shoulder and the high risk of lymphedema, the more so if combined with radiotherapy, the appearance of such a mutilation is shocking and may be exaggerated by sacrifice of the costal cartilages if a medial thoracic nodal cleareance has been done. The appearance of this fleshless hemithorax, whose skin is plastered directly on the outline of the rib cage, and where the shoulder appears retracted, is very striking (fig. 38).

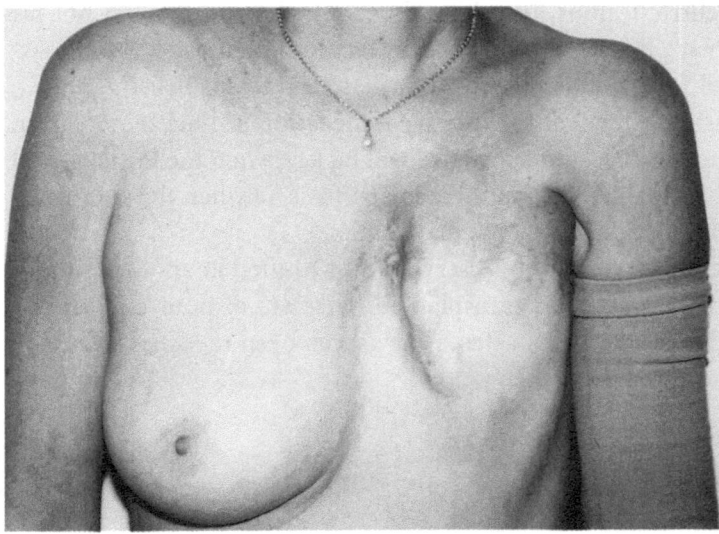

Fig. 38. Outcome of a Halsted operation : absence of pectorals, irradiated skin stuck to the rib cage, chondrocostal pseudarthrosis following medial thoracic nodal clearance, lymphedema.

Fortunately, while such procedures have added to our knowledge, particularly as regards lymphatic drainage, and especially in relating the prognosis to the degree of nodal invasion, advances in oncology and associated treatment have shown that (apart from deep tumors adherent to the muscle plane, or when recurrences require extended excisions) it is unnecessary to perform initial ablation of the pectoral muscles, and finally that medial thoracic nodal clearance may advantageously be replaced by high-energy radiotherapy.

Modified radical mastectomy

A new era opened with Patey's modified radical mastectomy, which sacrificed the breast and pectoralis minor and included nodal clearance at Berg's three stages (below, behind and above the pectoralis minor).

The procedure still conforms with the principle of a block resection, removing skin, mammary gland and axillary nodes in continuity, with an ellipse of skin excision whose main axis is horizontal or slightly oblique downward and inward; however, both pectoral muscles are now preserved and the nodal clearance ceases at the start of the second stage (except, of course, if there is palpable invasion). Thus, respect for the pectoralis minor allows preservation of the nerve supply of the pectorals, which is important not only for their function but also for their nutritional state.

While the classical accounts describe skin sacrifice extending to at least three fingerbreadths from the tumor, the size of the excisional ellipse has often become less.

This may be explained by the present-day decline in the indications for mastectomy associated with advances in conservative management.

The extent of skin sacrifice, relative or absolute, depends on three factors :
- the indication for mastectomy,
- the size of the lesion and its position in relation to the areola,
- the size of the lesion in relation to the remainder of the breast and to its skin envelope.

If the mastectomy is indicated for a small infiltrating intracanalicular carcinoma or for multicentric lesions, the skin ellipse may be constructed not far from the nipple-areolar plaque, since this has in fact to be removed. If the mastectomy is performed for a bulkier lesion (many surgical teams insisting on a 3 cm margin), the excision will be more extensive if the lesion is more remote from the areola. Finally, the residual skin substance will be less when the initial global volume of the breast is small and when there is no ptosis, ie when the skin envelope is not excessive in relation to its glandular content.

The nipple-areolar complex is not preserved to be grafted at another site for subsequent reconstruction. Areolas transplanted twice are of poor quality and often discolored, and secondary "metastases" have even been reported at the site which temporarily harbored the areola.

Operative technique

Mastectomy

The patient is positioned supine, with the arm free in the operative field or fixed to a stand, the elbow flexed to 90° and the shoulder in anteflexion (but not exceeding 90° of elevation to avoid the risk of stretching the brachial plexus). This position is the best for relaxing the lower border of the pectoralis major, so facilitating the dissection at the stage of axillary clearance.

After incision of the excisional ellipse, stripping of the gland is performed flush with the subcutaneous fatty tissue, while avoiding being too superficial so as not to risk skin necrosis, but also without being too deep since the dissection would then become more difficult and hemorrhagic and would risk leaving a not inconsiderable amount of the gland. Although there is no superficial fascia here, since it passes behind the gland at the level of the inframmary fold, this plane of dissection is quite easy to identify and to preserve throughout the stripping.

The dissection is pursued superficially as far as the limits of the gland, ie to the inframammary crease below and to expose the muscle fibers of the pectoralis major medially and above.

The deep aspect of the gland is then freed from the parietes from within outward. Preservation of the perimysium of the pectoralis major and the fascia which covers and extends inward the digitations of the serratus anterior is important particularly when immediate reconstruction is envisaged, to ensure continuity of the compartment intended to contain the prosthesis.

It remains to free the axillary tail of the gland, concluding with axillary nodal clearance, which is facilitated by this block excision.

Axillary nodal clearance

Without intending to resume in detail the technique of nodal clearance, we must stress several points.

Axillary clearance is aimed at removing all the cellular and nodal tissue situated in the triangular space bounded above by the axillary vein, behind by the latissimus dorsi and medially by the serratus anterior (fig. 39). The dissection is facilitated if three landmarks are located at the outset :

1) the upper landmark : the anterior aspect of the vein is easily freed once the clavi-pectoro-axillary aponeurosis has been breached. The axillary vein has a virtually transverse course when the arm is in simple abduction, without any great degree of anteflexion. The initial approach to the vein is also important in identifying and thus preserving the origin of certain nerves and pedicles : the long thoracic nerve (of Bell), the nerves to the pectorals (lateral and medial) and the 2nd intercostal perforant, or intercosto-humeral nerve of Hyrtl, which anastomoses with the accessory branch of the medial brachial cutaneous nerve (intercosto-brachial), situated lower than the vein and roughly parallel to it; this should be preserved if possible, to maintain normal sensation at the inner aspect of the upper arm. As well as the pedicle of the serratus anterior, the lateral thoracic (external mammary) vessels must be identified and isolated, but are not ligated until the end of the dissection. The subscapular pedicle (subscapular artery and

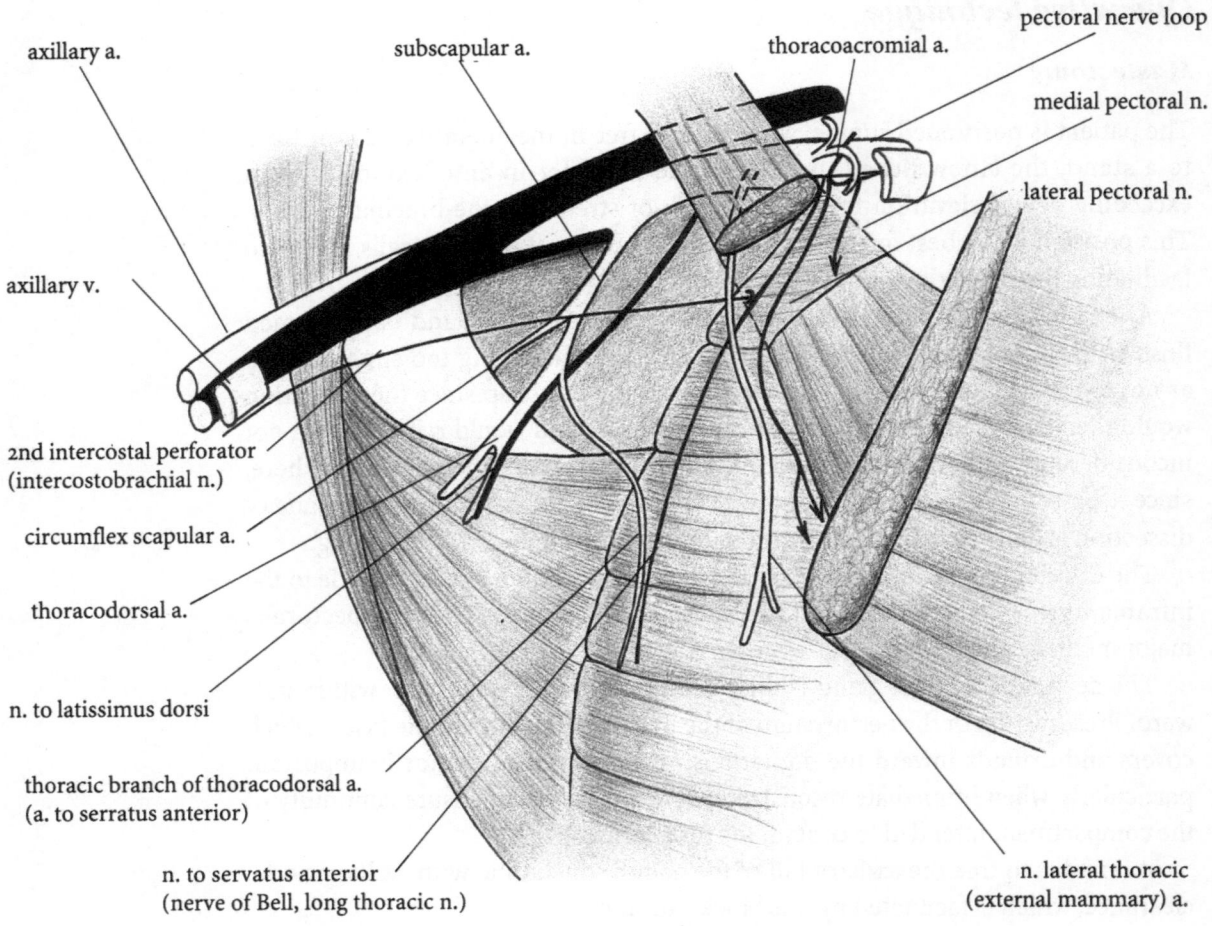

axillary a.

subscapular a.

thoracoacromial a.

pectoral nerve loop

medial pectoral n.

lateral pectoral n.

axillary v.

2nd intercostal perforator
(intercostobrachial n.)

circumflex scapular a.

thoracodorsal a.

n. to latissimus dorsi

thoracic branch of thoracodorsal a.
(a. to serratus anterior)

n. to servatus anterior
(nerve of Bell, long thoracic n.)

n. lateral thoracic
(external mammary) a.

Fig. 39. Nerves and arteries to be identified during nodal clearance

vein), deeper and more posterior, is not usually visible at this stage of the dissection, but if there is a risk of injuring it (in a very fatty axilla), it may be exposed at its emergence at the start of the dissection, which gives a good idea of its position and general direction once the anterior border of the latissimus dorsi is freed;

2) the lateral landmark, ie the anterior border of the latissimus dorsi, is freed by stripping the skin and subcutaneous tissue from the mastectomy incision superficially from within outward until the muscle is found;

3) the medial landmarks, the digitations of the serratus anterior, the lower border of the pectoralis major, and the chest wall are exposed by freeing of the deep aspect of the mammary gland in the last phase of the mastectomy.

When nodal clearance forms part of the same operative procedure as the mastectomy, it becomes simple, with the assistant holding the operative specimen, to perform the dissection in continuity from below upward, ascending progressively to the dihedral angle formed by the latissimus dorsi and the serratus anterior as far as the apex of the axillary fossa. As the dissection proceeds the long thoracic nerve and the vascular pedicle of the serratus anterior will be encountered medially, behind the inferior scapular pedicle, and the dissection ends laterally and medially at the apex of the axilla after the assistant has placed the arm in abduction and anteflexion to relax the pectoralis major. Care is taken after having freed the lateral border of the pectoralis minor to safeguard the lateral pectoral nerve, responsible for innervation of the most lateral bundles of the pectoralis major. The specimen is orientated before being sent for histologic examination by marking the limit of the dissection with a thread. Hemostasis is carefully checked, particularly at the perforating vessels at the inner ends of the intercostal spaces, at the inferior border of the pectoralis major muscle, and in the axillary region. Two suction drains are inserted, one in the axillary region and the other in front of the muscle plane, and closure is carried out.

Closure of the superficial layers (fig. 40)

Care at this stage will facilitate subsequent reconstruction. The margins of the incision should be approximated without tension, if need be by stripping the inferior margin at the level of the thoracic and abdominal aponeurosis.

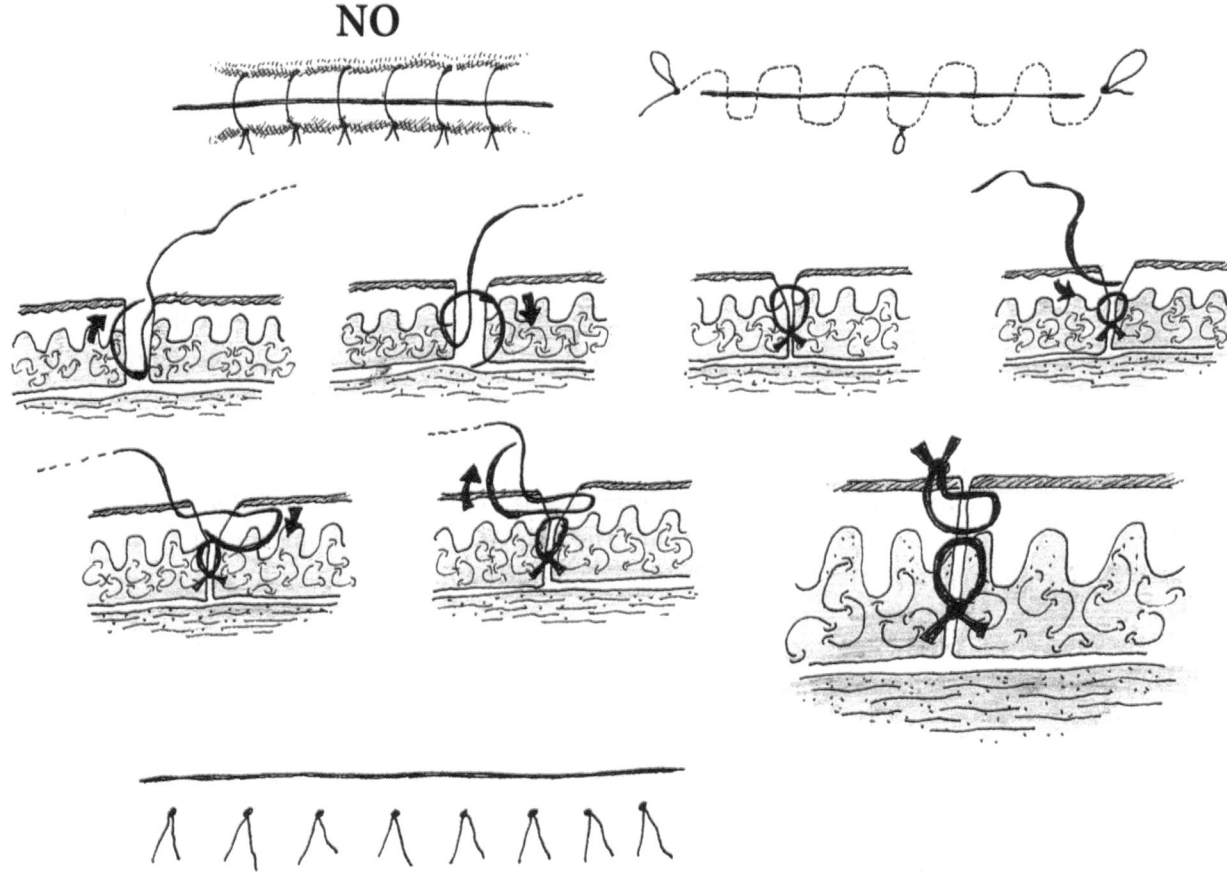

Fig. 40. Different suture techniques
– 1 left : interrupted stitches that grasp the entire skin very tightly are inadvisable since they give rise to unpleasant scars, the so-called "birdcage-ladder" (left); right : a continuous intradermal suture is preferable, made in the superficial dermis after having correctly apposed the deeper dermis by...
– 2 deep inverting dermal sutures (placing the knot in depth) made with slowly absorbed undyed material
– 3 if a further stage is desired after intradermal suture, it is also possible, after some deep dermal tacking sutures designed to stabilise the two margins, to use these "false" Blair-Donatti sutures which grasp only the full thickness of the dermis on the side opposite needle entry and give a minor scar defect, provided the needle is brought out very close to its point of entry; they also ensure excellent apposition of the margins
– 4 final appearance of this type of suture

The firm and resistant plane is that of the dermis, not the subcutaneous layer. Stitches inserted in the subcutaneous fatty tissue have no hold and do not relieve the tension on the scar, which will stretch. The two margins of the wound are initially apposed by interrupted inverting and absorbable tacking sutures seizing the deep dermis. These sutures should be close enough (about every cm) for the two margins to be perfectly in contact with each other before suture of the superficial dermal layer. The most inconspicuous scar is obtained by a continuous intradermal suture of monofilament nylon or rapidly absorbable material.

The superficial layer may also be sutured with interrupted monofilament nylon, provided the suture material is fine and the stitches are inserted vertically without too wide a grasp of the skin on either side of the scar and without too tight a closure.

For this purpose, the stitch that gives the best apposition, especially when the dermis is thick, is the sort of "false stitch" of Blair-Donatti (fig. 40), which grasps only the dermis of the side opposite the point of penetration and emerges only on the side of the knot.

The use of thick and very tight sutures does not lead to good healing, as is widely but incorrectly believed, but on the contrary leaves indelible "birdcage-ladder" markings, very unattractive and detrimental to the cosmetic appearance of the reconstruction. The only way to get rid of these is to excise the scar over the entire breadth of the sutures, which means a loss of the tissue stock available for reconstruction.

Dressing is made with tulle gras, dry pads and elastic bandages, with the addition of absorbent pads to produce moderate compression of the axillary fossa.

Whatever the indication, the mastectomy must be done primarily in the context of the malignancy, without reservations regarding skin conservation and without thought of the implications for a possible subsequent reconstruction. Plastic surgery is now rich in resources in this field and can supply supplementary skin substance in the form of a flap or increase the available tissue stock by the device of skin expansion. The only consideration influencing the plastic surgeon relates to the direction of the scar (the scar easiest to conceal and most favorable to reconstruction is transverse or slightly oblique downward and inward) and, especially, the care given to closure of the superficial layers.

It should never be forgotten that reconstruction after partial mastectomy is always more difficult of performance, and more often a source of imperfect results, than reconstruction after total mastectomy.

Important points

- Skin excision is a function of the size and site of the tumor;
- a scar that is transverse or oblique downward and inward is more favorable to a reconstruction than a vertical scar;
- the pectoral muscles, subscapular pedicle, and the nerves to the latissimus dorsi and serratus anteror can and must be respected;
- drainage lessens inflammatory reaction and promotes good healing;
- closure must be made carefully, approximating the wound margins without undue tension, and skin suture must be meticulous.

References

Bricout N, Servant JM, Banzet P (1987) L'abord chirurgical esthétique du sein, Congrès de Chirurgie, Paris

Glicenstein J. Abcès et tumeurs bénignes du sein, Encycl Méd Chir, Paris, Techniques Chirurgicales, 4. 3. 07, 41950

Hourtoulle FG. Chirurgie des tumeurs du sein, Encycl Méd Chir, Paris, Techniques Chirurgicales, 3.23.02, 41970

Petit JY (1991) Cancer du sein, Chirurgie diagnostique, curative et reconstructrice Medsi/Mc Graw-Hill

Surgical treatment of gynecomastia

Gynecomastia is a benign disorder, but one with profound psychological effects, even if the thoracic deformity is not very severe, which are in themselves an indication for surgical intervention as the only effective solution for idiopathic gynecomastia resistant to 3-6 months of medical treatment; in any case, the latter seems to have an effect only on gynecomastia of recent appearance and moderate degree.

It may be isolated or form part of an adipogynecomastia in an obese patient, the distinction being made by mammography.

Before deciding on operation, it is essential to exclude :

– temporary gynecomastia, essentially limited to a retroareolar prominence appearing in the pubertal period and disappearing in a few months in the majority of cases. Operation is indicated only if the phenomenon persists and resists medical management;

– an endocrine, tumoral or drug origin, the primary treatment of which is that of the relevant cause or medication.

A complete investigation must be carried out, directed to the detection of :

– an endocrine syndrome;

– hypogonadism, either isolated or part of a malformational syndrome such as that of Klinefelter;

– a testicular or adrenocortical tumor;

– the ingestion of certain drugs : estrogens, antiandrogens (for treatment of prostatic carcinoma in men), spironolactone, cimetidine, digitoxin, isoniazid, certain forms of chemotherapy inhibiting the synthesis of testosterone (bisulfan, vincristine, nitrosurea), certain psychotropic agents (tricyclic antidepressants, phenothiazines, amphetamines, diazepam, reserpine, metoclopramide, and certain drugs of abuse : hashish, cannabis).

If the disorder is iatrogenic, stopping the medication leads to regression of the gynecomastia. If a hormonal or drug cause has already been dealt with, the only effective treatment of a persistent gynecomastia is surgical, and the essential aim is to correct the dysmorphism leaving an unobtrusive defect which does not indicate that a breast operation has been performed.

Usual technique

The patient is positioned in dorsal decubitus or half-seated, the outlines of the gynecomastia having been carefully depicted in ink.

The classical incision, adequate with an areola of normal size, is an inferior or inferolateral hemiareolar incision (fig. 41). If this exceeds half the areola, there is a risk of contractile scarring which may lead to deformity of projection of the nipple. Through this incision the subcutaneous plane is reached and scissor dissection is begun superficially, from the entire periphery of the areola to the boundaries of the gland. It passes, as usual, at the level of the ridges of Duret, so as to respect the immediately subcutaneous tissue and not to damage the blood-supply.

When the entire surface of the gland has been freed to its periphery, having respected the areola, retroareolar glandular resection is performed with the scal-

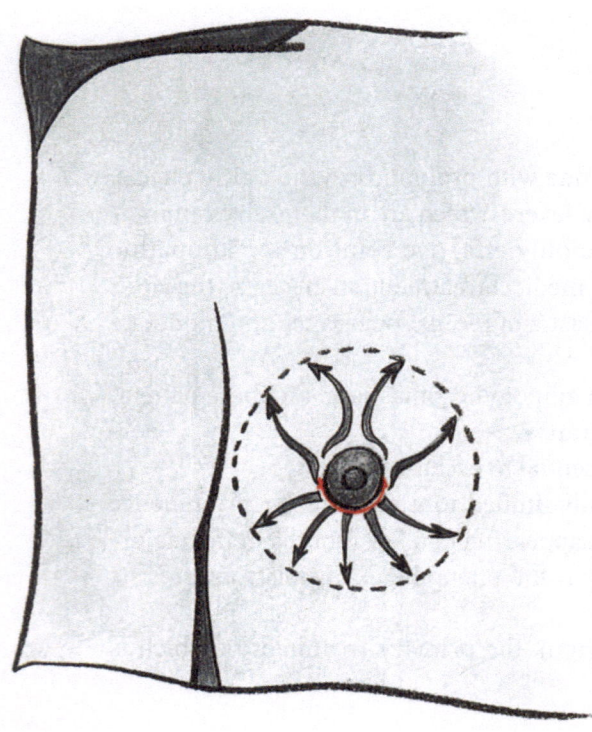

Fig. 41. Beginning with an inferior hemiareolar incision, the dissection is initially made in centrifugal manner up to the peripheral limit of the gland

pel, retaining a thin disk of glandular tissue 0.5 cm in depth behind the areola. The preservation of a little glandular tissue at this site prevents the later development of an unnatural domed depression.

After the stage of retroareolar freeing the deep stripping is performed, which is simpler to do if the parietal plane at the level of the inframammary crease is first located, and this is easier once the lower border of the pectoralis major has been crossed. This stage ends with peripheral section of the breast tissue.

Scrupulous hemostasis is then ensured, a suction drain is inserted, and the wound closed with fine absorbable inversion sutures for the deeper dermis and a superficial intradermal continuous suture of monofilament nylon or rapidly absorbed material. A compression dressing is applied, using tulle gras, dry pads and adhesive elastic bandages.

This technique usually gives a good result, provided certain precautions are taken, ie to respect the thickness of the subcutaneous fatty layer so that the zone where the excision has been made is no less thick than the adjacent tissues, and to preserve surplus tissue behind the areola to avoid any depression of the latter.

Variants

Certain variations of this classical technique have been suggested: radial incisions have been described, as have glandular resections combined with reduction of the skin envelope, but this has the disadvantage of adding visible thoracic scarring.

Again, skin resection as such is generally pointless; even if the skin does appear somewhat redundant after the dissection, it is of good elastic quality and can readapt subsquently on the chest wall.

An axillary approach is inadvisable. Although it allows easy access to any axillary extension of the gynecomastia, it is sited too far from the areola for proper dissection of the deep aspect of the gland, where it is more adherent, and for demarcating the thickness of the residual plaque. Also, hemostasis is more difficult with this route.

It has been suggested that gynecomastia might be treated by liposuction. This may possibly have some effect on an adipomastia, but in view of the firmness of the glandular tissue of true gynecomastia, the efficacy of such a procedure is dubious.

A more useful variant is possible, especially when the areola is small and reduction of the skin envelope is desired. The procedure begins with periareolar removal of the epidermis to a periphery between 1 and 3 cm on average from the areolar margin. A transcutaneous incision is then made on the inferior half of the de-epthelialised area and the dissection is carried on as before, and is facilitated by the wider approach, which also makes hemostasis easier. The sutures are placed in two layers, burying the dermal ring as in a mammoplasty.

References

Dufourmentel Cl (1928) L'incision aréolaire dans la chirurgie du sein. Bull Mem Soc Chir Paris 20 : 9-14

Reynaud JP, Gary-Bobo A,Merlier C, Selam JL, Bringer J (1983) Aspects techniques de la cure chirurgicale des gynécomasties. Ann Chir Plast Esth 28/4 : 383-387

Verges B, Putelat R (1989) Les gynécomasties. Le Concours médical 111/14 : 1171-1176

Webster JP (1946) Mastectomy for gynecomastia through a semi-circular intra-areolar incision. Ann Surg 124 : 557-565

Hypertrophy and ptosis

General considerations

Although it is practical in terms of definitions to make a distinction between mammary hypertrophy and ptosis, this becomes artificial as soon as a breast of abnormal morphology is studied since the two phenomena are usually associated, or have been, and the clinical effect of the one is inseparable from that of the other.

Every degree can be observed with the passage of time, and with hormonal influences and variations in general physical morphology, from simple juvenile hypertrophy, which will eventually lead to ptosis, to the breast devoid of glandular content, where the flaccid skin envelope evidences a preponderance of ptosis, developing once pregnancies, ageing and loss of skin elasticity have had their ill-effects even if the patient is not actually elderly.

Hypertrophy

Definition

Mammary hypertrophy is evidence of a pathologic process where the breast is increased in size beyond normal proportions.

This definition verges on the imprecise, since it allows some room for subjectivity as regards the bounds of hypertrophy; we have seen that the so-called "normal" breast is itself difficult to define, and varies with the tastes of individuals and historical periods, not to mention geography.

It seems much more sensible not to seek to define mammary hypertrophy in absolute terms, but to allow for the height of the patient and her overall and particularly thoracic build, and then, in relation to this, to consider the criteria we have laid down for the breast, particularly its base.

If we consider that the volume of a normal breast lies within 200 and 350 ml, hypertrophy exists once the upper limit is obviously exceeded :

– from 400 to 600 ml, hypertrophy is labeled moderate;

– from 600 to 800 ml, hypertrophy is labeled considerable;

– from 800 to 100 ml, hypertrophy is labeled major;

– beyond this, it is regarded as very great and above 1500 ml it is termed gigantomastia.

This gives a somewhat theoretic idea of breast hypertrophy, since in practice one does not resort to unpleasant and imprecise volumetric measurements.

What matters as regards breast reduction is what is left and not what is removed, stressing once again the importance of the concept of residual mammary volume.

An approximate idea of the degree of hypertrophy, to be recorded in the operative protocol, is given by the weight of the resection specimen; this is useful to know after resection of the first breast to guide the procedure on the other side, allowing for any possible asymmetry. It is relatively imprecise in absolute terms since the density of the breast varies, though only moderately, according to the proportions of gland tissue and fat, but this density is usually the same in both breasts of the same patient, except in certain cases of glaring asymmetry.

Physiopathology

Although the influence of hormonal factors (estrogens, progesterone and prolactin) on breast development at puberty and during pregnancy is relatively well-known, nothing is known about why this physiologic process can become pathologic and result in established hypertrophy.

One can only propose, and without proof, the very vague notion of an abnormal tissue receptivity for these different hormonal factors.

Thus, in the absence of a precise etiology, there is no medical treatment for breast hypertrophy and the sole solution lies in surgery.

In the young girl there is a distinction to be made between so-called glandular hypertrophy, where the breast is firm, and so-called fatty hypertrophy, where it is much softer, a difference confirmed at mammographic and histologic examination. We have found that hypertrophy of the glandular type occurs more readily in young girls whose height-weight ratio has not varied significantly in the pubertal period, whereas young girls with marked overweight at the time of puberty tend to have so-called fatty hypertrophy, the glandular tissue being present mainly in the retroareolar region, even if they subsequently regain a normal height-weight ratio. From this an important practical point may be deduced : it is necessary to be vigilant to avoid rapid weight-gain unrelated to growth in this period of reproductive life.

There is no relationship between breast hypertrophy of whatever type and the quality of milk secretion. It is even to be remarked that women with hypertrophy often do not make good milk-producers, which may perhaps be explained by the histologic finding that the resected tissue is very often dystrophic.

Clinical examination

History

Besides the height, weight, previous surgical, medical or gynecologic history and the administration of hormonal therapy, the age at appearance of the hypertophy must be ascertained (it usually accompanies the onset of puberty), as well the rapidity of its development (which is one of the factors influencing the quality of the skin) and whether the hypertrophy is stabilised or not.

This factor is significant in deciding on operation. It is important to the quality of the morphologic result and the extent (in length) of the scar to operate as soon as possible, before the skin envelope has suffered too greatly from the stretching produced by the over-development of the breast.

Thus, breast hypertrophy may be operated from the age of 15 years, provided only that breast growth has stabilised.

The size of the brassière should also be noted, and the depth of cup, while informing the patient that size is essentially relative to chest measurement and will vary only slightly after operation, the decrease being mainly evident as regards the depth of cup.

These measurements are also useful in choosing the size of brassière the patient will be asked to wear after hospitalisation, since it has to be worn day and night from the outset. We usually advise the purchase of a so-called "sports" type of brassière, with good support and fastening in front (for easier application) and with premolded unsewn cups (more comfortable and adapting well to the operated breast whatever the size of the residual breast base). The size (between 85 and 95 French, 32 and 36 USA and UK, 70 to 80 International) depends on general body morphology, for a B cup depth, which becomes adapted — with some variations permitted by the elasticity of this type of brassière — to the residual breast volume usually obtained.

Examination of the breast

This begins with assessment of breast shape, the degree of hypertrophy and of any associated ptosis, and the state of the skin and of the gland.

Special importance attaches to the state of the connexions betwen skin and gland (can the skin be pinched in front of the gland?) and to how plastic the gland tissue is. The firm gland of a young girl is easy to remodel as it is supple, whereas caution is required with the rigid gland of a 50-year-old woman, the irregular consistency of which is indicative of what is generally known as mastosis, and which corresponds to sclerosis of the supporting tissue in addition to clinical, radiologic and histologic mammary dystrophy. This type of gland may reserve some surprises when it comes to the actual stage of remodeling.

As will be seen, the breast itself shares the "responsibility" for the quality of the result, though other factors certainly relate to the surgeon and the patient.

The morphologic examination should include special attention to the base of breast implantation, particularly its lateral and medial limits, and to the more or less curved shape of the inframammary crease.

This implantation base has to be reduced in proportion to the anterior projection but such reduction has its limitations, associated with thoracic build and the degree of general obesity.

Excessive reduction of the base in a woman who is overweight (and whom it is better to try to persuade to slim down before operation by explaining what is at stake, ie the restoration of breast size in harmony with the general figure) carries a risk of producing an over-pronounced crease at the junction of the outer quadrants of the breast and the lateral chest wall. This crease marks the separation from an unpleasant lateral ridge situated above and lateral to the outer end of the infra-

mammary scar, which then protrudes beyond the crease. Reduction of the base is also limited when the inframammary fold is rendered transverse by an excess of abdominal fat in a woman with a short thorax.

Reduction of the breast base is also difficult, and limited, when there is a synmastia, ie when there is no inner boundary between the two breasts, the glandular tissue bridging the sternum. This must be taken into account in the breast reduction, since the decrease in size will be evidenced predominantly in the anterior projection. It is better, in this special case, to leave a residual breast size somewhat larger than usual, as a residual volume that is relatively too small will be marked in this case by a breast that is too flat.

Synmastia is a relatively rare anomaly, but there may be a transverse fold at the lower part of the intermammary sulcus which joins the two inframammary folds. This sulcus is a sign of excessive stretching of the skin envelope due to the hypertrophy.

It is important to note this at the preoperative examination and to point it out to the patient, since it cannot be corrected once it is well established except by taking the inframammary scar across the midline. It is better, in our opinion, to extend the scar (which is of excellent quality in this site because of its direction) rather than to allow this sulcus to remain, particularly since it will become the more obvious once the shape of the breasts has been rendered satisfactory.

One should also look for the presence of a fatty ridge at the anterior part of the axillary fossa. When this is well-marked, this ridge is separated by a sulcus from the axillary prolongation of the breast proper. Though this is not an accessory axillary gland, it does need correction to harmonise the morphologic result as it will be more visible, and displeasing, after correction of the hypertrophy.

Finally, the position of the areola in relation to the axis of the breast should be noted, its dimensions, the state of nipple sensitivity, and the presence of any asymmetry. Slight asymmetry is common, the larger breast being usually the left, though there is no explanation why this should be so.

There is a practical value in noting this asymmetry. Even if it exists naturally, this is no excuse for perpetuating it, and to correct the asymmetry more easily it is better to begin the operation with the smaller breast, since it is simpler to adapt the resection of the other breast rather than the other way round.

When ptosis is marked, the asymmetry, which then involves both envelope and content, is more difficult to assess, especially as the proportions between skin and gland are not necessarily the same on both sides. Hence the importance of techniques without a preestablished design which can adjust the skin envelope to the residual mammary volume as required (fig. 42).

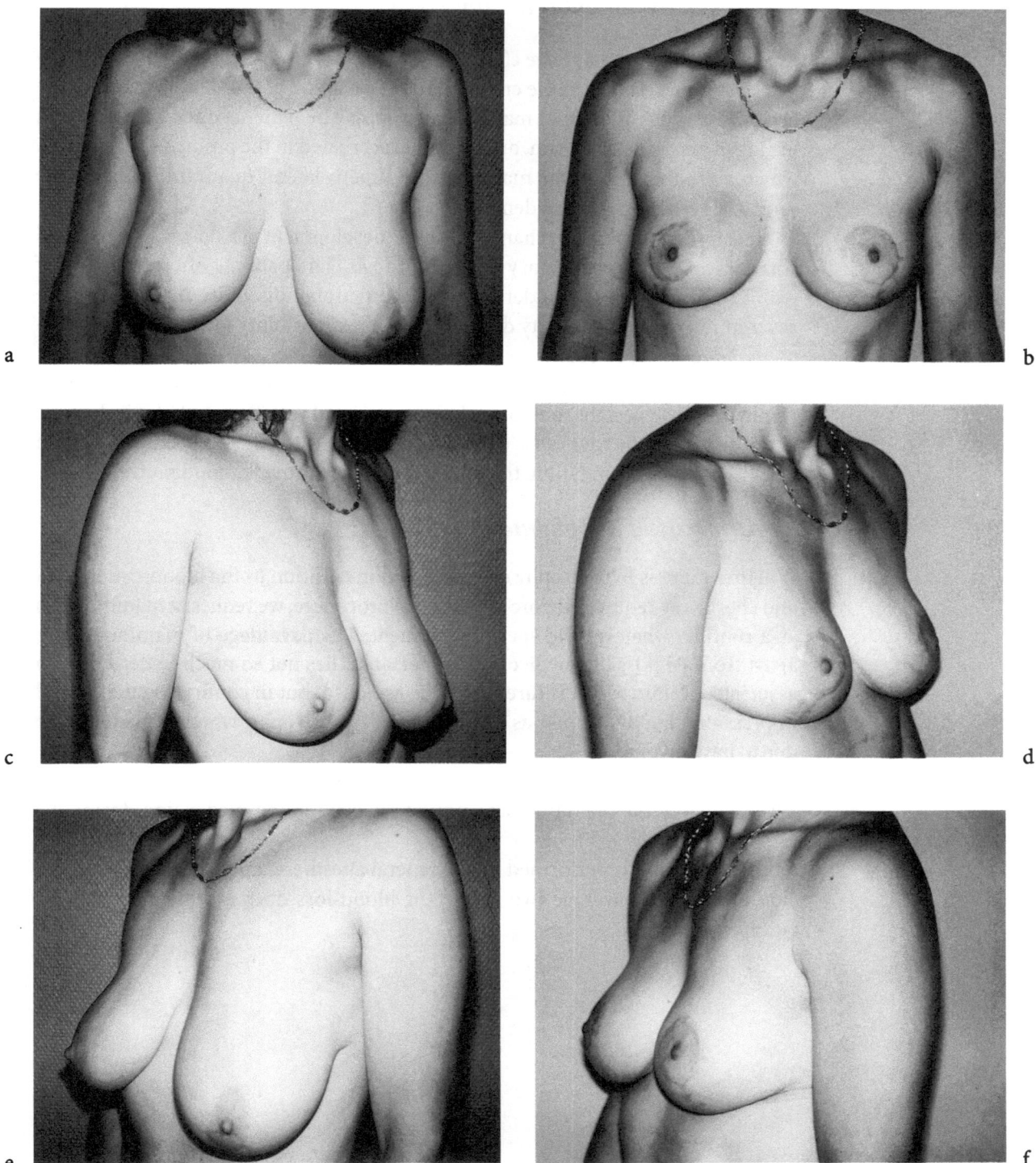

Fig. 42 a-f. Mammary asymmetry : distance from suprasternal notch to areola 27 cm right, 29 cm left, reduced to 18 cm. Resection of 150 g right and 300 g left. Result at 1 year : shape stabilised, scars globally moderately hypertrophic

Repercussions of hypertrophy

Breast hypertrophy may have effects which are :
– local (maceration in the crease, signs of irritation at the shoulders due to the brassière straps) in cases of major hypertrophy. The patients often complain of a feeling of permanent tension, or of pains, exacerbated in the premenstrual period, which are either diffuse or mainly in the supero-lateral quadrant, which is the region of greatest glandular density;
– regional, on spinal mechanics, with the development of a dorsal kyphosis and sometimes of a compensatory lumbar lordosis. The patients often complain of pain in the back and shoulders. This is a functional disability that justifies the assumption by social security departments of responsibility for the surgical treatment of breast hypertrophy;
– general : many young patients exhibit overweight accompanying the hypertrophy, this over-weight sometimes being associated with the psychological effects of the disorder. Whether cause or consequence, it is nevertheless useful to insist on weight-loss before operation, the prospect of which provides good motivation.

Preoperative assessment

Whether there is hypertrophy or ptosis, and in addition to the blood-count, ECG and chest Xray required before any surgical procedure, we request a mammogram as a routine, whatever the age of the patient. The advantage of mammography, apart from its possible medicolegal importance, lies not so much in detecting an associated lesion, which is rare below the age of 30, but in confirming the clinical impression already formed as to the type of hypertrophy, whether glandular or due to fatty involution.

We also specify that the patient should stop any contraceptive treatment at least 3 weeks before the operation, and not take aspirin-based medication during the previous week.

The operation is performed under general anesthesia and controlled hypotension and lasts on average two hours; the blood-loss does not therefore call for autotransfusion.

Ptosis

Definition

Ptosis of the breast is an acquired condition in the great majority of cases, the result of disproportionate excess of the breast envelope (the skin) in relation to its content (the gland).The container becomes too large for the content, either because the skin is overstretched or because the content has decreased in volume, without the container having succeeded in adjusting, because of loss of the skin's elasticity and capacity for contraction.

Physiopathology

We have seen that the sole factor important to support of the breast is represented by its connexions with the skin, and is therefore closely dependent on skin quality and that of the ligaments of Cooper.

Because of the action of gravity, ptosis is a virtually unavoidable physiologic phenomenon, but it will develop at varying rates depending on various factors :

– the bulk of the breast and the extent of its anterior projection, which to some extent determine breast "overhang" ;

– the skin quality : whether the dermis is thick or thin (differences exist betwen women even in youth); it tends to become thinner with age, such physiologic ageing being also accompanied by weakening of the supporting connective tissue ;

– variations in size of the breast :

• local, associated with the different stages of reproductive life,

• general, episodes of weight-gain and weight-loss.

These local or general variations are more injurious if they occur rapidly in time and at close intervals, for they then impair the recuperative capacity of the skin.

They are also more harmful when they occur under the influence of hormonal factors (hormonal flooding of pregnancy, the transient hyperadrenocortical activity of puberty). In fact, as well as the influence of these hormonal factors on augmentation of the breast content, they promote the development of radial stretch-marks over the entire breast, evidence of an irremediable loss of elastic fibers throughout the breast envelope.

These striae are to be distinguished form the finer markings which are localised entirely to the base of the breast, and are particularly connected with the effects of gravity; these are less unfavorable as they do not indicate total loss of elasticity of the breast content.

Analysis

Ptosis occurs as soon as the thoraco-mammary angle decreases and falls below 90°, and is accompanied by a change in the form of segment II which, normally convex, becomes first straight and then concave.

The extent ot the ptosis may be measured in the standing patient by the distance separating the horizontal plane tangential to the inframammary crease from the tangent to the most dependent point of the lower pole of the breast (fig. 43). However, this measurement reflects only one of the aspects of the ptosed breast and must be incorporated in a wider analysis which takes account of the position of the areola.

This is the basis of the classical distinction (J.P. Lalardrie) between glandular and cutaneous ptosis, a distinction which, though somewhat artificial since the two phenomena may be associated, has some didactic value.

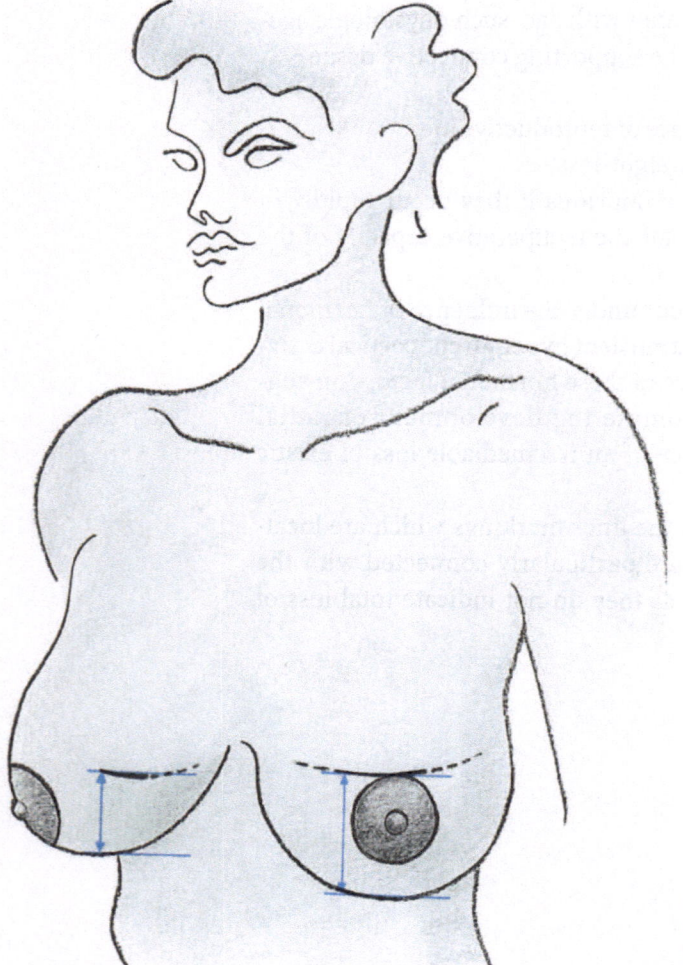

Fig. 43. Assessment of severity of ptosis by measurement of the distance between the tangent transverse to the inframammary crease and the most dependent point of the breast

Glandular ptosis

This is due to decrease in volume of the content, ie to glandular involution, in an initially normal or even hypertrophic breast. Theoretically, the skin is not involved, but this is rare once marked hypertrophy exists.

This loss of volume is marked by a decrease in anterior projection, the nipple-areolar plaque falling back towards the thoracic plane. The skin being unaffected, segments II and III change their shape but do not elongate. The descent of the nipple is due only to the loss in curvature of segment II, which becomes straight (fig. 44).

Surgical correction may be envisaged from two aspects.

If the skin retains good elastic quality, ie if the glandular ptosis is absolutely isolated, and if the skin envelope is of moderate dimensions and satisfactory shape, with a well-centered areola, correction can be achieved merely by the insertion of an implant which does no more than restore the loss in size of the content. The scar defect is minimal, since no skin reduction procedure is necessary; the scar corresponds only to the route of access needed for implantation.

If provision of an implant is not contemplated, a glandular procedure is indicated, such as a spiral "rolling-up" procedure. But this is necessarily accompanied by a reduction of the breast base (the only way of restoring anterior projection with unaltered volume). It is quite rare to be able to dispense with a skin reduction procedure designed to stabilise the glandular procedure, which is known not to have any stabilising value in titself in the long term.

More often, when there is glandular ptosis justifying surgical intervention, there is generally an associated skin ptosis. The problem is then whether or not to provide an implant to ensure that breast size is adapted to the morphology of the patient, and of an adequate reduction of the skin envelope. The scar will be longer when residual breast size is small, and shorter when volume has been increased. If breast size is inadequate and not adapted to the general body build, the outcome is worse if accompanied by scars, but the long-term results of implantation are not always trouble-free .This is why the advantages and disadvantages of the various possible methods must be carefully explained to the patient.

Skin ptosis

Here, involvement of the container, ie of the skin envelope, predominates and is evidenced by elongation of segments II and III (fig. 45).

It is rare for this not be associated with some change in content.

In a breast of normal size it is due to physiologic ageing of the skin envelope, a phenomenon which may develop very early as it depends mainly on the quality of the skin.

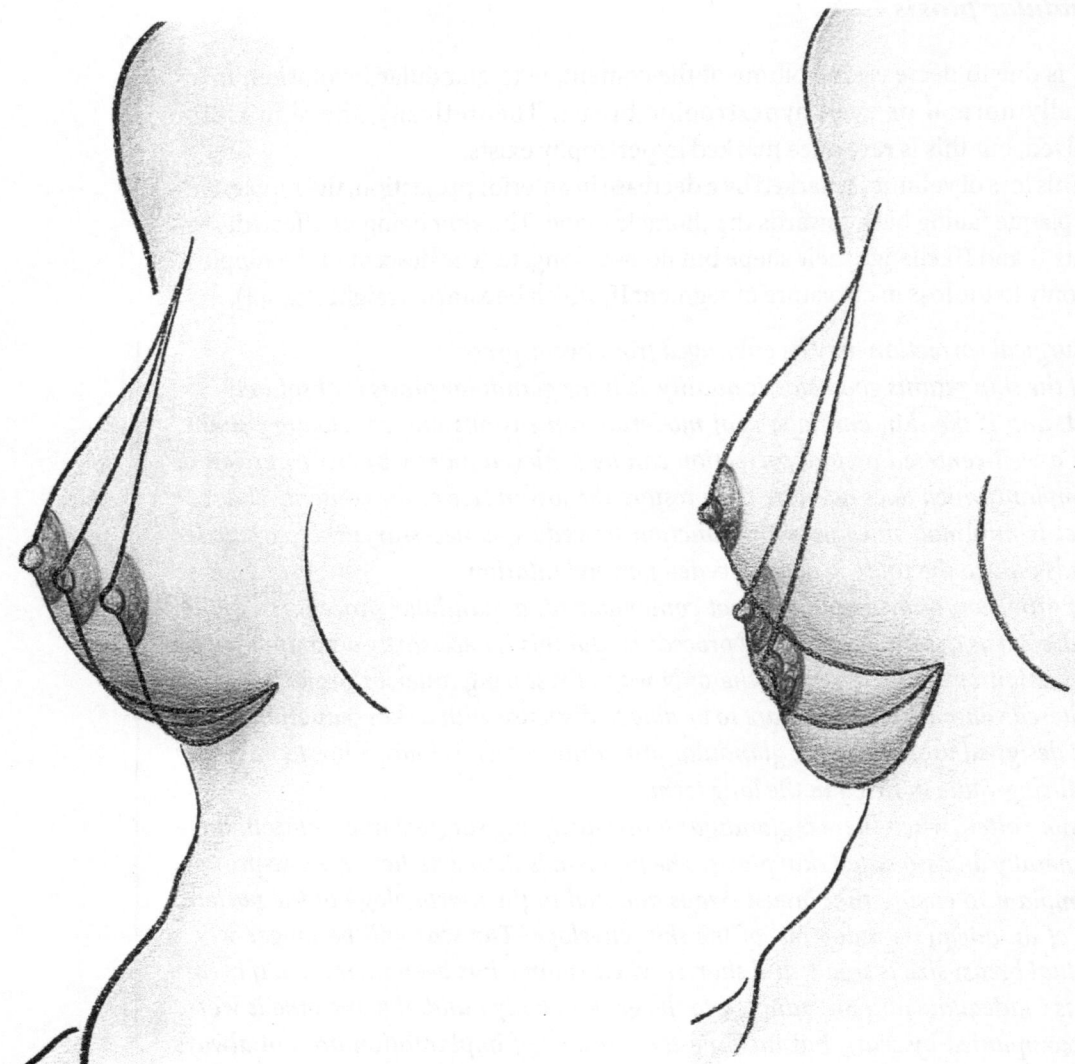

Fig. 44. Glandular ptosis : segments II and II are not elongated and the nipple has fallen back

Fig. 45. Cutaneous ptosis : segments II and III are elongated and the nipple has descended more than it has fallen back

This situation, acquired at a varying number of years after puberty, is to be distinguished however from the special case of breasts which may be considered as suffering from "congenital" ptosis; at puberty, whether or not there is any hypertrophy, the skin envelope develops exaggeratedly as if it had been programmed without reference to the glandular surge.

This skin overdevelopment relative to glandular size results in a segment II relatively much longer than segment III, with the areola directed downward and situated in dependent position at the lower pole of the breast.

As opposed to the two preceding situations, ptosis in a hypertrophic breast is due to the supplementary and permanent stretching produced in the skin by the weight of the gland, a stretching that worsens with physiologic ageing.

This distinction between cutaneous and glandular ptosis remains to a great extent a matter of artificial definitions since the majority of cases of ptosis are mixed, with one factor — cutaneous or glandular — more or less predominating.

More recently, F. Vandenbussche has suggested another classification of ptosis, in the context of "dysmorphism due to excess of the skin envelope".

Dysmorphism due to excess of the skin envelope

On this basis, a distinction is made between :
– early ptosis without hypertrophy, due either to an anomaly of skin elasticity or to a constitutional defect in development of the skin sac, characterised by pendulous breasts with the nipples facing downward and situated at the lower pole of the breast from the outset. These two anomalies share their early appearance, simultaneous with pubertal development, and differ in that the elasticicity of the skin is poor in the first case whereas it is preserved in the second, and that it is actually a matter of anomalous programming of the shape of the breast content;
– ptosis accompanying breast hypertrophy, an inevitable consequence of the effect of gravity in the long term as affecting the excess of content over container;
– acquired ptosis due to glandular or adipose shrinkage, or to loss of weight.

Whatever classification is used, it is necessary to analyse the relative importance of the different factors in ptosis, particularly the condition of the skin (dermal thickness, presence of striae, quality of the gland-skin connexions, shape of the skin envelope), and the state of the gland (size, plasticity), not forgetting the position of the nipple-areolar plaque, since these will influence the surgical indications.

Conclusion

Whatever the relative importance of the glandular and cutaneous factors, the objective of a mammoplasty is :
– to restore a residual breast volume in harmony with the general build of the patient (whether this is by adequate reduction of glandular volume in hypertrophy, whether or not ptosis predominates, or by addition of an implant when the volume seems inadequate despite the local possibilities of glandular reduction) ;
– to readapt to this the skin envelope, hence the importance of study of the skin. The more the ptosis is of cutaneous origin, with a thinned dermis and numerous diffuse striae, the less one may rely on it for the quality of the result; more skin will need to be resected and the scars will be relatively longer;
– and finally, to center the nipple-areolar plaque correctly and to preserve its sensation.
None of these factors can be dealt with in isolation.

References

Bricout N, Chavoin JP, Flageul G, Ohana J, Ricbourg B (1989) Hypertrophie mammaire. Rapport du XXXIVe Congrès de la Société Française de Chirurgie Plastique, Reconstructrice et Esthétique, Paris

Georgiade NG, Georgiade GS, Riefkohl R (1990) Aesthetic surgery of the breast. Ed. Saunders, ? city

Lalardrie JP (1987) A propos de la ptose mammaire. Interview recueillie par Flageul G. Ann Chir Plast Esth

Lalardrie JP, Jouglard JP (1973) Chirurgie Plastique du Sein. Masson, Paris

Vandenbussche F (1987) Les ptoses mammaires. Communication du LXXXIXe Congrès Français de Chirurgie, Paris

Surgical treatment of hypertrophy and ptosis

It seems inopportune to distinguish betwen the surgical treatment of hypertrophy and that of ptosis. In practice, in the great majority of cases, due to the simultaneous development, though in variable proportion, of the skin envelope and of the gland and to the secondary ill-effects of gravity, hypertrophy is usually associated with ptosis in varying degree.

Progress of a hypertrophic breast towards ptosis is also favored by stretching of the skin envelope, inevitable with the passage of time, the loss of skin elasticity (striae of the prepubertal period or of pregnancy) and changes in the breast content (variable proportions of gland and fat, depending on the degree of global overweight and on fatty involution after pregnancy and lactation).

As regards isolated ptosis, and whether the size of the breast is adequate or not, the principles of re-adjustment of the skin envelope to the residual breast volume, ie of container to content, are the same as those in hypertrophy once breast size has been restored to proper proportions, if need be by the addition of an implant.

Modern techniques of mammoplasty have afforded security in terms of vascularity and allowed variations designed to improve results in terms of morphology.

Current debate centers essentially on the scars , the only real remaining problem posed by mammoplasty, and more precisely on their position, length and quality. Now that security, shape and symmetry are problems resolved in principle, current practice tends to minimise their extent of the scars and if these are to be least obvious, they must be properly sited, as short as possible and of good quality.

But the debate may continue indefinitely if one insists on comparing like with unlike factors, for the position of the scars is closely dependent on the technique employed, their length much less so. This, the factor most discussed in current arguments, depends not only on the amount excised but also on the skin.

The length of the scars reflects correct adjustment of container to content, ie adaptation of the skin envelope to the residual breast size.

Whatever the technique, the absolute length of the scar, for equal excisions and equal residual breast volumes, will be longer when the necessary skin excision is considerable and when the skin has lost its elasticity.

While the actual presence of scars is an obligatory defect in any surgical procedure, in the particular case of mammoplasty they bear witness not only to the procedure performed, but also to the period, since the development of the concept of mammoplasty has adapted to technical progress. It may be useful here to briefly retrace this development.

Evolution of ideas

The initial objective was to reduce the breast and to correct the ptosis. The first concern was vascular in nature : to preserve a sufficient blood-supply for the glandular residue so as avoid its necrosis and damage to the nipple-areolar plaque, while obtaining a satisfactory shape. Possible problems created by the scars were a lesser concern.

The second stage, once the vascular and morphologic problems had been resolved, was to position the scars better so as make them less obvious.

The third stage was the freedom provided in the mode of glandular resection, and in positioning the scars, by extensive de-epithelialisation and the avoidance of cutaneo-glandular cleavage.

With the vascular and morphologic problems resolved, and with different modes of resection allowing numerous technical variants, current developments relate to the length of the scars. However, to concentrate on this factor in isolation, without taking account of the overall unity that should be the outcome of a mammoplasty, is there not a risk of arriving at an impasse, or even taking a step backward ?

Evolution of ideas and requirements

It is not our intention to resume the entire history of mammoplasty, which would be tedious, but simply to summarise the main lines of this development insofar as they are useful for understanding the treatment of breast hypertrophy.

Biesenberger's technique (1928)

The first technique to be employed routinely and satisfactorily was that of Biesenberger, and we shall briefly review here its principal features in the variation described by Gillies and MacIndoe in 1936 (fig. 46):

• the nipple-areolar plaque is first reduced and de-epithelialised with the peri-areola by Schwartzmann's maneuver. This procedure, described in 1930, is intended to protect the blood-supply of the areola and the nipple (and especially their venous drainage). This is a simple de-epithelialisation and not a nipple-bearing flap (fig. 47);

• the gland is then split widely from the cutaneous plane, since the dermo-glandular connexions are preserved only medially, using a vertical approach or one slightly oblique downward and outward, passing from the areola to the infra-mammary crease (fig. 47);

• the lower pole of the breast is freed behind from its adhesions to the plane of the pectoralis major muscle in order to allow subsequent glandular rotation;

• the glandular resection, of varying extent, is made at the outer quadrants by an incision commencing at the upper pole of the breast and extended vertically up to 2 cm from the reduced nipple-areolar plaque, skirting it and then continuing obliquely downward and outward or vertically according to the degree of hypertrophy (fig. 48);

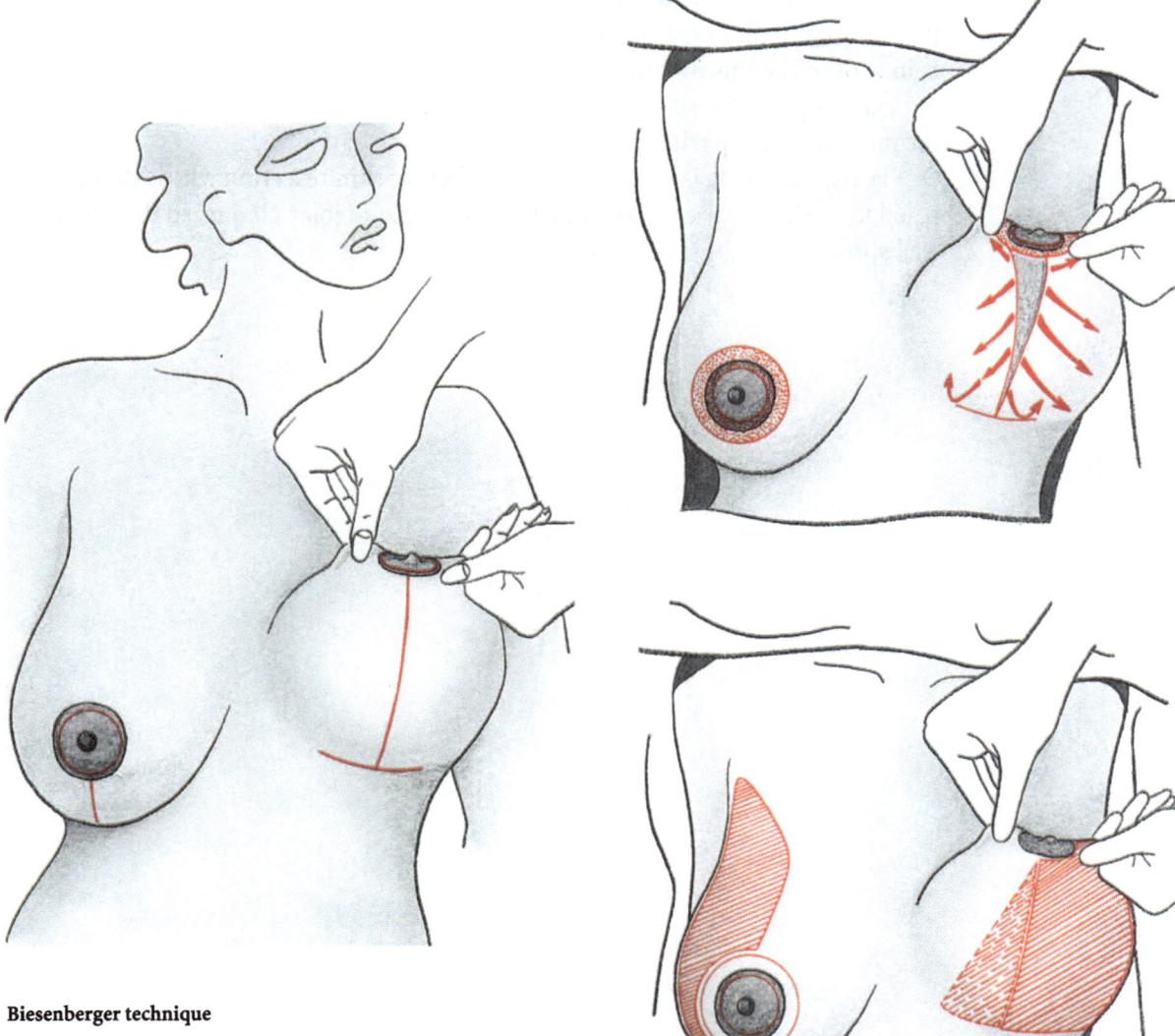

Biesenberger technique

Fig. 46. Tracing the skin incisions

Fig. 47. Zone of de-epithelialisation *(right breast)*, skin incisions and cutaneo-glandular cleavage *(left breast)*

Fig. 48. The zone of glandular resection involves mainly the outer quadrants, but may possibly be extended a little medially into the inferomedial quadrant

• the remaining glandular stump (fig. 49), freed from its posterior attachments, is rolled up and sutured on itself to reconstitute the convexity of the breast (fig. 50) and possibly anchored to the axillary prolongation of the gland if this has been preserved in order to better maintain the outer convexity;

• the skin envelope is applied to the glandular residue and its adjustment is made with the aid of a curved clamp (fig. 51). This reveals all the difficulty of maneuvers with a clamp, since it must not be placed too vertically (the nipple will then be too high, the breast base insufficiently reduced and the breast not properly centered) or too horizontally (the nipple will be projected too far forward, the breast base relatively over-reduced in relation to the anterior projection and the breast exposed to secondary ptosis due to tilting over of the nipple). One must also ensure that the lower end of the clamp is well applied to the chest wall at the level of the inframammary crease; the skin margins are resected to the inner limit of the course of the clamp, and then the inferior horizontal resection is performed, taking care to place the scar well into the inframammary crease, possibly tethering the margins to the parietes;

• lastly, the areola is exteriorised by a circular skin resection whose diameter is equal to or slightly greater than that of the nipple-areolar plaque, so that it can be well spread out (figs. 52 and 53).

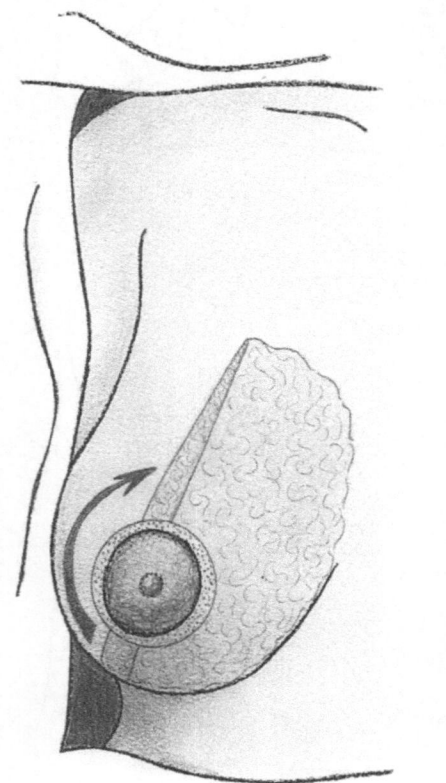 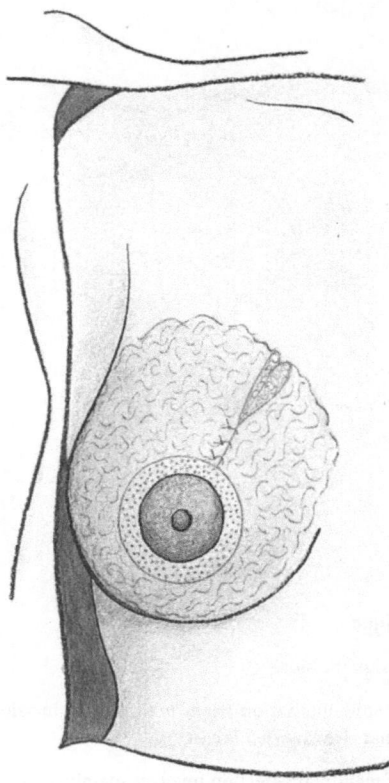

Biesenberger technique

Fig. 49. The remaining gland is rolled up on itself

Fig. 50. The rolled-up gland is sutured

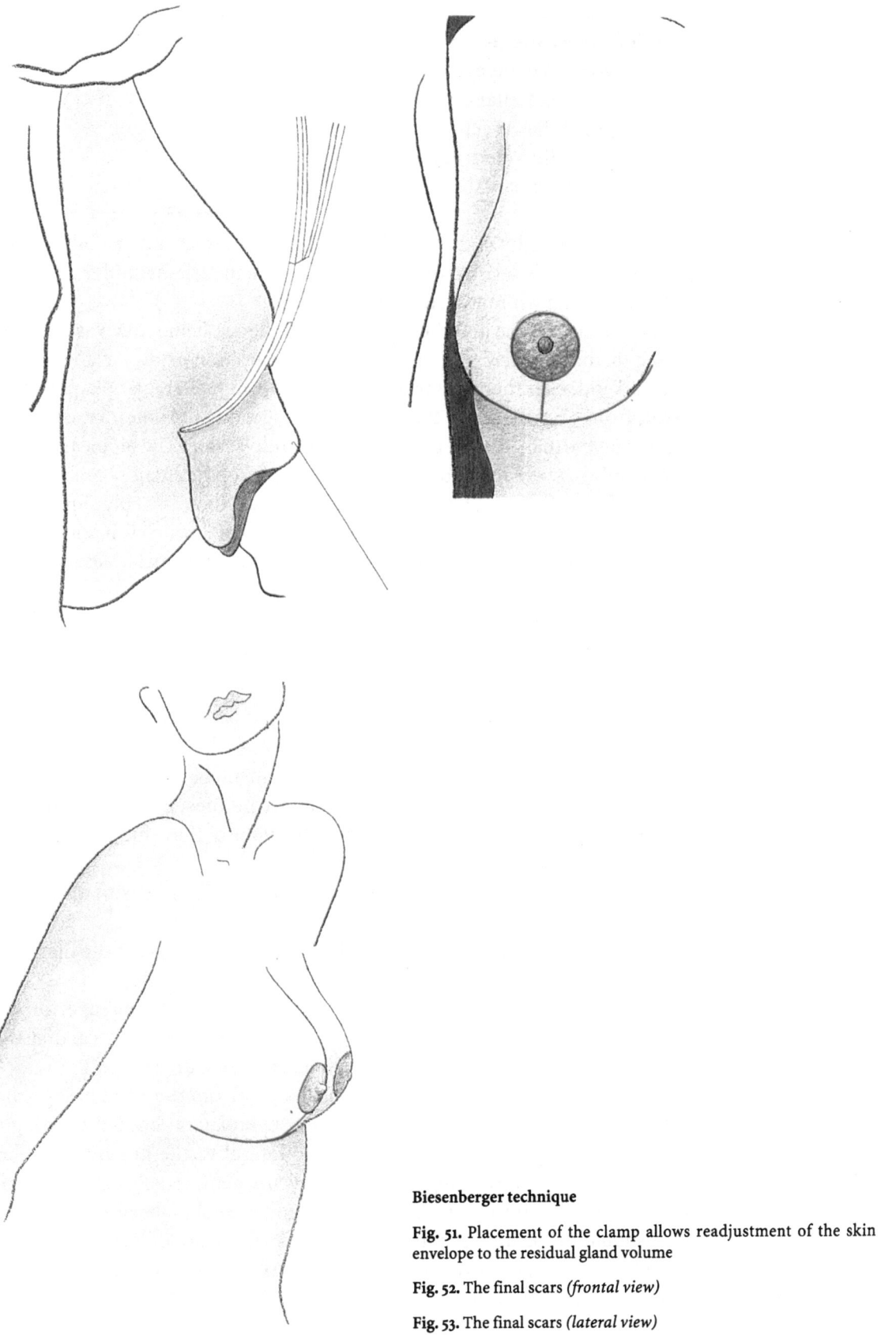

Biesenberger technique

Fig. 51. Placement of the clamp allows readjustment of the skin envelope to the residual gland volume

Fig. 52. The final scars *(frontal view)*

Fig. 53. The final scars *(lateral view)*

This technique therefore combines :
- Schwartzmann's maneuver,
- intercutaneo-glandular cleavage.
- variable glandular resection,
- independent adjustment of the skin envelope,
- final exteriorisation of the nipple-areolar plaque

At that time the quality of the morphologic result and its relative stability made this the first undeniably satisfactory technique, at least in cases of moderate hypertrophy. But it was not without certain disadvantages :

- the glandular residue and the nipple-areolar plaque being now vascularised only by the medial thoracic plexus, any anatomic variation or over-vigorous dissection could endanger their survival. Necrosis of the nipple-areolar plaque might even result from obstruction of the venous drainage, due to somewhat excessive traction during the maneuver of coiling up the glandular flap. The nipple therefore not infrequently necrosed, as did the cutaneous angles of the anchorage;

- the need to safeguard the entire medial thoracic blood-supply limited the resection possibilities; this may not exceed 3/5 of the gland, which is inadequate in major hypertrophy. In this case, moreover, the size of the residual breast compromised the stability of the result;

- the cutaneo-glandular cleavage favored secondary glandular ptosis, since the nipple-areolar plaque remained in place, with unrolling and excessive elongation of segment III.

The oblique method (1961)

At the Hôpital Saint-Louis in Paris, Claude Dufourmentel and Roger Mouly, dissatisfied with the "not negligible" scar defect of the Biesenberger technique, described in 1961 the technique of mammoplasty by the oblique method. Its main features are as follows :

• it is a technique with a preestablished design of the excision, with the following characteristics:

- the circular areolar incision is marked out so as to decrease the diameter of the areola;

- the ellipse of skin resection is drawn between two points, one superior, situated a little above and medial to the nipple, the other inferior, situated at the intersection of the inframammary crease and the anterior axillary line;

- the margins of the ellipse, which is shaped like a quarter of an orange, are drawn with the breast retracted medially by its superolateral border, drawing a virtually straight line which passes above and lateral to the areola; a similar maneuver, but this time displacing the breast outward, allows tracing of the inferomedial margin of the ellipse which passes below and medial to the nipple;

- it should be ensured that both ends of the ellipse are quite symmetric in relation to the midline; however, if asymmetry exists, the ellipse will be wider on the bulkier or more ptosed side.

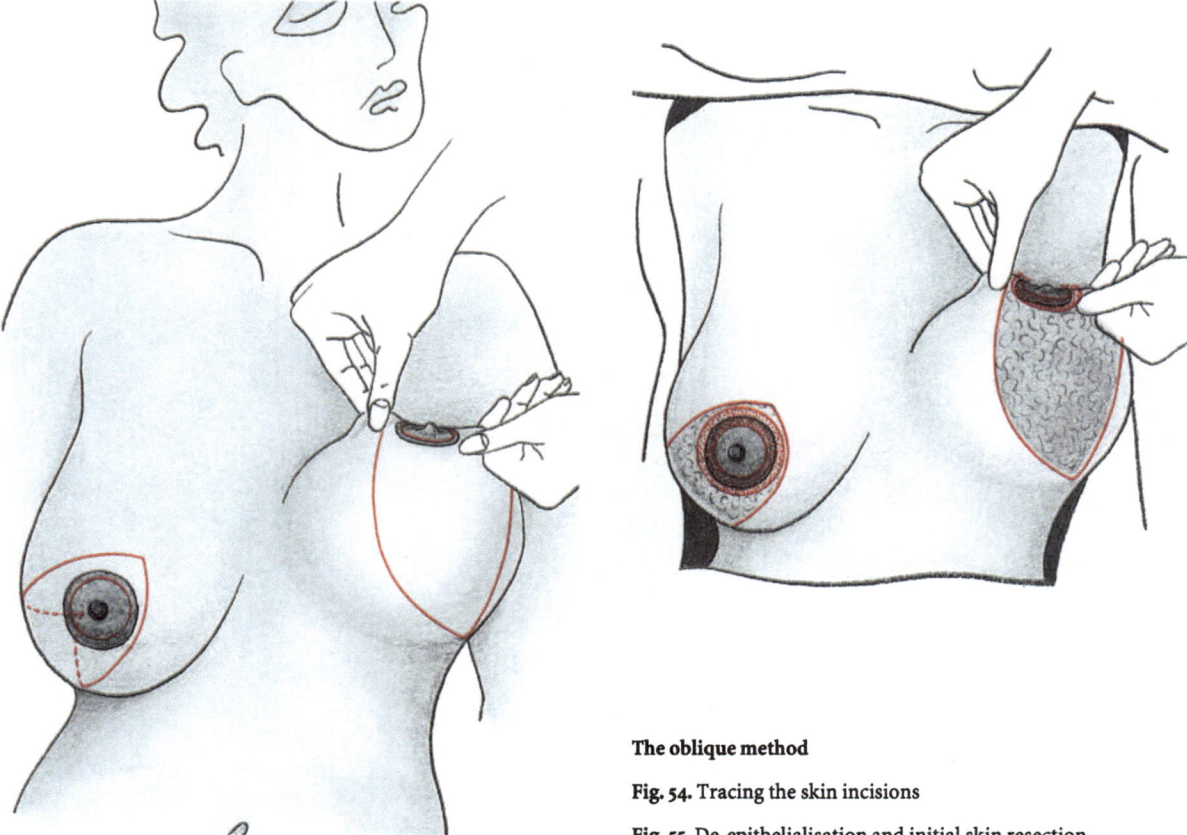

The oblique method

Fig. 54. Tracing the skin incisions

Fig. 55. De-epithelialisation and initial skin resection

• The periareolar incision respects the deep dermis, and a peripheral de-epithelialisation protects the areola, constituting a Schwartzmann's maneuver (fig. 55).

• The skin of the ellipse is initially resected, save at the areola (fig. 55).

• The skin margins are widely freed to a more or less equal extent on each side, working at the level of the gland to preserve the blood-supply to the skin. Laterally, this dissection ascends as far as the axillary tail.

• The gland being freed at its outer border, the dissection is carried to its deep aspect, the posterior stripping not transgressing the lateral half of the gland.

• The resection is performed in the outer half, but preserving the stump of the axillary tail (fig. 58).

• The skin is redraped over the gland and sutured with embedding of the nipple-areolar plaque. Very often, because of breast reduction and the coiling maneuver applied to the gland residue, the inferolateral end of the suture slightly transgresses on the inframammary crease.

• Lastly, the nipple-areolar plaque is exteriorised (after having performed the same procedures on the other side) by a circular excision made quite symmetrically, and placed slightly below the apex of the breast cone (figs. 59 and 60).

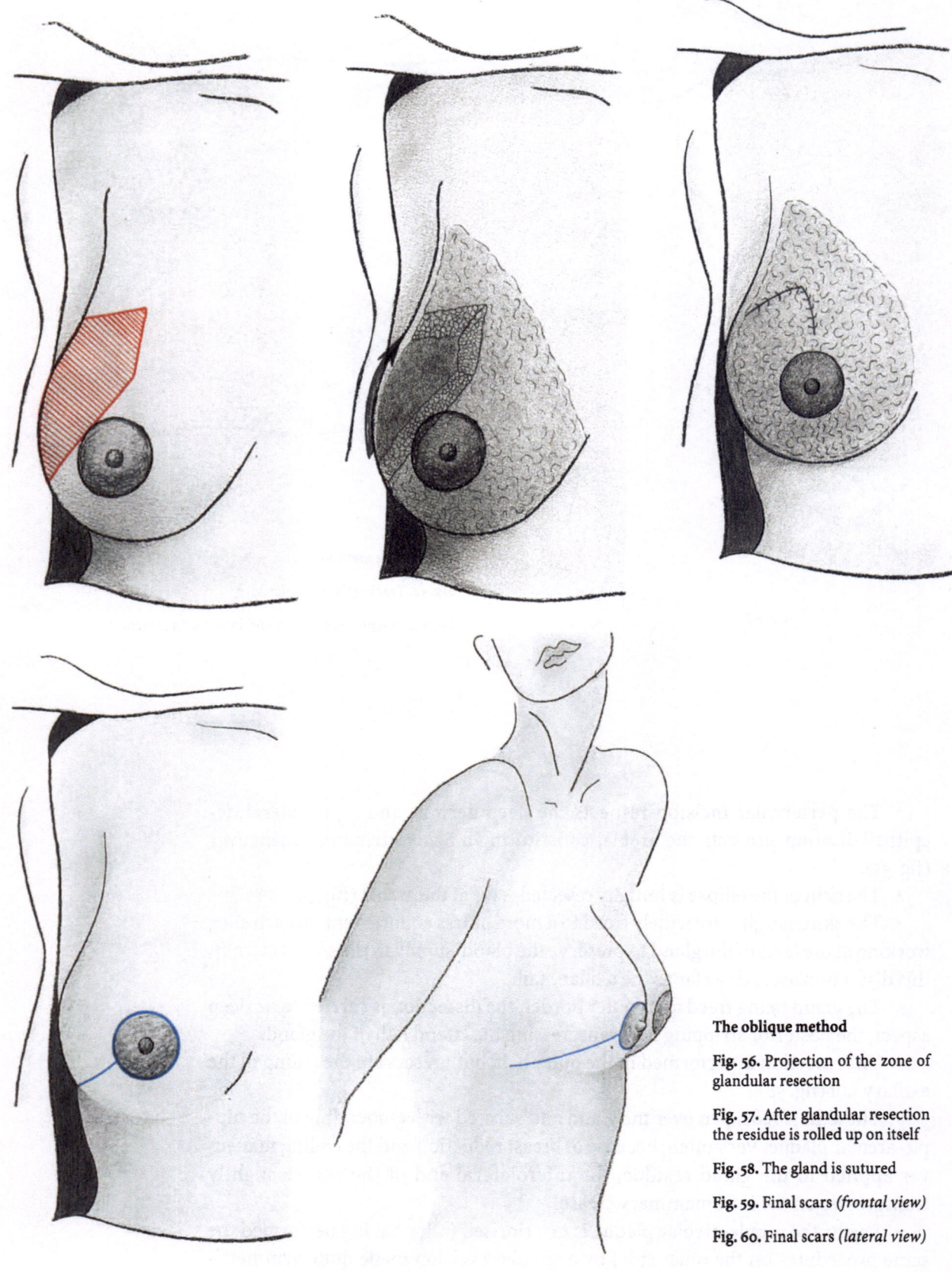

The oblique method

Fig. 56. Projection of the zone of glandular resection

Fig. 57. After glandular resection the residue is rolled up on itself

Fig. 58. The gland is sutured

Fig. 59. Final scars (*frontal view*)

Fig. 60. Final scars (*lateral view*)

To sum up, this is also a technique with:
- intercutaneo-glandular cleavage,
- Schwartzmann's maneuver,
- and lateral resection as in the Biesenberger technique.

But the oblique method differs in:

- its lateral approach,
- suspension by the axillary tail (the value of which in long-term stabilisation, like that of any isolated mammoplasty procedure, remains debatable),
- the oblique scar.

However, the vascular insecurity associated with the cutaneo-glandular stripping remained the same.

A fundamental turning-point was reached with the achievement of survival of the nipple-areolar plaque on a dermal flap. Schwartzmann had done this in 1936, using a medial pedicle, but it was forgotten for many years.

This nipple-bearing flap was rediscovered with a base that varied with its author:

- Strombeck, in 1960, isolated the nipple-areolar plaque on a double transverse pedicle,
- while Skoog, in 1963, confined himself to a lateral pedicle,
- however, it was Pitanguy, in 1961, realising the undeniable advance afforded by the avoidance of cutaneo-glandular stripping, who isolated the nipple-areolar plaque on a superior pedicle and performed a "boat-keel" resection.

Strombeck's technique (1960)

This was published for the first time in 1960, but the modified version dates from 1972.

The axis of the breast is drawn from the middle of the clavicle through the nipple. On this axis a nipple point is determined which is situated at a minimum of 22 cm from the suprasternal notch; this point is situated virtually opposite the inframammary crease (fig. 61).

A template is then applied (derived from those of Wise) whose axis corresponds to that of the breast. Two models of template exist, one for medium degrees of hypertrophy and ptosis and the other for more severe cases.

The size of the areola is reduced. Two lines joining C and B, A and D determine the de-epithelialised nipple-bearing "bucket-handle" flap, which has a double transverse pedicle. BC passes at least 2 cm above the areola, AD at least 1 cm.

The breast is mobilised inward and then outward, and after having marked the inframammary crease with ink, the line AD is prolonged so as to rejoin the crease at A' and D' (figs. 62 and 63).

The dermo-glandular bridge ABCD is de-epithelialised (Fig. 64) and the future areolar site is incised with excision of a cylinder of gland and skin down to the pectoral plane (fig. 65). The inferior glandular excision is made after incision of A'D'. The inferior skin resection is performed after construction of the subareolar vertical. The glandular excision may be pursued to the deep aspect of the dermo-glandular bridge (fig. 66).

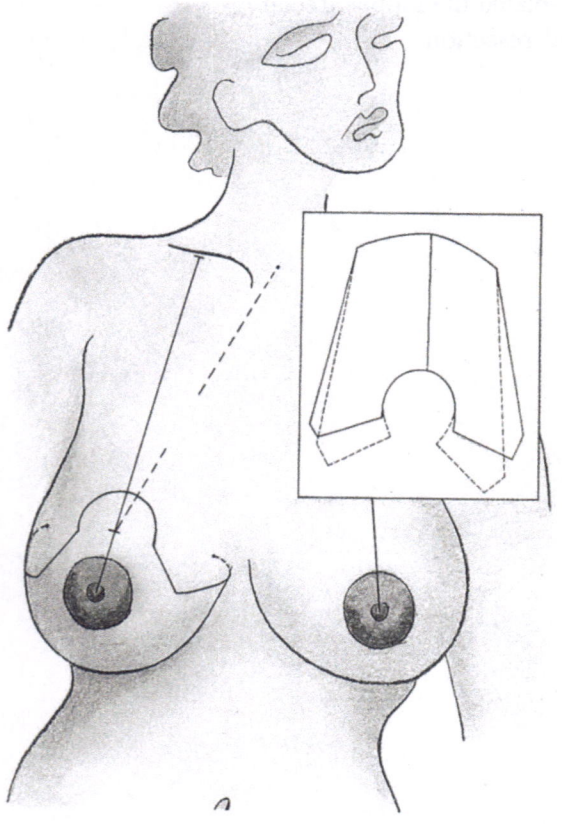

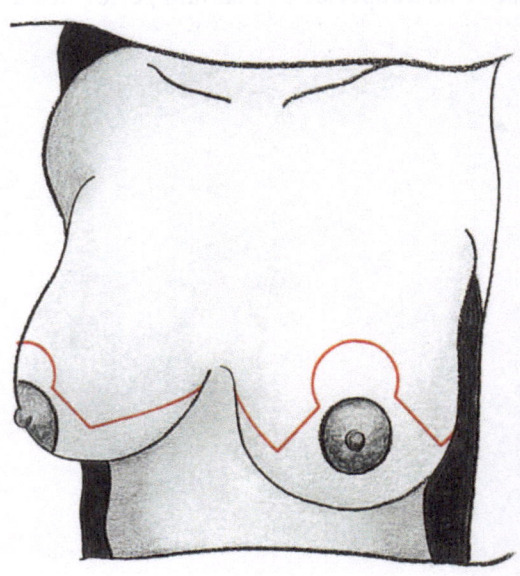

Strombeck's technique

Fig. 61. Landmarks and template

Fig. 62. Skin incisions (*frontal view*)

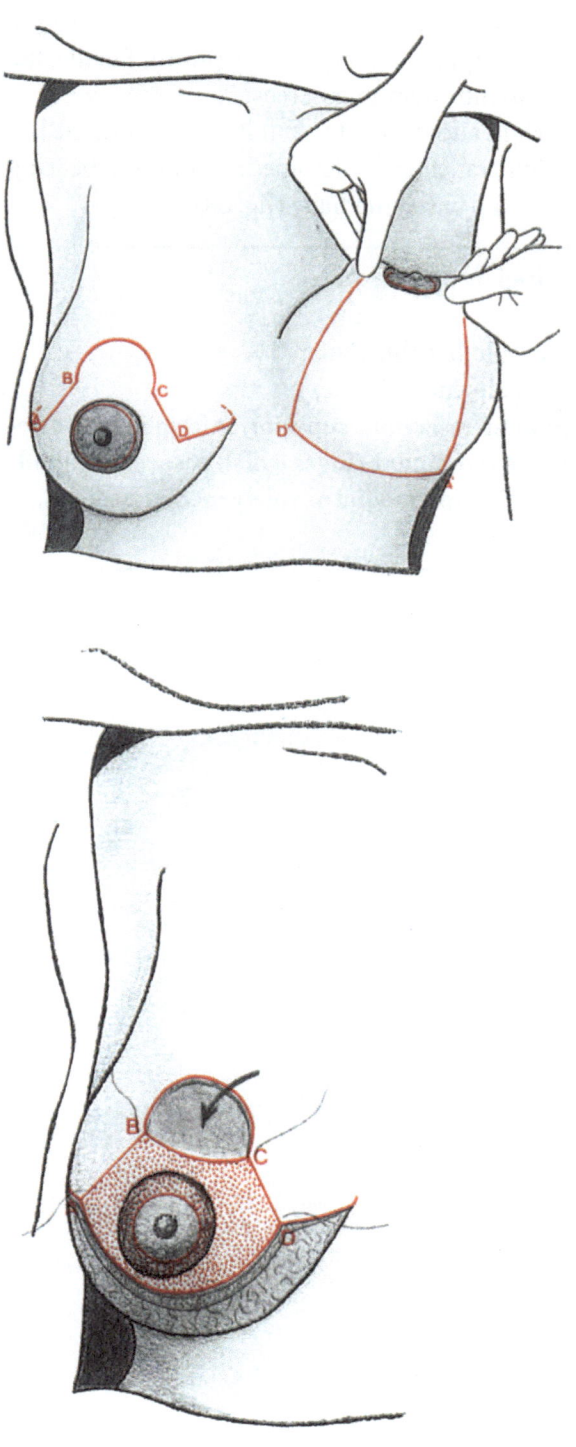

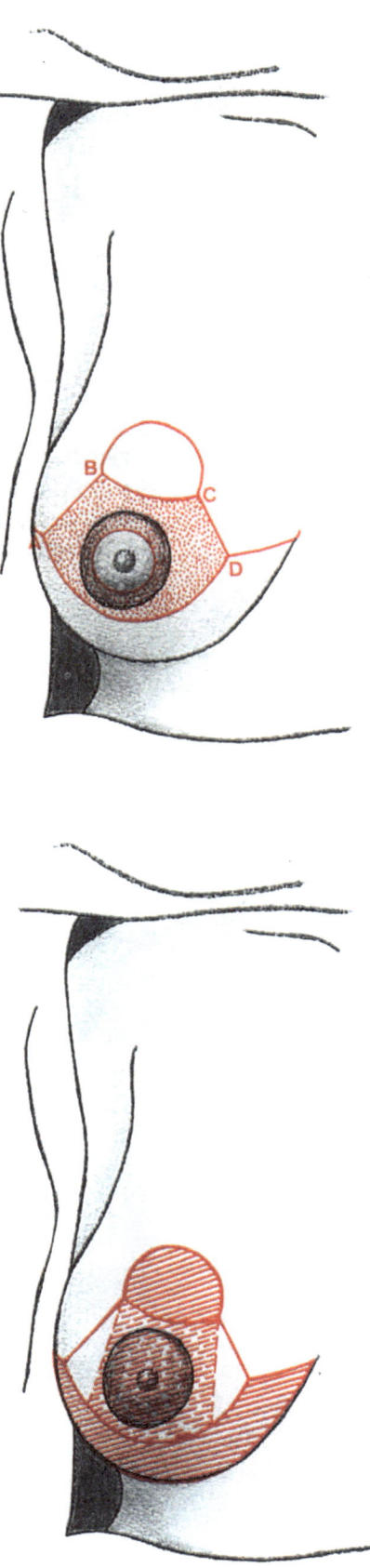

Strombeck's technique

Fig. 63. Skin incisions *(frontal view)*

Fig. 64. De-epithelialisation of the nipple-bearing flap

Fig. 65. Excision of the dermo-glandular cylinder and incision of the nipple-bearing flap

Fig. 66. The glandular resection opposite the upper part of the gland and cylinder *(continuous lines)* may be prolonged behind the nipple-bearing flap *(interrupted lines)*

The vertical suture is made to approximate A and D by fixing them to the crease, and then B and C, bringing the nipple-areolar plaque upward. Finally, the sutures are completed at the areola and inframammary crease.

If the nipple-bearing flap is too rigid and difficult to put into position, the lateral pedicle may be sectioned, which transforms the bipedicled nipple-bearing bucket-handle flap into a unipedicled flap based medially (fig. 68).

Strombeck's technique is characterised by:
  – the use of a template,
  – a bipedicled "bucket-handle" nipple-bearing flap.
  – which may become unipedicled at its medial base,
  – a so-called "hour-glass" glandular resection, superior, inferior and posterior, leaving in place the lateral dermo-glandular bridges which ensure the blood-supply of the areola and nipple via lateral and medial or solely medial pedicles,
  – avoidance of cutaneo-glandular cleavage.

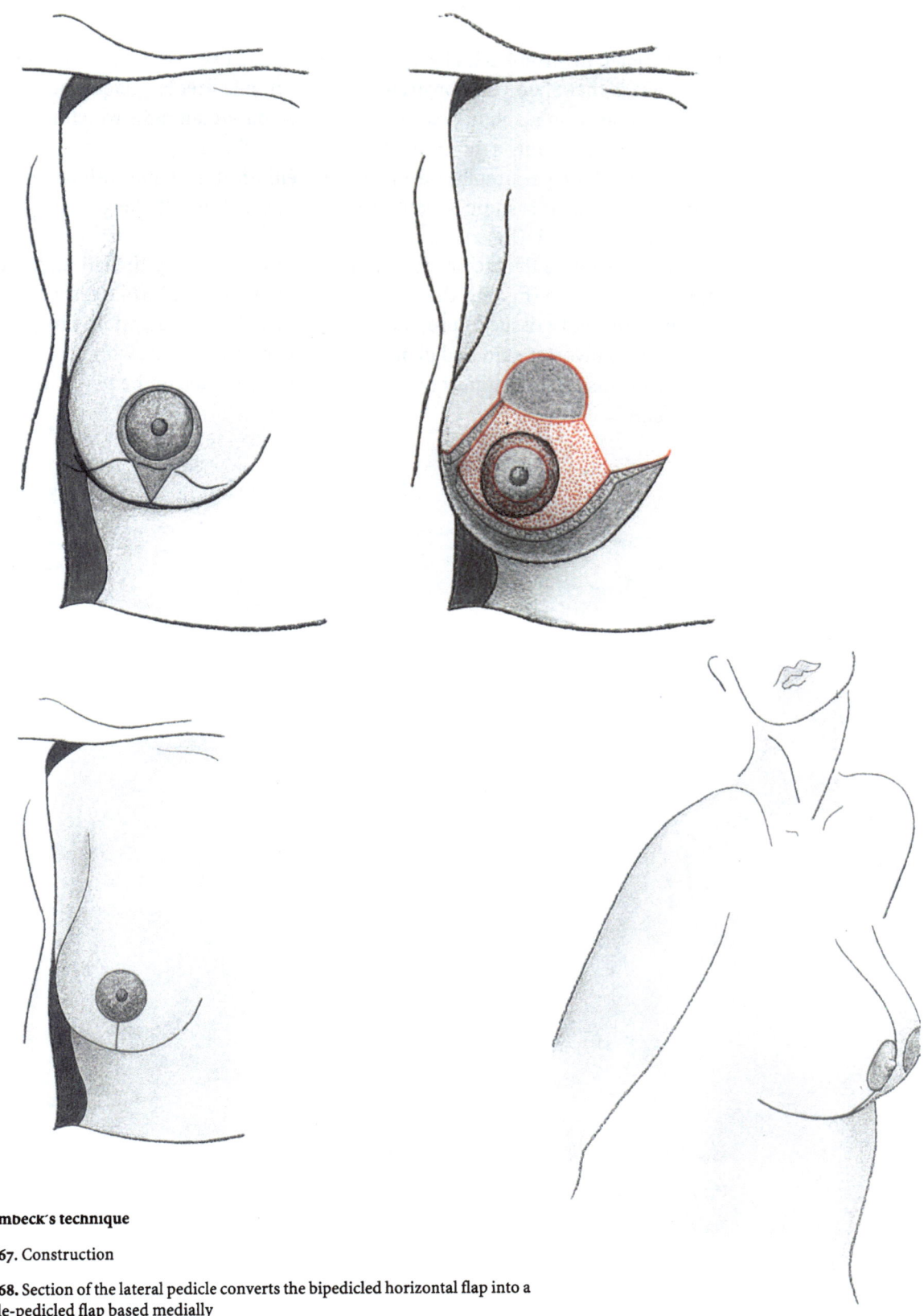

Strombeck's technique

Fig. 67. Construction

Fig. 68. Section of the lateral pedicle converts the bipedicled horizontal flap into a single-pedicled flap based medially

Fig. 69. Final scar (frontal view)

Fig. 70. Final scar (lateral view)

Skoog's technique (1963)

This is related to Strombeck's technique in that it also uses a template, but the great difference is that Skoog demonstrated that the nipple-areolar plaque can survive from the outset on a single pedicle, in this case based laterally, which is dermoglandular but with only a minor thickness of glandular tissue.

The line of the periareolar skin incision is elliptical in shape with its long axis transverse, so as to assume a circular shape after closure. Its height AB (or CD) does not exceed 7 cm (fig. 71).

After incision of the areolar ellipse and incision and de-epithelialisation of the nipple-bearing flap (fig. 72), the latter is split from the gland while respecting the subcutaneous fatty tissue to preserve the subdermal vascularisation. The glandular resection involves skin and gland together (figs. 73 and 74), without any stripping. If it is insufficient, it may be cautiously supplemented at the posterior aspect of the gland.

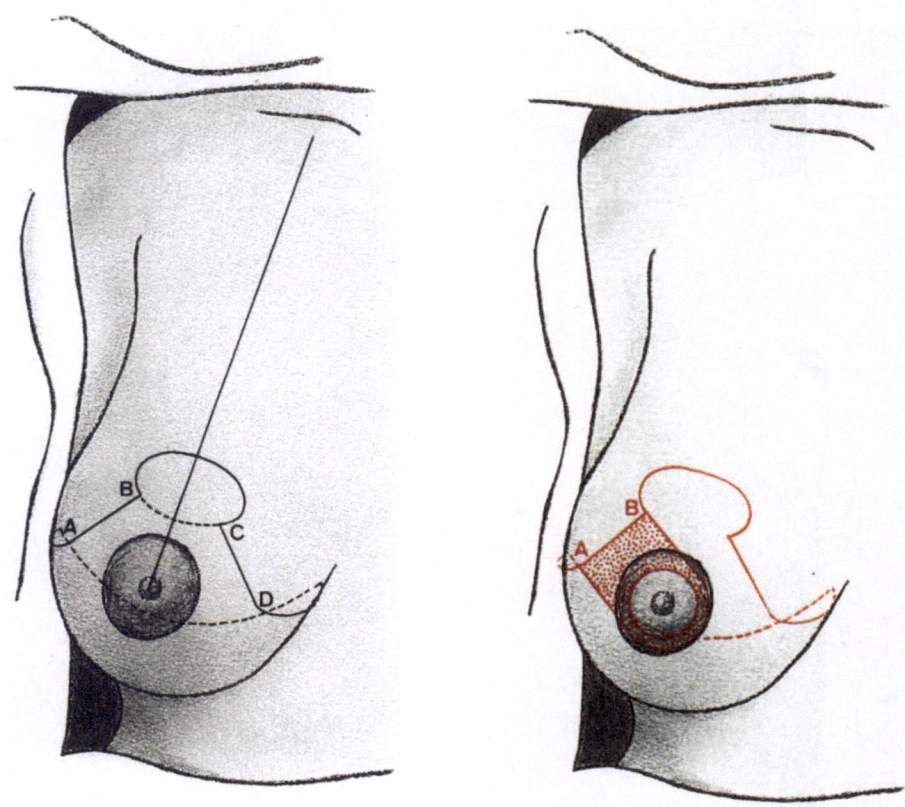

Skoog's technique

Fig. 71. Preoperative tracings

Fig. 72. De-epithelialisation and skin incisions

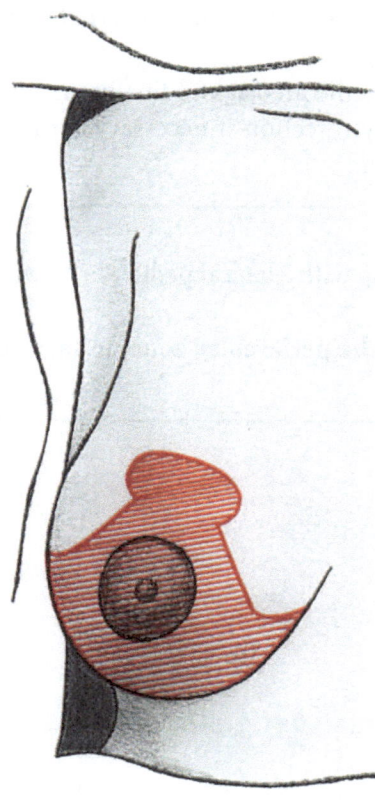

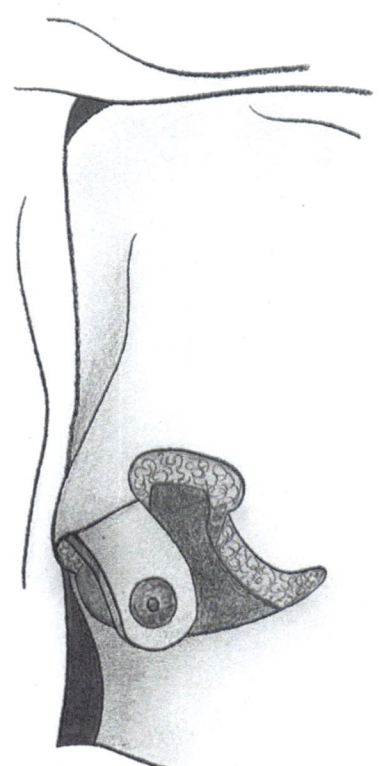

Skoog's technique

Fig. 73. Projection of the zone of glandular resection

Fig. 74. The glandular resection

The nipple-bearing flap is positioned after a limited stripping (2 cm) of the skin margins from the areola to lodge the flap (fig. 75).

The subareolar vertical is tacked down, as is the areola, and finally the inframammary suture is made after supplementary resection if necessary, ensuring that this suture is placed in the crease (figs. 76 and 77).

Skoog's technique is characterised by:
  – a thin, de-epithelialised nipple-bearing flap with a lateral pedicle,
  – a one-piece cutaneo-glandular resection
  – cutaneo-glandular stripping limited to the periareolar zone, to facilitate postioning of the nipple-bearing flap.

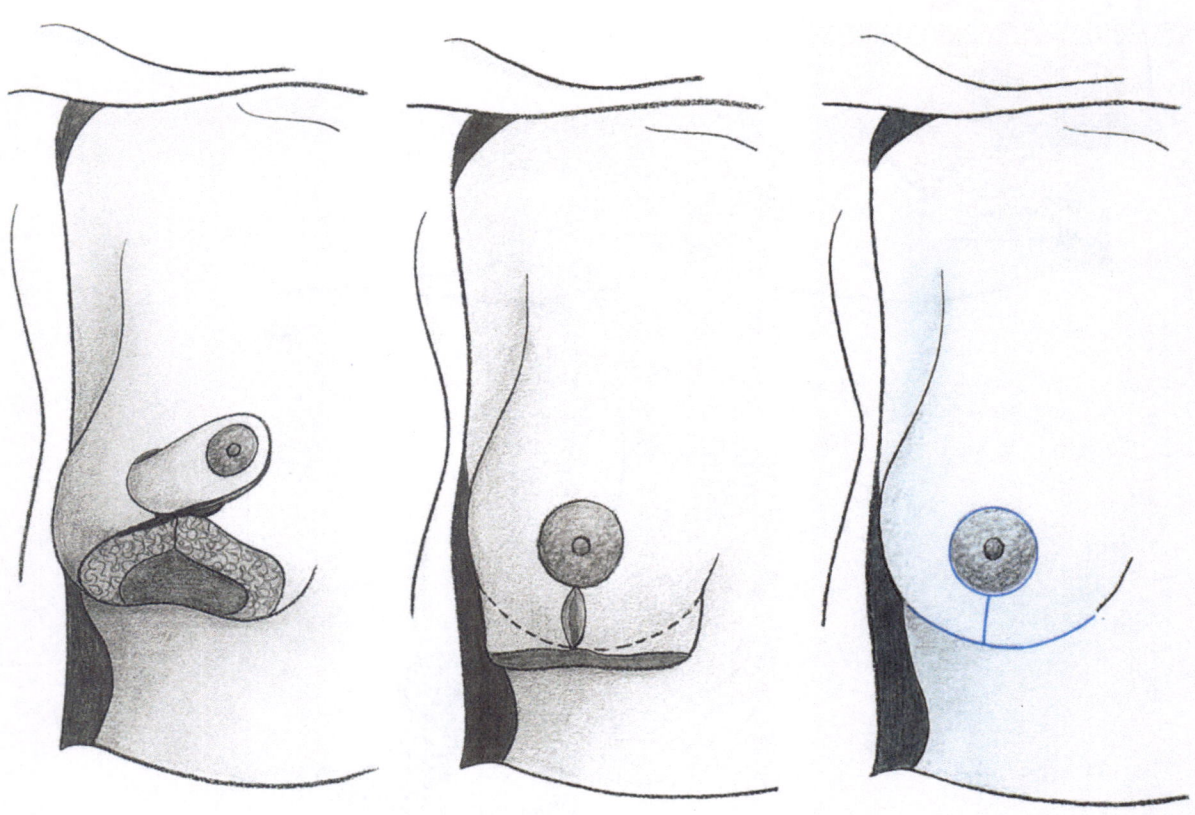

Skoog's technique

Fig. 75. Placement of the nipple-bearing flap

Fig. 76. Suture of the areola, construction of the subareolar vertical and supplementary glandular resection in the inframammary crease

Fig. 77. Final scars

Pitanguy's technique (1961)

This is performed with the patient in the semi-seated position.

It will be recalled that this position is the one that best permits peroperative assessment of the convexity and distribution of glandular volume of the operated breast, and that it is necessary whenever the chosen technique does not depend on, and is thereore not subject to, a preestablished design.

The axis of the breasts, passing through the nipple, is drawn from the middle of the clavicle.

A nipple point A is situated on this axis, slightly below the projected level of the inframammary crease (located by a finger placed under the breast at the middle of the fold and slightly elevating it). B and C are located in terms of the amount of tissue to be resected, without being placed higher than the nipple. The distances AB and AC must not exceed 6 to 7 cm. B' and C' are located at the level of the crease (BB' + CC' = B'C') (fig. 78).

The areola is reduced to a diameter of 4 to 4.5 cm; the de-epithelialisation of the triangle BAC extends below to at least 2 cm from the nipple (fig. 79).

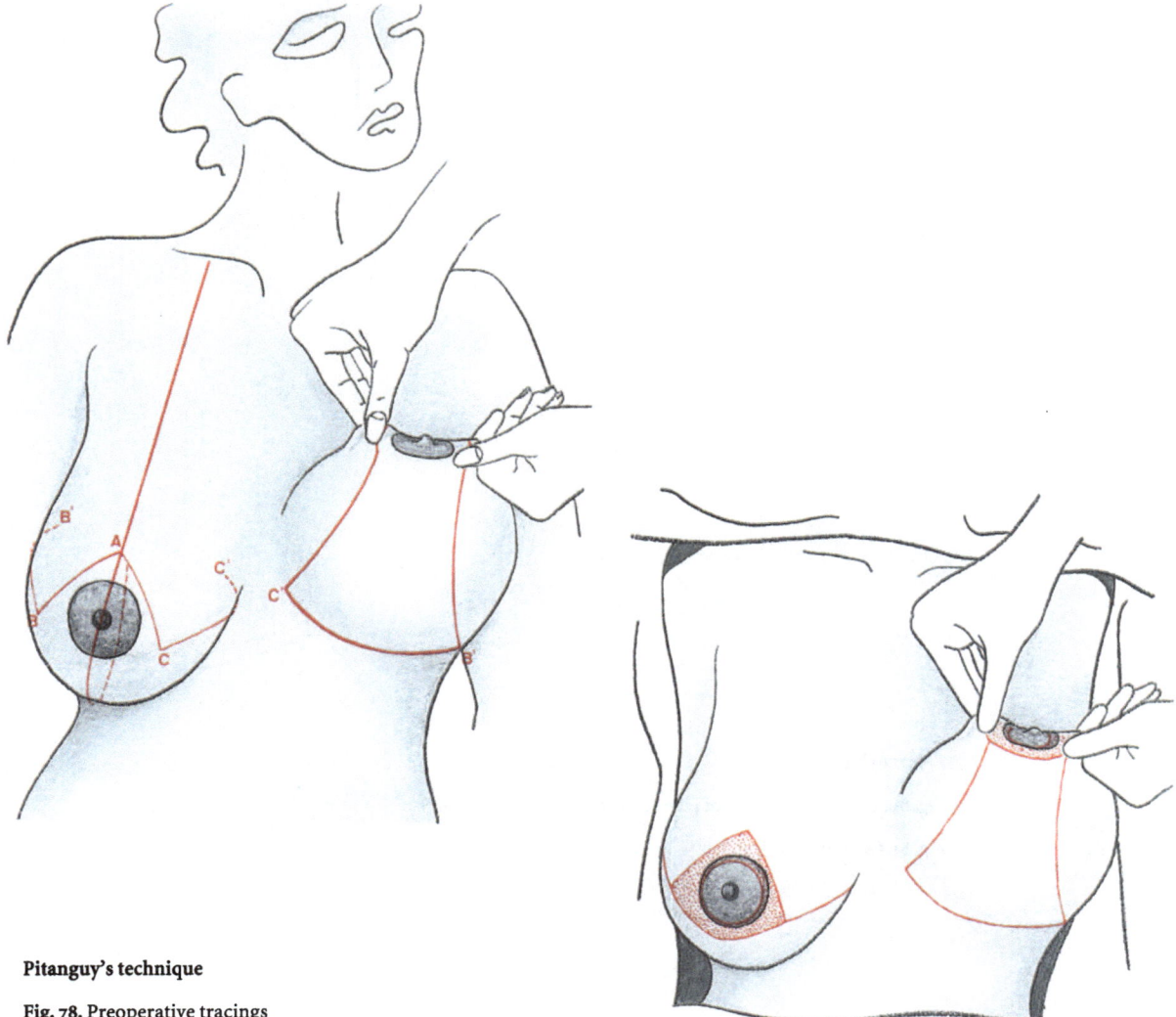

Pitanguy's technique

Fig. 78. Preoperative tracings

Fig. 79. De-epithelialisation and skin incisions

A hook placed at A elevates the gland. The skin and gland are incised freely as far as the pectoral plane along BB' and then BC, to the lower limit of the de-epithelialised zone, in such a manner that this resection of skin and gland en bloc has the shape of an "inverted boat-keel" (fig. 80).

The author's advice is to resect the gland simultaneously before reconstruction to ensure symmetry.

The gland sections are approximated by some tacking sutures (fig. 81), which projects the nipple upward; the gland may be fixed to the pectoral plane at this stage. If there is a lack of skin reduction in relation to the residual gland volume, the skin may be stripped along the margins of the incision and the excess resected, but this stripping must not extend beyond that to be resected, so as not to infringe the principle of avoidance of cutaneo-glandular cleavage.

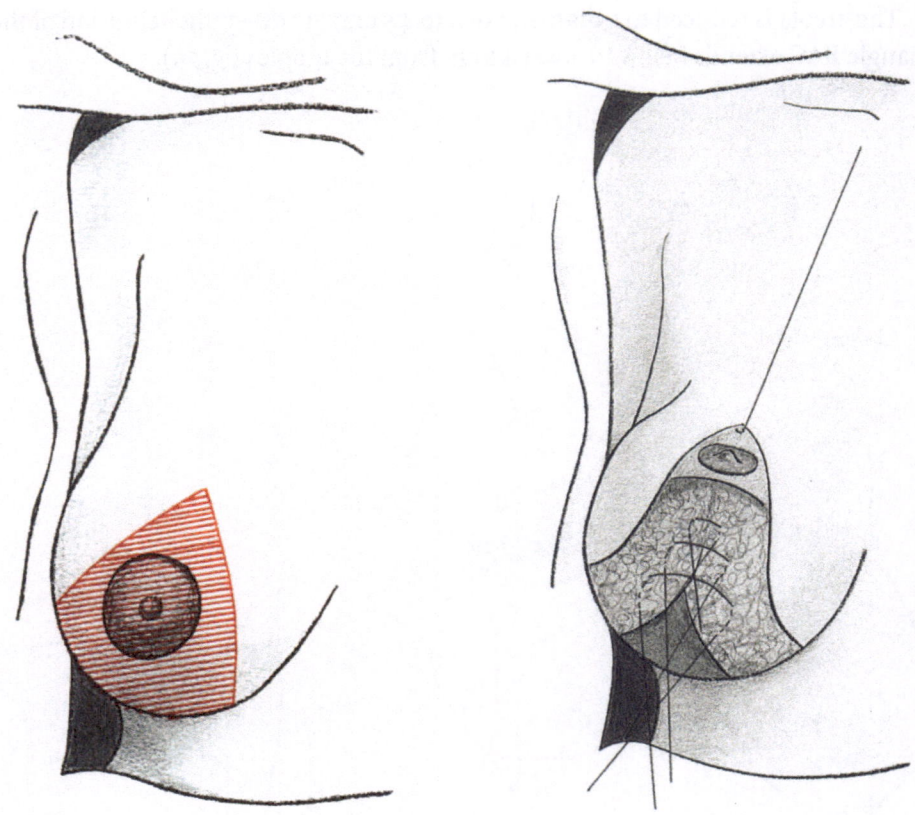

Pitanguy's technique

Fig. 80. Projection of zone of glandular resection *("boat-keel")*

Fig. 81. Glandular suture

The sutures are made at the subareolar vertical and the inframammary zone, and finally the areolar zone is determined according to the shape and projection of the reconstructed breast, which involves some minimal periareolar stripping to facilitate placement of the areola.

The technique of Pitanguy is based on :
   – **an "inverted boat-keel" resection,**
   – **avoidance of cutaneo-glandular cleavage,**
   – **preservation of the medial and lateral vascular pedicles.**

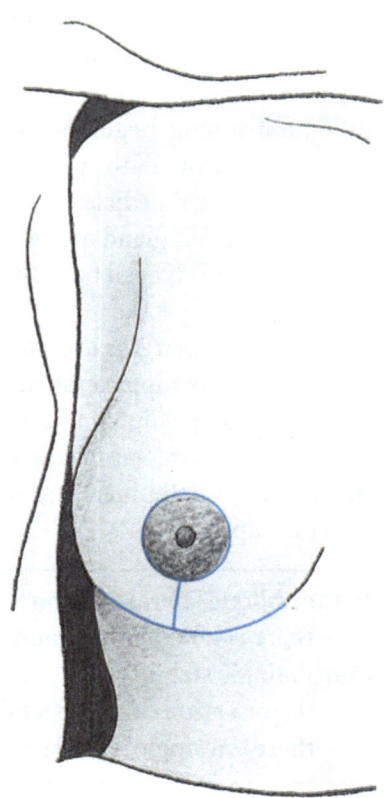

Pitanguy's technique

Fig. 82. Final scars

The oblique lateral method

These considerations led Claude Dufourmentel and Roger Mouly to modify their technique; in 1965 the oblique method became the oblique lateral method :

• the skin tracings are comparable, the lower point of the ellipse being situated at the intersection of the anterior axillary line and the inframammary crease, ie above the most dependent point of the fold. The upper point of the ellipse is situated on a line from the suprasternal notch to the nipple, but at more than 2 cm from the peripheral margin of the areola;

• the greater the hypertrophy, the more rounded is the upper end of the ellipse. If there is any doubt as to the breadth of the ellipse, it is better to draw it a little narrower and to rectify this during the procedure;

• the entire surface between the areola (reduced to 4-5 cm in circumference) and the skin incisions up to 1 cm from the inferolateral pole of the areola is de-epithelialised (fig. 83);

• the stripping, begun below and laterally, can be pursued to the deep aspect of the gland, in front of the pectoralis major muscle, but always safeguarding the vessels of the medial pedicle;

• skin, fat and gland are resected en bloc at the level of the skin incisions, supplementing this if need be with resection at the deep aspect of the gland starting at each margin (fig. 84);

• the gland margins are sutured in two layers, superficial and deep, the skin is sutured and the nipple embedded after making a very slight subcutaneous stripping to house the nipple-bearing dermo-glandular flap;

• the nipple-areolar plaque is exteriorised as before at the end of the procedure, this helping to eliminate the skin which had been stripped to lodge the nipple-bearing flap.

In the oblique lateral method :

– there is no cutaneo-glandular cleavage, thus ensuring vascular security and morphologic stability),

– the resection can be extended further at the deep aspect of the gland,

– there is a single lateral scar (except, of course, for the periareolar scar).

In cases of pure ptosis without hypertrophy, and with an upper segment devoid of glandular tissue, it becomes necessary to perform a "snail-shell" reduction. But since there is no cutaneo-glandular cleavage, this coiling-up cannot be made laterally. The reduction is made by means of an inferolateral dermo-glandular flap, slid under the superolateral margin.

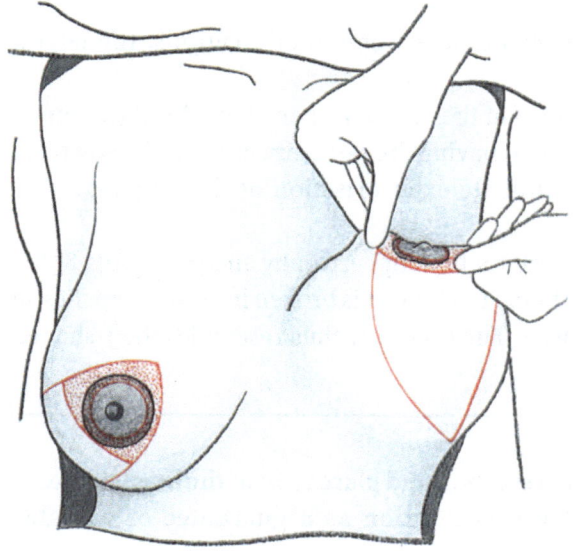

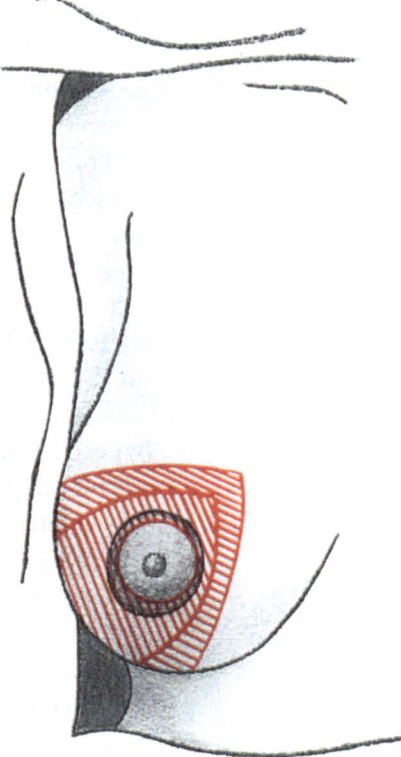

Oblique lateral method

Fig. 83. Skin incisions and de-epithelialisation

Fig. 84. Projection of zone of glandular resection

The lateral method

Finally, in 1973, this technique became, with some modifications, the lateral method:

• the new areolar site is determined at the outset, its peripheral limit (designed with a metal ring which can be opened) having the same size as the reduced areola (this avoids the embedding and ultimate exteriorisation of the nipple-areolar plaque) (fig. 85);

• the "snail-shell" rolling-up is used for both hypertrophy and ptosis (fig. 86);

• if the oblique lateral scar risks being too long, it is broken into two branches so as not to transgress on the chest-wall. The final scar thus resembles the J-shaped scar described by Elbaz (fig. 87).

The lateral method combines:

– **preestablished design for skin resection and placement of the areolar site,**

– **respect for the subdermal vascularisation as a guarantee of vascular security,**

– **"snail-shell" rolling-up,**

– **an oblique lateral scar.**

From its inception this technique has met with considerable success, both in France and elsewhere, because of the security afforded by safeguarding the subdermal vessels and the final position of the scar.

But it still had its limitations:

– it is a satisfactory technique for moderate hypertrophy and ptosis, because of the morphologic result obtained for a moderate scar defect (the "valley" between the breasts is spared);

– but the morphologic outcome is much less satisfactory once there is severe hypertrophy, whether or not associated with a predominant ptosis stretching the skin envelope;

– in practice, the absence of uniform glandular resection, in particular the virtual impossibility of resecting as much under the medial quadrants as under the outer, leads to a breast shape which in our opinion bulges too much medially compared with the more flattened lateral segment, and this defect becomes worse with the effects of time and gravity;

– on the other hand, the limited de-epithelialisation also decreases the possibilities of skin reduction and of adaptation of the skin envelope to residual breast size.

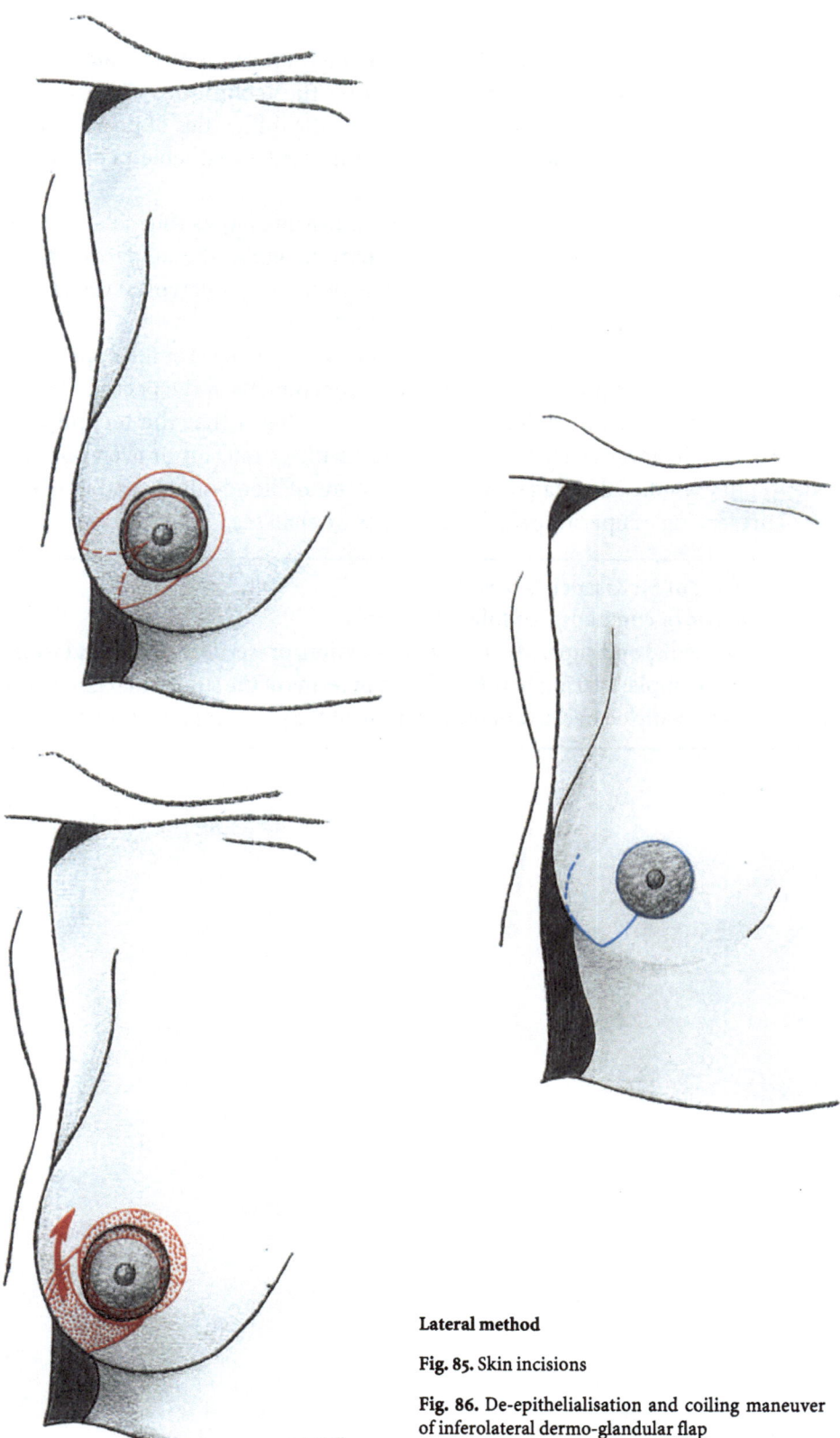

Lateral method

Fig. 85. Skin incisions

Fig. 86. De-epithelialisation and coiling maneuver of inferolateral dermo-glandular flap

Fig. 87. J-shaped scar

McKissock's technique (1972)

The technique of McKissock, more or less contemporaneous with the later version of Dufourmentel and Mouly, and inspired by the techniques of Skoog and Strombeck (figs. 88 and 89), sought to get rid of the difficulties of positioning of the horizontal dermo-glandular flap and was still based on a double-pedicled flap, but this time vertical (fig. 90).

The upper, supra-areolar, part of the nipple-bearing flap is thin so as to assist its ascent and plication. Its lower, subareolar, part maintains the subdermal vascular continuity with the crease derived from the perforating intercostal vessels. It is embedded by approximation of the lateral flaps.

The glandular resection (fig. 91) is made laterally at the level of the upper quadrants if necessary, but preserves the posterior attachments at the pectoral level in the central zone. To this extent, it may be considered that the technique of McKissock is the forerunner of the techniques with an inferior or even posterior pedicle, but with the advantage over these in terms of blood-supply and morphology of preserving a superior pedicle (fig. 92) as we shall see.

The technique of McKissock is based on :
  – avoidance of cutaneo-glandular cleavage,
  – lateral, medial and superior glandular resection, preserving the central zone,
  – a vertical nipple-bearing flap, bipedicled in terms of the subdermal circulation but actually tripedicled because of preservation of the posterior attachments.

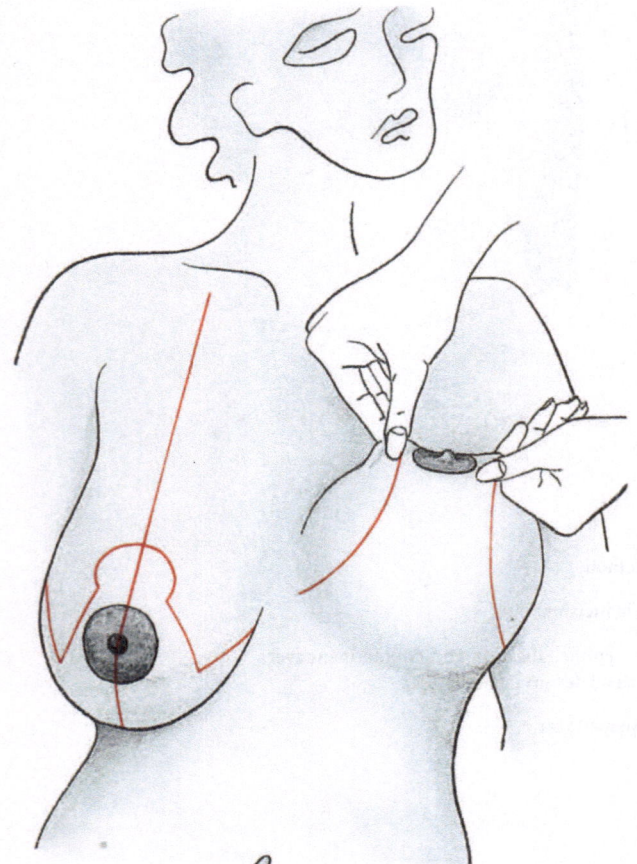

McKissock technique

Fig. 88. Preoperative designs

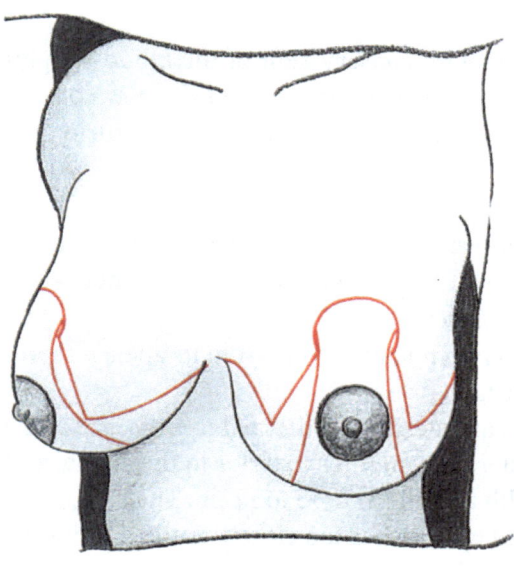

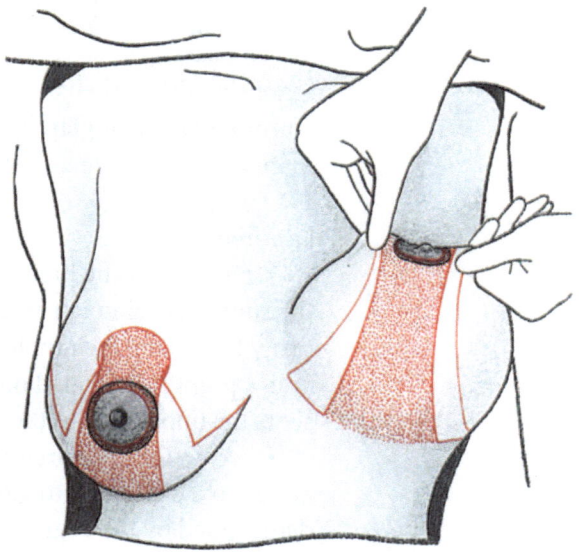

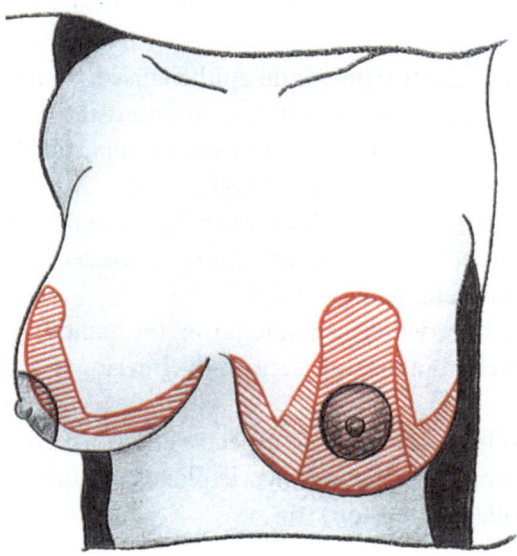

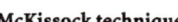

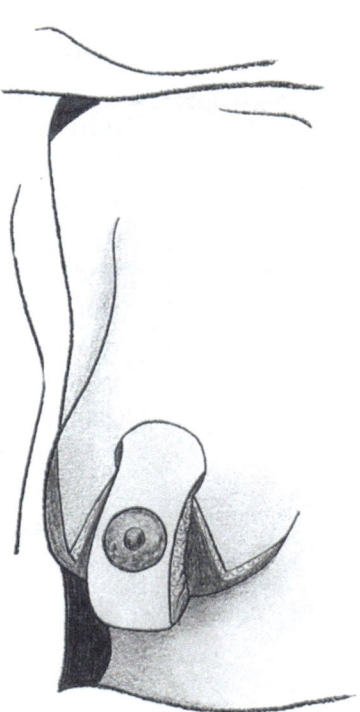

McKissock technique

Fig. 89. Tracing of skin incisions

Fig. 90. De-epithelialisation and incisions

Fig. 91. Projection of zone of glandular resection : this extends to the lower, outer and inner parts of the gland and under the upper part of the flap, but leaving a wide medial and inferior dermo-glandular bridge

Fig. 92. The vertical dermo-glandular bridge after glandular resection

The dermal vault technique (1972)

Extensive de-epithelialisation (and therefore conservation of the blood-supply) and uniformity of glandular resection are the two key-notes of the new concept manifested in the dermal vault technique, pioneered in 1972 by J.-P. Lalardrie.

Technique

• The axis of the breast is traced starting from a point situated 5 cm lateral to the suprasternal notch and extending to the inframammary crease, but not necessarily traversing the nipple if this is eccentric;

• a point A is located on this axis, between 14 and 15 cm from its apex; it represents the upper pole of the denuded surface;

• two concentric circles are drawn : an interior one that reduces the size of the areola to a circle of 4 to 4.6 cm diameter; and another, exterior to the areola, and determined by the degree of ptosis, with a diameter of 10 to 14 cm. The danger lies in designing a circle that is too big and approaches too closely to the midline, so that skin is lacking at the end of the procedure. In determining this circle it is helpful to employ the maneuver used by Biesenberger, ie displacing the breast inward and then outward, and taking care not to come closer than 9 cm to the midline. If need be, to join point A, this circle can be reduced in diameter and ovalised in the vertical direction (fig. 93);

• the entire zone situated between the two lines is de-epithelialised. This procedure, performed more easily on a breast stretched by a mammostat, must be superficial enough to respect the subdermal plexus, but not so superficial as to risk inclusions responsible for secondary epidermal cysts (fig. 94);

• the breast is drawn upward and the skin is split along its axis from the inferior border of the de-epithelialised zone as far as the inframammary crease. The incision is made boldly down to the glandular plane (fig. 95);

• the skin and subcutaneous tissue are then separated from the gland from the extremities of the horizontal diameter of the large circle to the inferior pole of the gland;

• the inferior pole of the gland is freed on its two aspects : anteriorly from the subcutaneous plane, posteriorly from the pectoral muscle plane, and quite far at each side (inner extremity and axillary extension) (fig. 96);

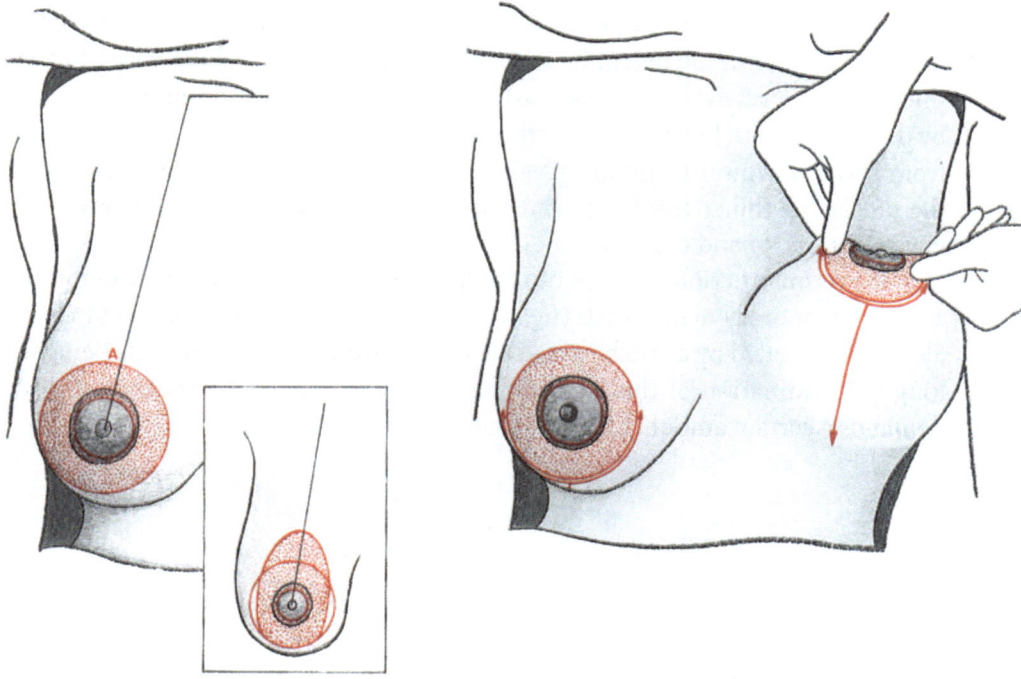

Dermal vault technique

Fig. 93. Preoperative tracings *(inset: in cases with marked ptosis the design is ovalised so as not to approach the midline too closely)*

Fig. 94. After de-epithelialisation : the skin incisions

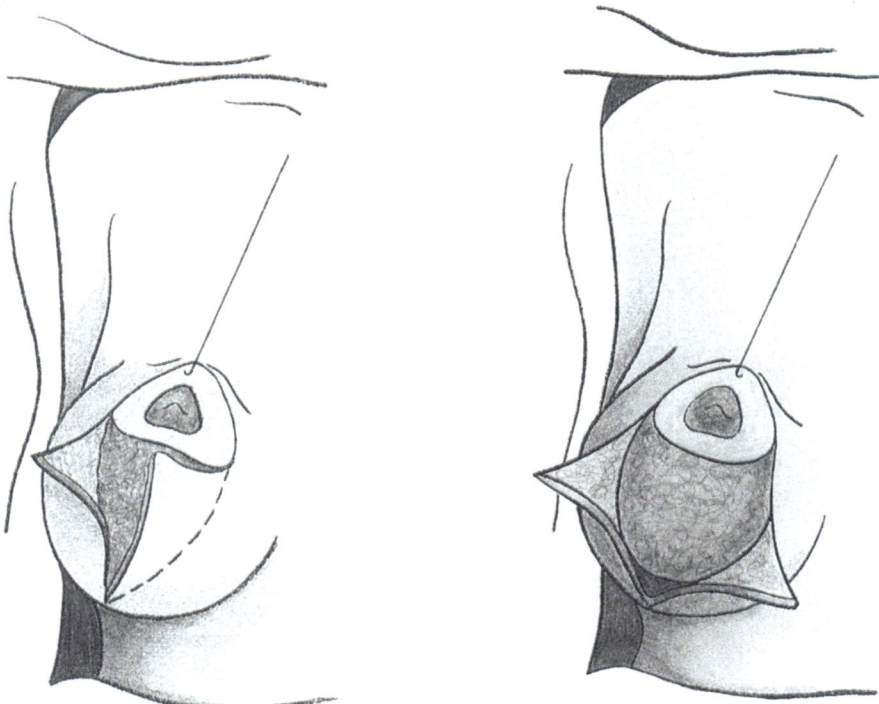

Dermal vault technique

Fig. 95. The two inferior skin flaps are stripped

Fig. 96. The lower pole of the gland is freed and its deep aspect stripped from the pectoral plane

• the glandular resection is then performed, commencing with an incision at the lower border of the de-epithelialised zone, creating a glandular slice 1 to 2 cm thick, and progressively elevating the breast. This resection, monitored constantly by the flattened left hand placed vertically behind the areola, is made progressively from above downward, and must leave a variably thick glandular layer (the more the ptosis, the thiner this layer), but one that is uniform beneath the entire skin envelope (figs. 97 and 98);

• the reconstruction is begun by attaching point A to the upper pole of the areola by a temporary nylon stitch (fig. 99). The two margins of the larger circle are also approximated by a stitch passed 6.5 to 7 cm from point A, the ends being left long (determination of this point B, also a tricky part of the technique, often demands a certain amount of feeling one's way) (fig. 100);

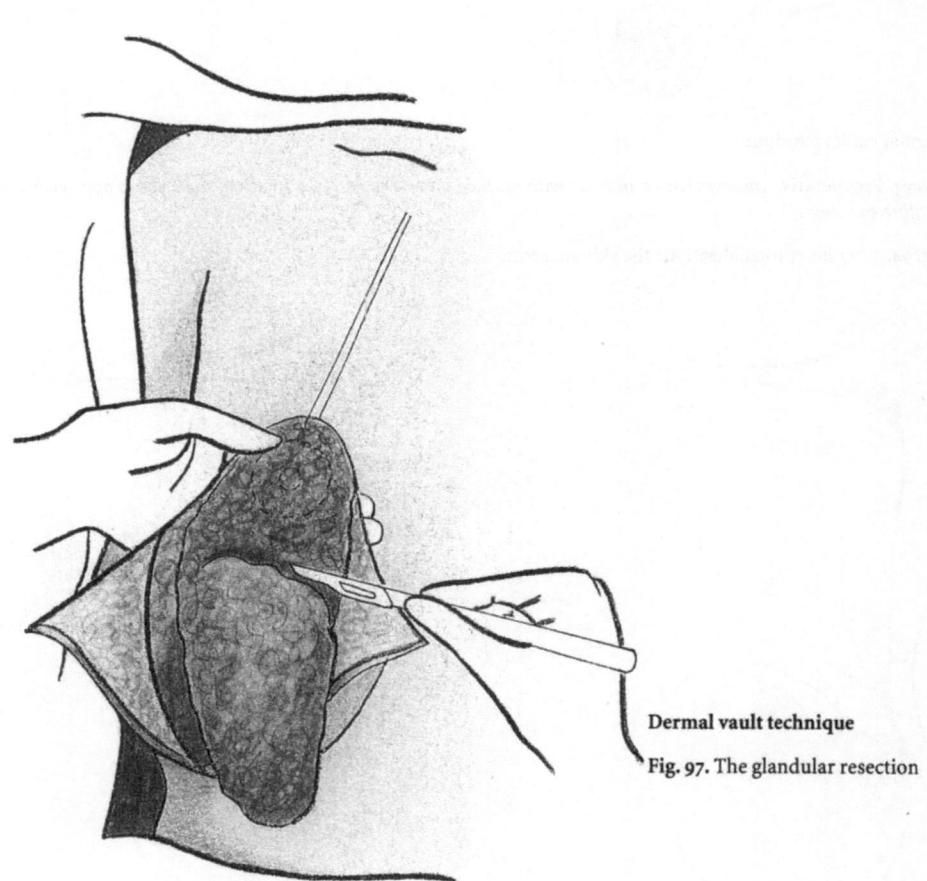

Dermal vault technique

Fig. 97. The glandular resection

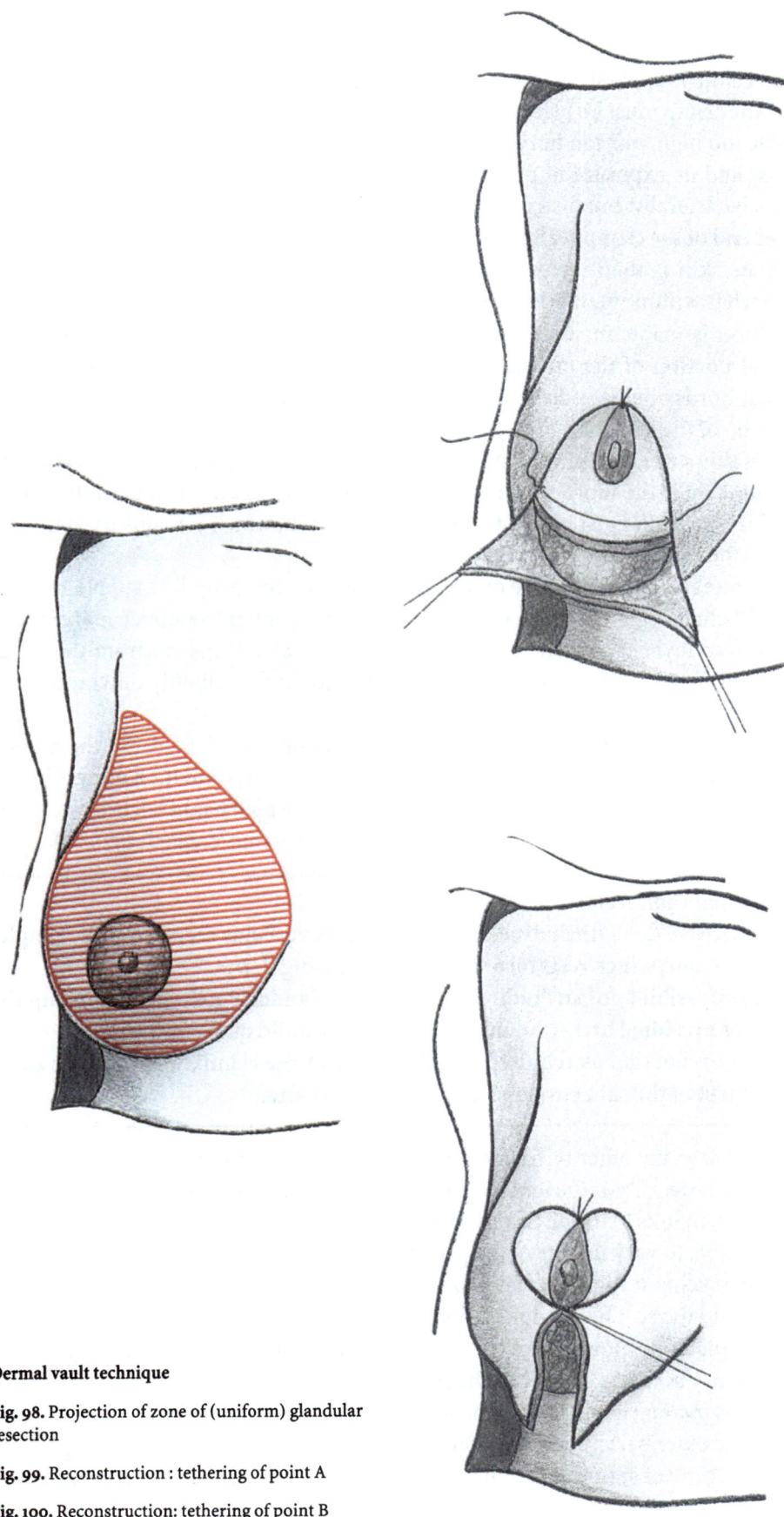

Dermal vault technique

Fig. 98. Projection of zone of (uniform) glandular resection

Fig. 99. Reconstruction : tethering of point A

Fig. 100. Reconstruction: tethering of point B

• the two inferior skin flaps are then approximated and pulled forward and fhe short clamp is applied (fig. 101);

• the clamp must be placed correctly, neither too vertically, to avoid leaving the nipple too high, nor too horizontally, to avoid excessive forward projection of the breast and its exposure to ptosis. It must also be checked that the tension is not excessive laterally, but distributed uniformly from above downward, and that the lower end of the clamp really reaches the thoracic plane;

• the skin is then incised along the track of the clamp, placing the incision somewhat within the marks, then it is sutured in two layers, and the horizontal resection is made, in such a way as to position the inferior scar strictly in the medial portion of the crease. The inferior scar is horizontal in its entirety, its medial border being reduced to the maximum by a "lift" effect outward on the lower lip of the incision;

• at this stage, the inframammary crease may be brought upward in relation to the chest wall (the more so when the breast has been reduced), but on the other hand the incision must be located in the crease itself, which remains fixed in relation to the cutaneous plane;

• it remains to position the nipple-areolar plaque correctly, by a supplementary de-epithelialisation (fig. 102) in a circle whose tangent at the upper margin is at point A and whose tangent at the lower margin is at 4 to 4.5 cm from the inframammary crease. The nipple-areolar plaque should face slightly downward and outward at the end of the operation;

• before final suture, the landmark stitch at point A is divided and the nipple-bearing dermo-glandular cylinder is exteriorised (fig. 103) and then reinvaginated without distortion, thus forming the "dermal vault" which has given ts name to the technique by reason of the dermo-dermal application thus created (fig. 104).

The dermal vault technique combines :

– extensive de-epithelialisation, guaranteeing vascular security of the nipple-areolar plaque, which rests on a wide nipple-bearing flap ;

– the possibility of an "unlimited" uniform glandular resection, allowing the choice of a residual breast volume adjusted to the build of the patient;

– skin reduction as required, thanks to use of the clamp, which allows exact adjustment of the skin envelope to residual breast size.

After so many other techniques, this was a new attempt to reduce the length of the scars, especially at the inner segment of the inframammary incision.

In fact, thanks to the distribution of the skin resections ensured by the clamp, it was possible to vary the site of the principal resection :

– by placing it high up; the maximum of skin was left in the inframammary region, and the scar here would be long;

– by placing it low down; the maximum was left in the areolar region: the inframammary scar was short, but the periareolar excision was extensive with a risk of serious incongruity between the length of the inner areolar circumference and that of the outer periareolar excision. This incongruity was responsible for puckering at the time of suture, which in time produced a more or less hypertrophic scar which widened inexorably.

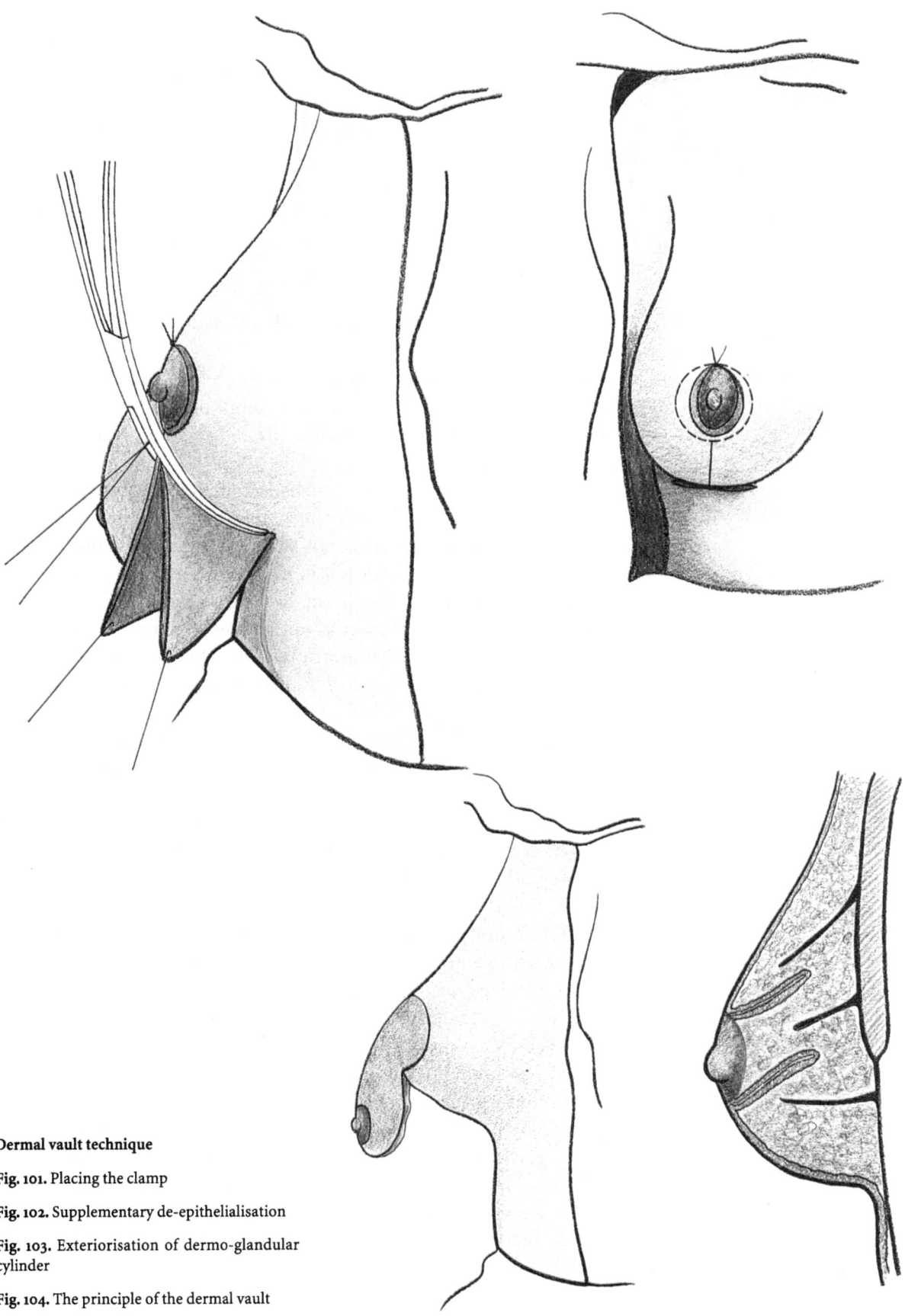

Dermal vault technique

Fig. 101. Placing the clamp

Fig. 102. Supplementary de-epithelialisation

Fig. 103. Exteriorisation of dermo-glandular cylinder

Fig. 104. The principle of the dermal vault

There was a choice :

• at the beginning it was a challenge; priority was accorded to shortness of the inframammary scar, and the result was marred by excessive enlargement of the periareolar scar, which temporarily discredited the technique;

• then the good quality of the periareolar scar was ensured by leaving a long inframammary scar;

• finally, a proper balance was reached. There was no longer a hypertrophic scar limited to the areola, indicative of localised incongruity. When hypertrophic scars do exist, they are on the three segments, which is evidence that the cause lies in the patient's skin.

However, the dermal vault technique is not without its difficulties, especially in performance :

• the absence of a preestablished design gives the technique its freedom but also causes some difficulties, especially if the inner limits of the circle of periareolar de-epithelialisation are not located very carefully and symmetrically, as also in the determination of point B;

• poor assessment of the circle of de-epithelialisation, if it is too large in relation to the size of the areola, leads to broadening of the areolar scar; if the relations between the outer circle and the areola are not identical on each side this leads to asymmetry of the areolae (this concerns not so much the size of the areola,which is relatively easy to assess, as the dimensions of the outer circle);

• freeing the gland presents no particular difficulties. It is easy to perform a glandular resection leaving a layer of uniform thickness beneath the entire skin envelope when the hypertrophy is marked and the skin envelope vast, for the breast opens up as the resection proceeds, monitored by the flattened left hand behind the gland. This resection is more difficult to perform when hypertrophy is moderate and without great skin stretching, since assessment of the residual glandular layer is more difficult, access being less extensive;

• placement of the clamp is also a tricky stage which calls for some experience, both in its orientation and in exerting uniform tension over the entire extent so as to reduce the breast base in symmetric fashion.

Overall, the dermal vault technique is an excellent one, but if it is to be fully mastered it calls for some amount of experience and a personal incorporation of the techniques of breast surgery.

In our view, it cannot be taught to a beginner at the outset, but with practice it is the first technique which has proved adaptable to all cases of hypertrophy, ptosis and associated asymmetry of different degrees, since the possibilities of glandular resection are not limited by a skin template or by the need to preserve a deep pedicle, and adjustment of the skin envelope to the residual glandular volume can be made as required. The most advanced use of this method, and one that finally demonstrates its absence of limitations, is in subcutaneous mastectomy, which requires, in addition to maximal glandular resection, an adequate readjustment of the skin envelope to the volume, in this case represented by an implant.

With some particular individual variants, it is currently the technique most widely employed, as shown by an enquiry made by the Société Française de Chirurgie Plastique, Réparatrice et Esthétique in 1989.

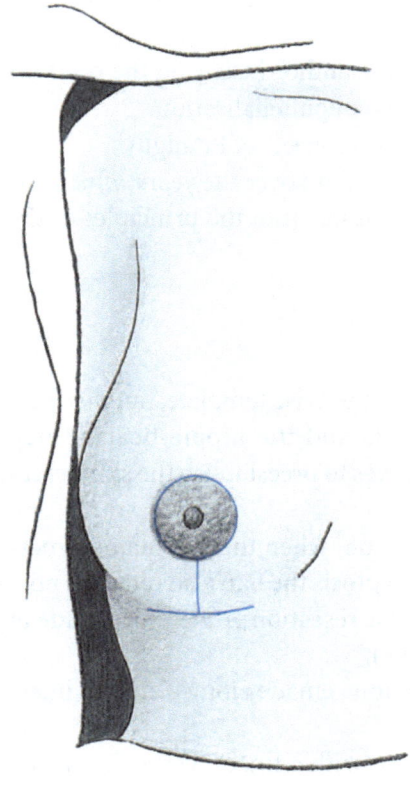

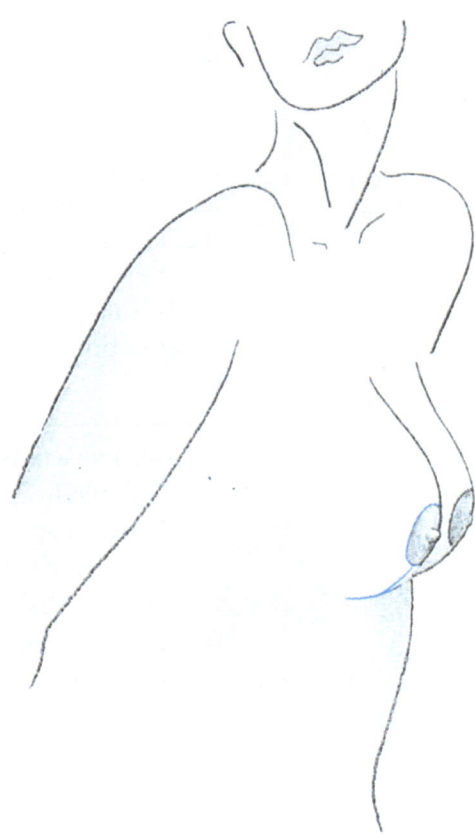

Dermal vault technique

Fig. 106. Final scars *(frontal view)*

Fig. 106. Final scars *(lateral view)*

Weiner's technique (1972)

This was proposed by its author to overcome the difficulties that may be presented by the placement of a nipple-bearing dermal flap, as in Skoog's technique or Strombeck's dermo-glandular flap. It is based on the use of a purely dermal nipple-bearing flap with a superior pedicle, which facilitates its plication and placement without distortion of the areolar site.

The design marks the axis of the breast starting from the middle of the clavicle and uses a Wise template.

The nipple-bearing flap is a dermal flap and the author insists on the need for careful and very superficial procedure during the de-epithelialisation.

The glandular resection is comparable to the "boat-keel" of Pitanguy.

It is useful to follow the evolution of Weiner's method over the years, which has led to modification of its technique which approximate it to the principles of the dermal vault.

The modified Weiner technique (1982 and 1990)

The breast axis is always available for placement of the Wise template, but this is no longer used except for designing the periareola and the nipple-bearing flap (fig. 107). The lower part of the pattern, which serves to preestablish the skin resection, is no longer traced.

The nipple-bearing flap remains dermal (fig. 108) when there is major hypertrophy, but in cases of moderate hypertrophy and ptosis the flap also retains a posterior glandular pedicle: in this case the glandular resection is therefore made at the sides, around the nipple-bearing flap (fig. 109).

The areola is constructed and the skin reduction is made along a curved intestinal clamp.

Resection of the lateral "dog-ears" is done last, with a final inverted T-shaped scar.

Thus Weiner's technique combines :

– a nipple-bearing dermal or dermoglandular flap,

– hence a superior pedicle (1972) or dermo-glandular pedicle (1982-1990),

– absence of cutaneo-glandular cleavage,

– preestablished skin resection (1972), later a resection adapted to actual requirements, using the clamp (1982-1990).

This technique may therefore be considered as derived from that of the dermal vault.

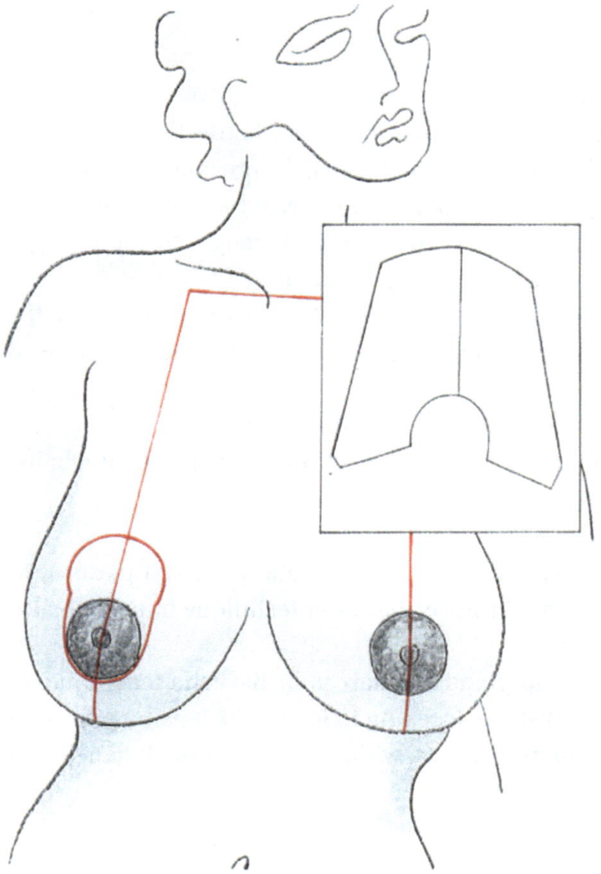

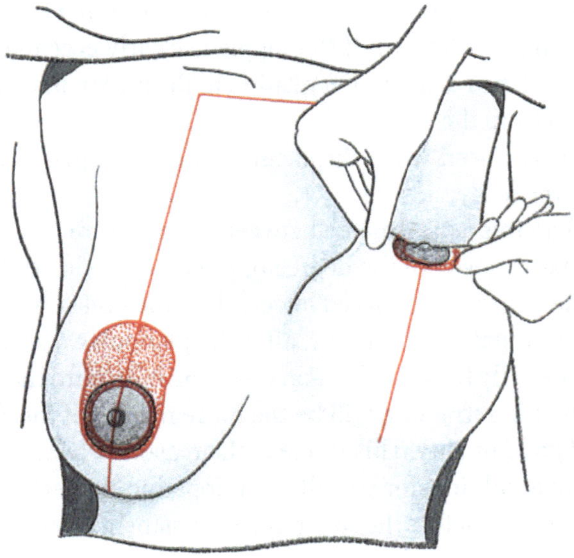

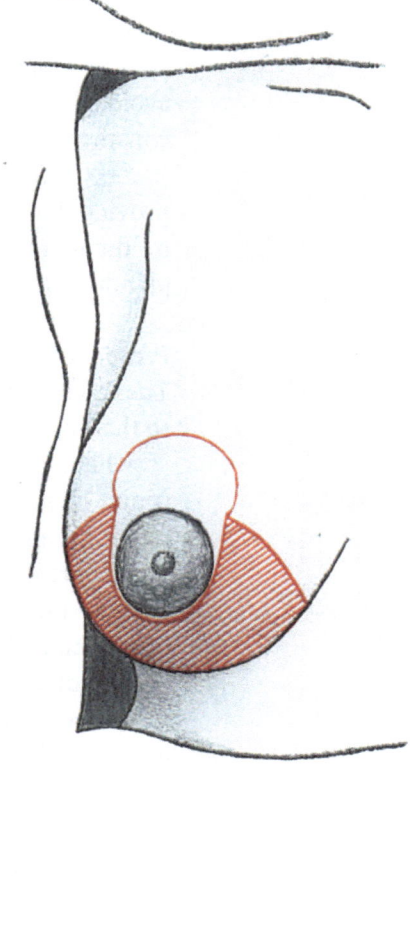

Weiner's technique

Fig, 107. Preoperative design (using the Wise template only for the periareola)

Fig. 108. The de-epithelialised nipple-bearing flap

Fig. 109. In the modified Weiner technique the glandular resection involves the lower half of the breast while preserving a posterior glandular pedicle for the nipple-bearing flap

The Saint-Louis technique

This technique, so named because developed in the department of plastic surgery of the Hôpital Saint-Louis, the former department of Claude Dufourmentel, sought to escape the pitfalls of an entirely preestablished design, and also the difficulties of a too liberal technique, since we needed to have a basic method with a minimum of easily determined landmarks, and one easily taught to the younger staff members under instruction in a hospital department.

It is just as useful in cases of moderate or major hypertrophy, whatever the degree of associated ptosis, and is ultimately of mixed parentage since it is derived from :
– the principle of a superior pedicle, as in the lateral method,
– and that of the dermal vault in its mode of resection, extensive depithelialisation and the final inverted T scar,
– while adding :
• a partly preestablished design which is not actually a fixed pattern, to avoid what may well be the freedom of the dermal vault technique but which also constitutes its entire difficulty,
• and a medially based dermo-glandular flap as in Baruch's technique, to provide the volume and stability of shape (seeking to lessen the tension exercised on the margins of the vertical subareolar scar, while facilitating the balancing of glandular resection).

Preoperative design
The tracings are made on the standing patient before she has been premedicated, so that she can hold herself quite upright.
• First, an axis is drawn from the suprasternal notch to the inframmary crease (point B) passing through the nipple (fig.110). If the nipple is clearly eccentric in relation to gland size, this axis will be recentered in relation to the breast, but without departing more than 1.5 cm from the nipple;
• the lower part of the axis is traced while displacing the breast upward and inward along its axis, and not vertically;
• a point A is then marked on this axis, situated between 17 and 19 cm from the suprasternal notch, a point that varies with the degree of ptosis and skin stretching, also with the height of the patient. It is placed lower when the breast is more bulky, the skin elastic and the woman tall. Actually, after the glandular resection this point "reascends" spontaneously because the skin envelope is disburdened of the mass stretching it and this skin retraction will be the more marked if the skin has preserved elastic fibers of good quality. This is one of the reasons why we consider it preferable to operate in good time for so-called :"idiopathic" hypertrophy — sometimes even at the age of 15 — before the skin pays a permanent price for its glandular burden;
• a point A' is located between 5 and 6 cm from point A (fig.111). A perpendicular to the breast axis is drawn through A' and on it are located two points, C laterally and D medially, situated between 4 cm (if A' is 5 cm from A) and 5 cm (if A' is 6 cm from A) from point A';

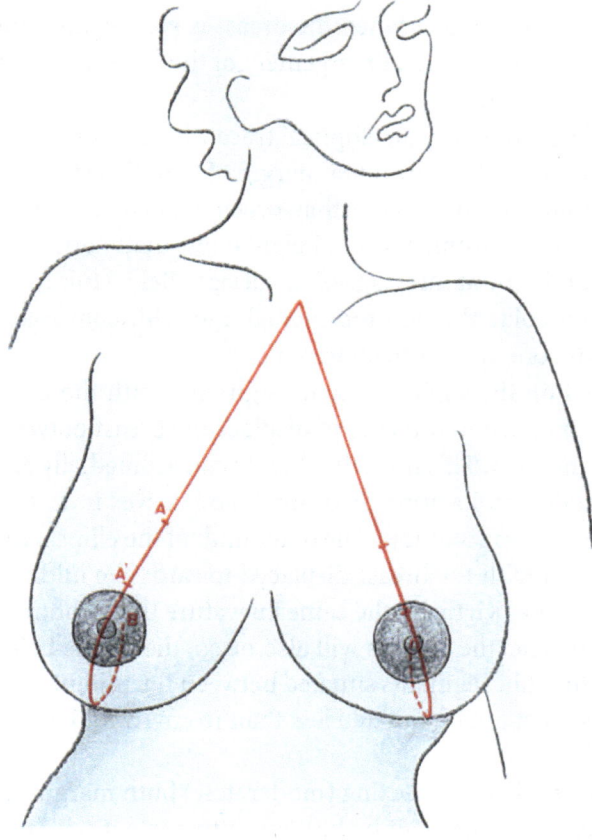

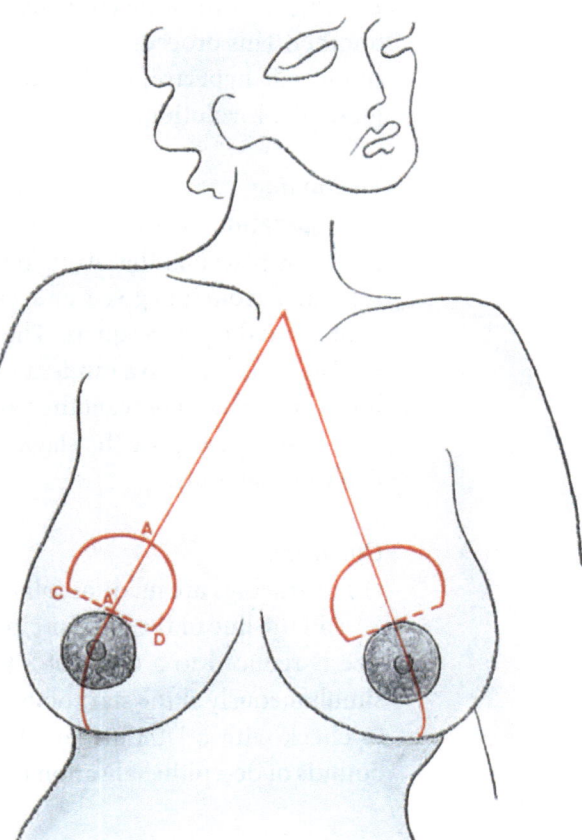

Saint-Louis technique

Fig. 110. Preoperative design : axes, points A and B

Fig. 111. Design of the periareola

• this line CD is the anatomic base of the future nipple-bearing flap, and varies between 8 and 10 cm. It will be made longer when the breast is ptosed since the nipple-bearing flap will be so much the longer. Enlargement of the base of the flap increases the vascular security at the areola;

• the points A, C and D are then joined by an elliptical trace which is simply the areolar circle open laterally. The tangents to the inner margin of the ellipse must be at the same distance from the mid-line and not less than 9.5 cm from it, and this is checked on the supine patient. Only in women whose height is less than 1.60 m can one approach to 9 cm from the midline at this stage of the design. Below this limit, there is a risk of ending with areolae that are too medial and with convergent breasts, an unpleasant defect and one very difficult to remedy;

• the tracings are completed on the supine patient, beginning with the inner limb of the ellipse. It is determined without trying to displace the breast outward as its weight will do this spontaneously. This line DB is barely convex medially and is practically parallel to the midline in its upper two-thirds and curves inward in its lower third to reach point B (figs. 112 and 113). The outer limb of the ellipse, CB, is drawn in a rounded movement with the breast displaced towards the midline, but without excessive traction. It has virtually the same curvature throughout its extent. If the breasts are asymmetric, the ellipses will also be so, the ellipse being wider on the bulkier side, but the skin segments situated between the midline and the inner border of the ellipses must not be situated less than 10 cm from the sternum;

• by displacing the gland upward and squeezing (moderately) both margins of the ellipse, it must be confirmed that they can be brought into contact with one another. This procedure is rather more difficult to perform on the firm taut breast of juvenile hypertrophy than on a breast that already exhibits skin stretching and glandular involution.

Positioning

The operation is conducted under general anesthesia with intubation and the patient is placed in the sitting position, with the arms beside the body but slightly separated from it to give free acess to the midaxillary line. The shoulders are horizontal and the pelvis square. The head is fixed to prevent cervical hyperextension.

The table is put in a moderate downward tilt, and then broken to raise the lower limbs slightly and prevent the patient sliding toward the foot of the table.

The drapes expose the clavicles (upper drape quite horizontal) and the midaxillary line laterally.

Operation

1) The tracings are made as follows :

• in the line of the areolar circle, with moderate spreading of the areola, whose size is reduced to a circle of 4 to 4.5 cm diameter, both areolae being designed simultaneously at the start of the procedure so as to be symmetrical. It is advisable to check with a Dufourmentel ring that the periareolar circle representing the bounds of de-epithelialisation is of proper shape;

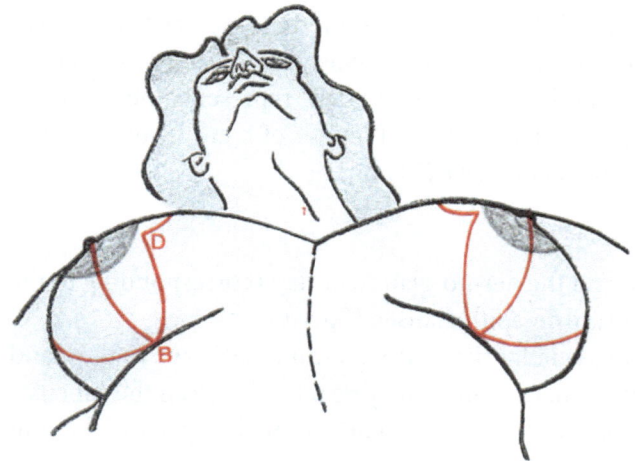

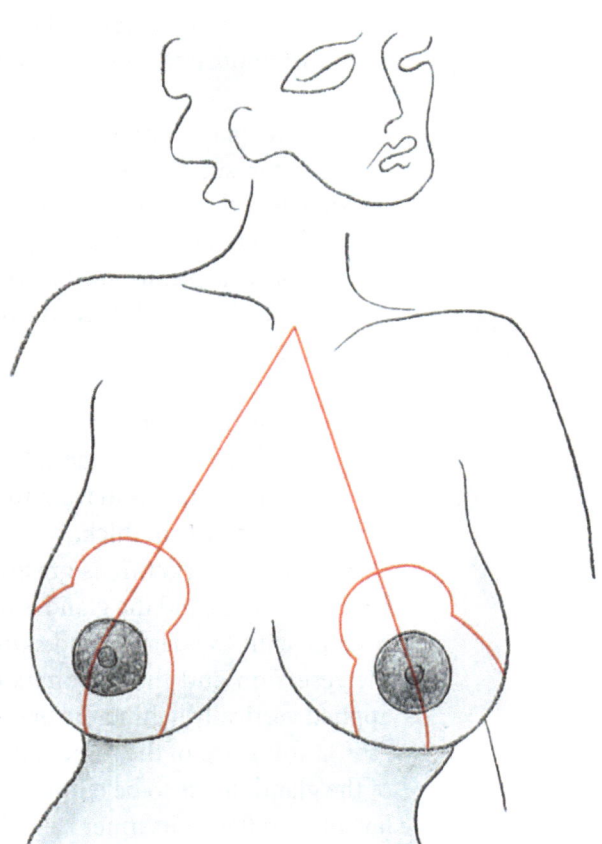

Saint-Louis technique

Fig. 112. Design of the ellipse is made on the reclining patient

Fig. 113. Appearance of the ellipse in the standing position

• design of the dermo-glandular flap, whose medial base DD' measures between 6 and 7 cm (this length decreases spontaneously to 5 cm after the glandular resection when the skin is under least tension); DD' represents the anatomic base of the future dermo-glandular flap. A final length of 5 cm is necessary to ensure proper nutrition and satisfactory size (fig. 114).

2) Dissection

• The nipple-bearing flap and the dermo-glandular flap (corresponding to the stippled area in the diagrams) are de-epithelialised (fig. 115);

• the skin and subcutaneous cellular tissue are freely incised down to the gland from D' to B and from C to B, so that stripping may be made between the subcutaneous fat immediately beneath and the gland, and not immediately under the skin (fig. 116);

• the dissection continues at B, diving into the depths to reach the parietal aponeurotic plane, and is then continued by simultaneous stripping of:

– the gland from the deep prethoracic plane and then the prepectoral plane, preserving the prepeectoral fascia. Tissue adhesion is relatively marked as far as the lower border of the pectoralis major, but stripping becomes easier and almost avascular once this border is left well behind, when it can be done with the finger. The most important zone for hemostasis is just below the lower border of the muscle;

– the gland and its entire axillary extension from the skin, taking care to preserve the subcutaneous fatty tissue in contact with the skin. This freeing in depth is less thorough medially so as to preserve the blood-supply of the future dermo-glandular flap. The prepectoral perforating intercostal branches from the medial thoracic plexus must be respected;

– the gland is also freed from the subcutaneous plane and the deep parietal plane from B to D'.

3) Glandular resection

• A bold incision is made at the lower border of the nipple-bearing flap, from D to C, passing about 1.5 cm from the lower border of the reduced areola and creating a gland slice 1 to 2 cm thick;

• the entire structure is grasped with two Kocher's forceps and held vertically by the assistant, and the gland is incised leaving a layer of constant thickness, continuous with the dermis and skin, while constantly monitoring the regularity of the resection and the thickness of the remaining gland with the flat left hand applied vertically behind the breast;

• at this stage of the resection, if the nipple-bearing flap is of definitive size, all of the gland that is to be eliminated is still integral with the future dermo-glandular rotation flap at its inner base DD';

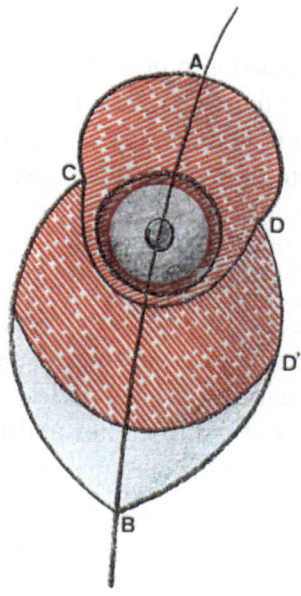

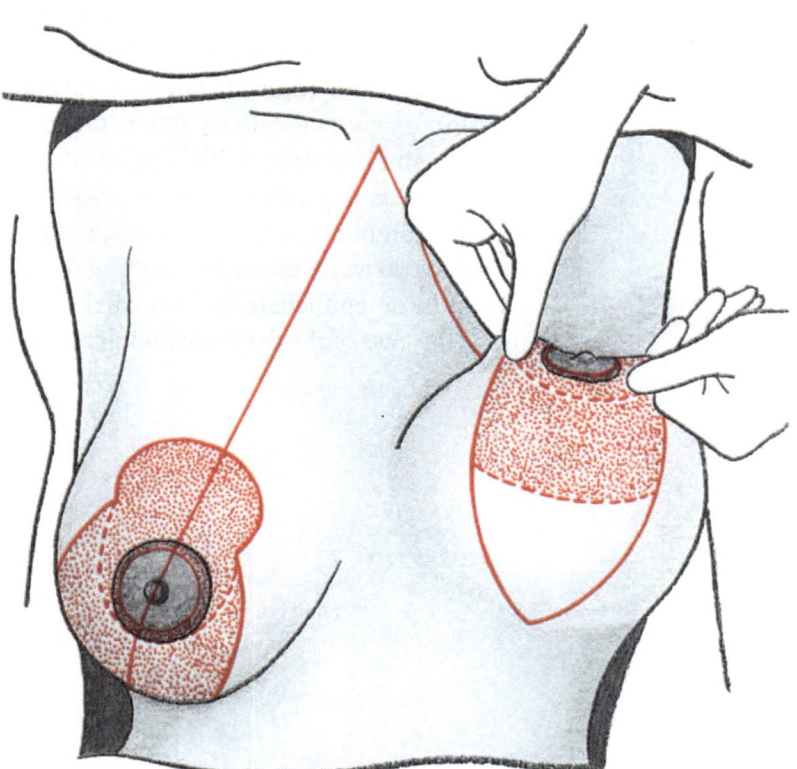

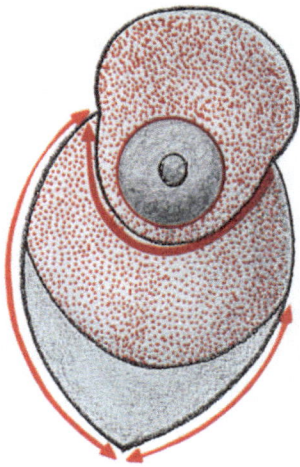

Saint-Louis technique

Fig. 114. The ellipse and the dermoglandular flap

Fig. 115. De-epithelialisation

Fig. 116. Skin incisions

• freeing is completed by separating the lower border of the de-epithelialised skin flap from D to C, and by performing the gland resection proper under the flap, from its distal end to its origin, leaving beneath the flap a glandular cushion which is rather thicker under its inner two-thirds than under the nipple-bearing flap (fig. 117). When the flap is rolledup it will serve to render the inferolateral quadrant convex.

4) Construction

• The periareolar circle is closed and then the areola is tacked down by 8 regularly placed dermal inversion sutures, giving U-shaped support to the peripheral side so as to compensate for the slight difference in size between the two circles;

• the vitality of the dermo-glandular flap is checked and its outer end is resected as required; then it is tethered at its extremities and the outer part of its lower border to the anterior aspect of the pectoralis major muscle. The most medial of these fixation sutures are placed virtually behind the areola, on the muscle, while the lowest suture is situated at the level of the anterior axillary line on the serratus anterior (fig.117). The vertical subareolar line is tacked down so as to measure 4.5 cm in length (without traction), and its lower extremity is then tethered to point B to resect both "dog-ears";

• if, at this stage, there appears asymmetry of shape associated with inequality of reduction of the breast base because of defective skin reduction, it can be corrected in two ways : either by resecting the skin on the outer slope of the subareolar scar, or by de-epithelialising its medial slope (but remaining very superficial, since this is the base of the dermo-glandular flap).

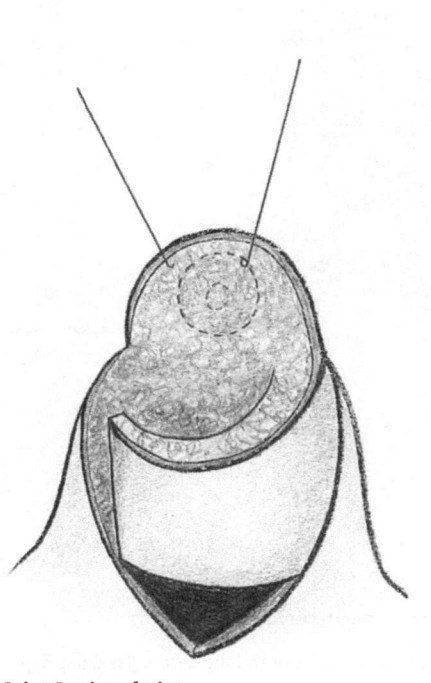
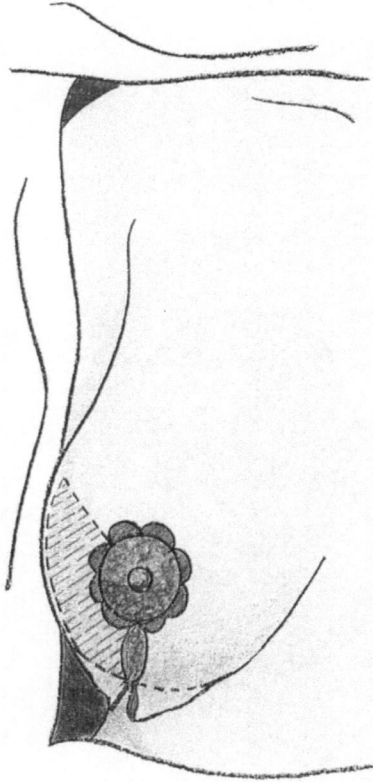

Saint-Louis technique

Fig. 117. After the glandular resection

Fig. 118. Position of the dermoglandular flap

It must be ensured that both vertical subareolar scars are symmetric in relation to the midline, for if they are not in the same direction the breasts will appear asymmetric even if they are alike in size and shape.

5) The final inframammary resection
• The ellipse of resection of the inner dog-ear places the slightly rounded scar in the crease;
• the outer dog-ear, on the contrary is resected so that the final scar is horizontal, without exerting traction on its upper border during this resection, which would have the disadvantage of ascending the scar too much secondarily and with the risk of a hypertrophic scar.

6) Sutures
After inserting a suction drain, the stitches are completed in two layers : inverting dermal sutures of fine slowly-absorbed material (4/0 at the areola, 3/0 in the inverted T scars), a superficial continuous intradermal suure of monofilament nylon (to be retained for bewen 3 and 4 weeks) at the areola, and continuous intradermal sutures of rapidly absorbed material at the limbs of the T. It is inadvisable to use rapidly-absorbed suture material at the areola, as the rapid disappearance of this suture, which is under centrifugal tension, risks broadening of the scar.

7) Dressing
This is done with tulle gras and pads and shaped with elastic hypo-allergenic adhesive strapping. It is left in place for 3 to 4 days and removed at the same time as the drains on the day the patient is discharged. The sutures are then protected by adhesive strips and showering is allowed daily with an antiseptic soap, the only constraint being the wearing of a moderately compressive elastic brassière, without undersewing of the cups, (a 'sports' type of brassière fastening in front, which is more comfortable), day and night for two months.

The Saint-Louis technique is based on :
– a preoperative design where the peripheral limit of the areola is slightly larger than the circle of the reduced areola to obtain good skin reduction and a breast of rounded shape. But this device must not be exaggerated beyond the elastic potential of the skin for fear of producing a defect (areolar puckering and broadening of the scar);
– a quasi-total freeing of the deep aspect of the gland from the deep plane by disinsertion of the axillary tail, but respecting the medial thoracic blood-supply to ensure the vitality of the rotation flap;
– uniform glandular resection preserving the same thickness beneath the skin and the denuded surfaces of the nipple-bearing and coiled flaps;
– coiling of the flap at its inner base in the snail-shell manner of Gillies, which gives the breast its curvature;
– a final inverted-T resection, which allows completion of the skin reduction and perfect adjustment of the skin envelope to the residual breast size as required.

This technique, for which no originality is claimed, may be considered as a synthesis of the evolution of certain ideas :

– the absence of cutaneo-glandular cleavage is the guarantee of vascular security;

– combined with an extensive de-epithelialisation (at both the nipple-bearing flap and the coiled flap) which is also the main factor in morphologic stability;

– while its role in supporting the rotation flap (although it is dermo-glandular) may be debatable in the long term, it is at all events a useful factor in constructing the size and the reduction of skin and dermis:

– this reduction is made in two stages ;

• areolar siting and breadth of ellipse, by preliminary design;

• final T resection as required makes it possible to avoid the pitfalls of an entirely preformed pattern, but also overcomes the problems that may be posed by an unconstrained technique like that of the dermal vault, the freedom of which confers great plasticity but has its own difficulties;

– the design is more a serie of landmarks serving as guidelines than an actual pattern.

Validity and limitations

• The reliability of the technique rests on the extensive de-epithelialisation and the absence of cutaneo-glandular cleavage, which prevents any risk of skin necrosis. It has been possible to use the technique on very long nipple-bearing flaps (up to a distance of 35 cm between the suprasternal notch and the nipple).

• The sole complication we have observed has been, in some cases, an induration of the extremity of the dermo-glandular coiled flap, palpable at the level of the areola and a little lateral to it.

• This eventuality may occur when the deep aspect of the gland under its medial border has been excessively freed and the extremity of the flap has been insufficiently resected before fixing it. Its length must not exceed twice its breadth. The radiologic image is that of an opacity of benign appearance suggestive of a process of cytosteatonecrosis, which is confirmed histologically.

• This method can be easily used in moderate and major hypertrophies (fig. 119), whatever the degree of ptosis, but it finds its limitations in minor ptoses without hypertrophy, where the width of the ellipse does not permit the construction of a worthwhile rotated flap.

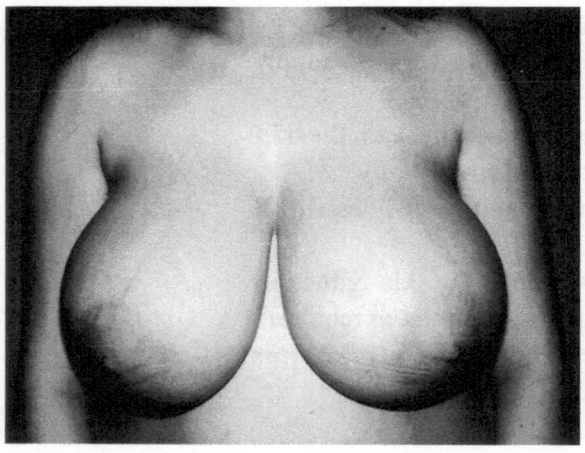
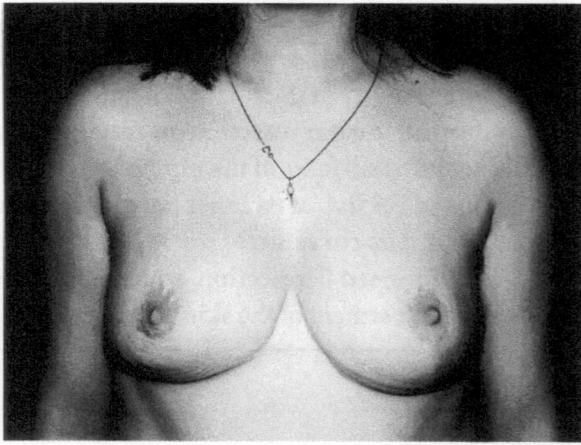

a

b

Fig. 119 a,b. 20-year-old : resection of 1050 g right, 1300 g left

• While the technique is equally well applicable to major hypertrophies, whatever the degree of ptosis, the scar defect is not negligible, particularly as regards the length of the horizontal scar (fig. 120), which is undoubtedly a little greater than is given by the dermal vault technique for an equivalent resection and quality of skin. This is probably due to the fact that the skin reduction opposite the subareolar vertical is largely determined by the design of the ellipse, and does not therefore allow for retraction of the skin envelope during the procedure — in cases of good skin quality with preservation of satisfactory elasticity — once the skin is relieved of the

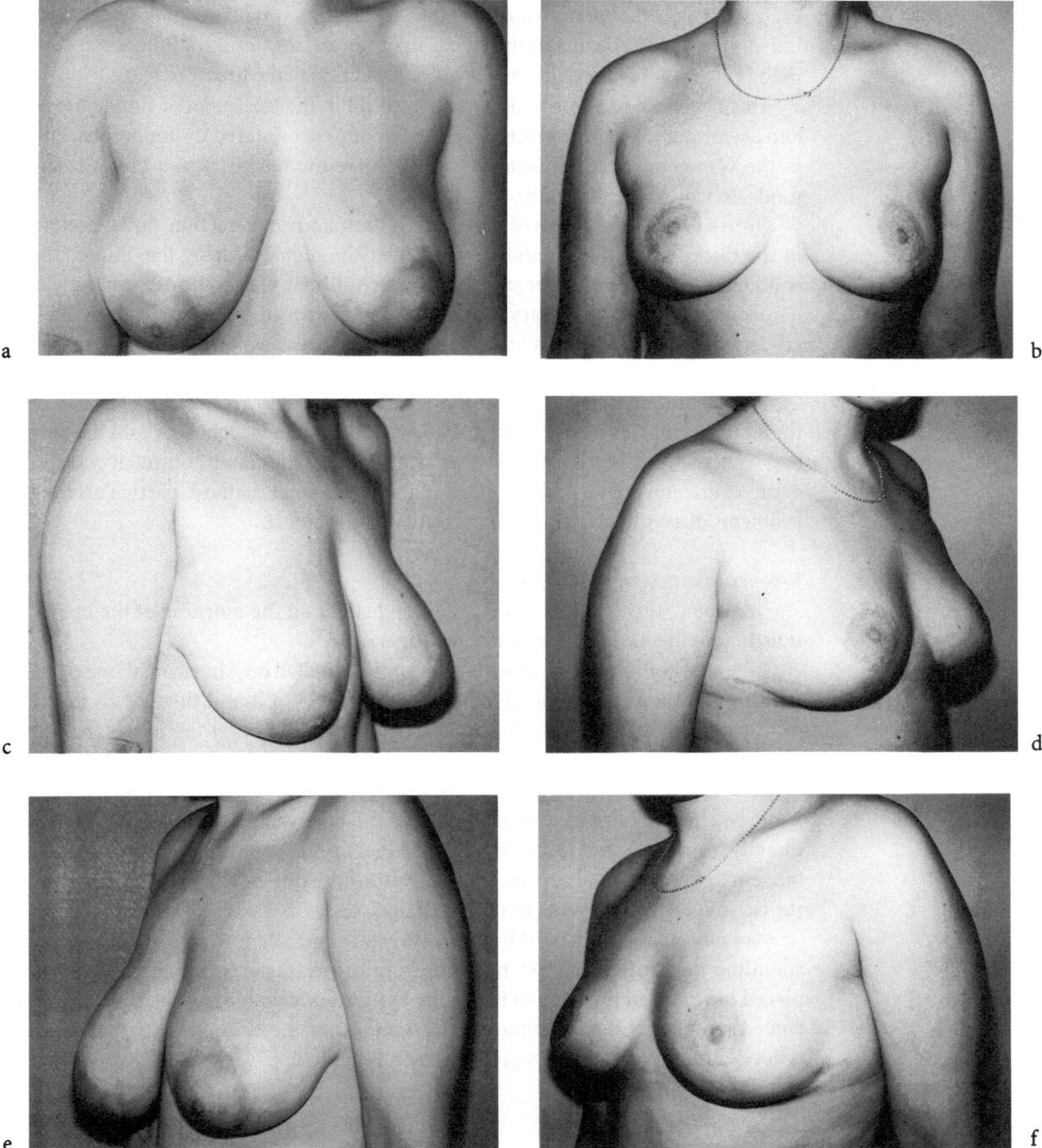

a
b
c
d
e
f

Fig. 120 a-f. 21-year-old : skin of moderate quality: resection of 460 g left, 520 g right

excessive weight of the gland. Only the techniques using a clamp can have this advantage, but once again we stress the fact that we have deliberately favored the easy achievement of a satisfactory shape at the expense of somewhat more extensive scarring, in order to have an easily taught technique at our disposal.

Personal experience

After having used the "Saint-Louis technique" for some years, which has allowed us to understand, teach and master the fundamental problems raised by mammoplasties (vascular security, extent of glandular resection, adjustment of the residual breast volume to the skin envelope), we have sought to make ourselves independent of the design of the ellipse in order to gain some additional freedom in the adaptation of the skin envelope and reduction of the breast base.

This degree of freedom is particularly useful in the treatment of simple ptosis and asymmetry, where the Saint-Louis technique encountered its limitations, and in the symmetrisation of reconstructions where the reconstructed breast is the model to which it is imperative to conform.

Once a proper evaluation of the extent ot the glandular resection, and therefore of the thickness of the glandular layer under the nipple-bearing flap and of the residual skin envelope, has been acquired and routinely mastered with experience, it no longer becomes necessary to use the coiled or "rolled-up" flap, since the main advantage of this was the readjustment of residual breast volume in cases of asymmetric resection beneath the nipple-bearing flap and the superior pedicle.

This technique, which also employs a clamp for assessment of the reduction of the skin envelope, is intermediate between the Saint-Louis technique and the dermal vault method, but it will be seen that, apart from the clamp control, it endeavors to overcome the possible pitfalls of the dermal vault method, particularly the problems of asymmetry of size and position of the areola.

Preoperative design

• As usual, this is made on the standing patient on the morning of the operation, before she has been premedicated (fig. 121);

• the axis of the breast is drawn from a point situated on a horizontal line passing through the suprasternal notch and 5 cm lateral to it and then down to the inframammary crease at B. This axis usually passes through the nipple, except when this is markedly eccentric in relation to the glandular mass;

• the sole precaution to be observed at this stage is to trace this line really horizontally, checking the level of the shoulders. The advantage over an axis drawn directly from the suprasternal notch is that the former is more vertical: the medial tangent to the future periareolar trace is a little more distant from the midline, and the risk of placing the areola too far medially is less;

• a point A is located on this axis, between 15 and 16 cm from its apex (corresponding to a distance of 16.5 to 18 cm from the suprasternal notch). Point A is placed lower when the woman is tall, the hypertrophy major and the skin elastic, since there is a risk of spontaneous reascent after the skin envelope has been relieved of the weight of the resected gland;

• a point A' is marked on the axis, between 5 and 6 cm at most from point A. The perpendicular to the axis is lowered to A' and two points C and D are marked symmetrically between 4 and 5 cm from point A' (the distance CD is 8 cm if A' is 5 cm from A, 9 cm if A' is at 5.5 cm, and 10 cm if A' is at 6 cm);

• the three points A,C and D are joined by a curve which is actually the same as the open circle of the future periareola. Moreover, the harmony of this line can be checked at the start of the operation with a Dufourmentel ring;

• when these lines have been completed, the patient is laid supine to check two points : that the tangent to the inner border of the periareolar trace is situated not

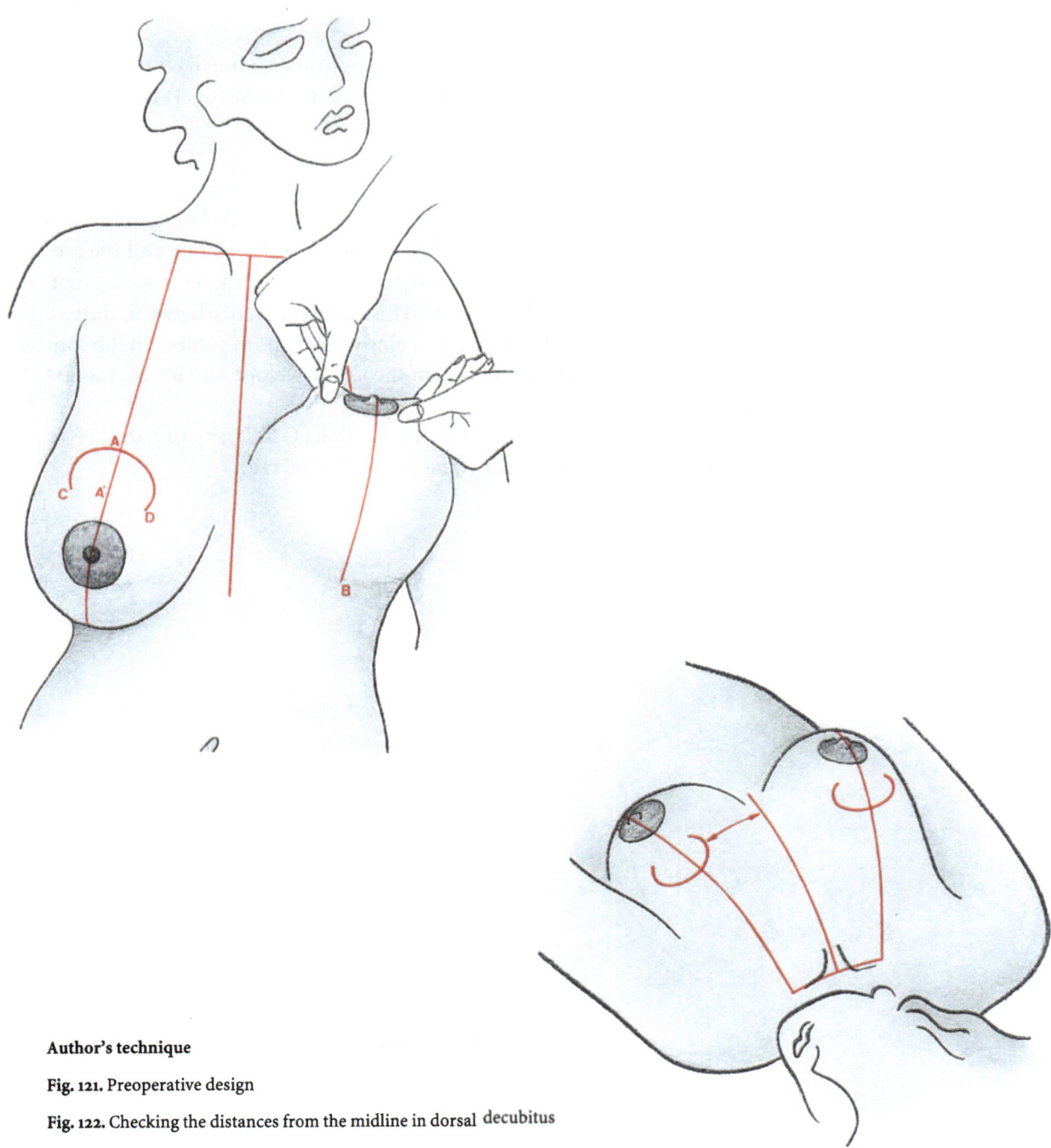

Author's technique

Fig. 121. Preoperative design

Fig. 122. Checking the distances from the midline in dorsal decubitus

less than 8-9 cm from the midline (depending on the skin elasticity and the degree of hypertrophy which variably stretches this segment in dorsal decubitus), and that points B are symmetrical, between 10 and 12 cm from the midline (fig. 122).

Positioning

The operation is performed under general anesthesia with intubation and controlled hypotension (which excludes any need for autotransfusion, whatever the degree of hypertrophy).

The table is tilted slightly so that the patient does not slide towards its foot, and the break is situated at the gluteal fold. The shoulders and pelvis are squared, the arms placed alongside the trunk and the head is immobilised to prevent any hyperextension of the cervical spine.

The operative field exposes the clavicles and suprasternal notch above and the midaxillary line laterally and just excludes the umbilicus below (fig. 123).

Procedure

1) The design is completed :

• The regularity of the periareolar trace is checked with the aid of a Dufourmentel ring (fig. 124). The assistant lightly spreads the nipple-areolar plaque and the areola itself is decreased by using a ring of very slightly lesser diameter (0.5 cm) than that used to check the external line (fig. 125). This small difference between the two circles is tolerable and will not result in puckering at the time of suture; on the contrary, it is useful for periareolar reduction of the skin envelope and for harmonising the shape of the breast;

• the nipple-bearing flap is drawn. The tracing links C to D, skirting the areola and passing 3 cm below the line of the reduced areola (fig. 126);

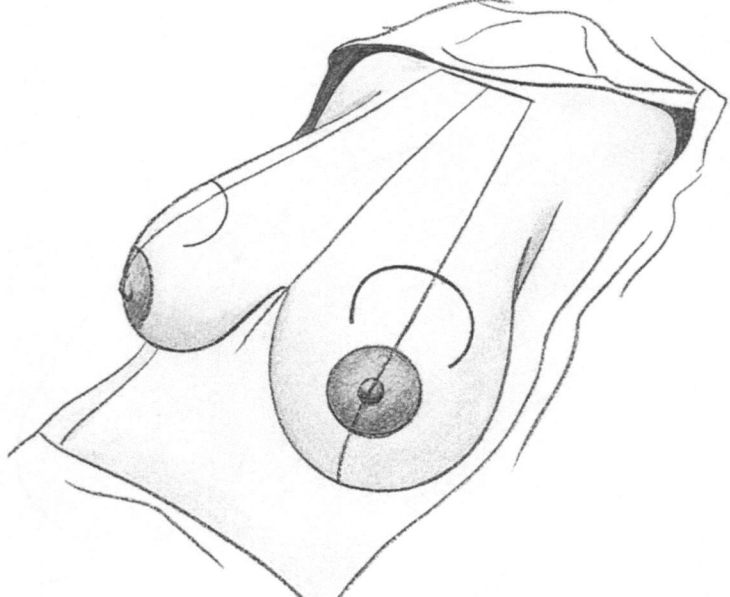

Author's technique

Fig. 123. Positioning the patient

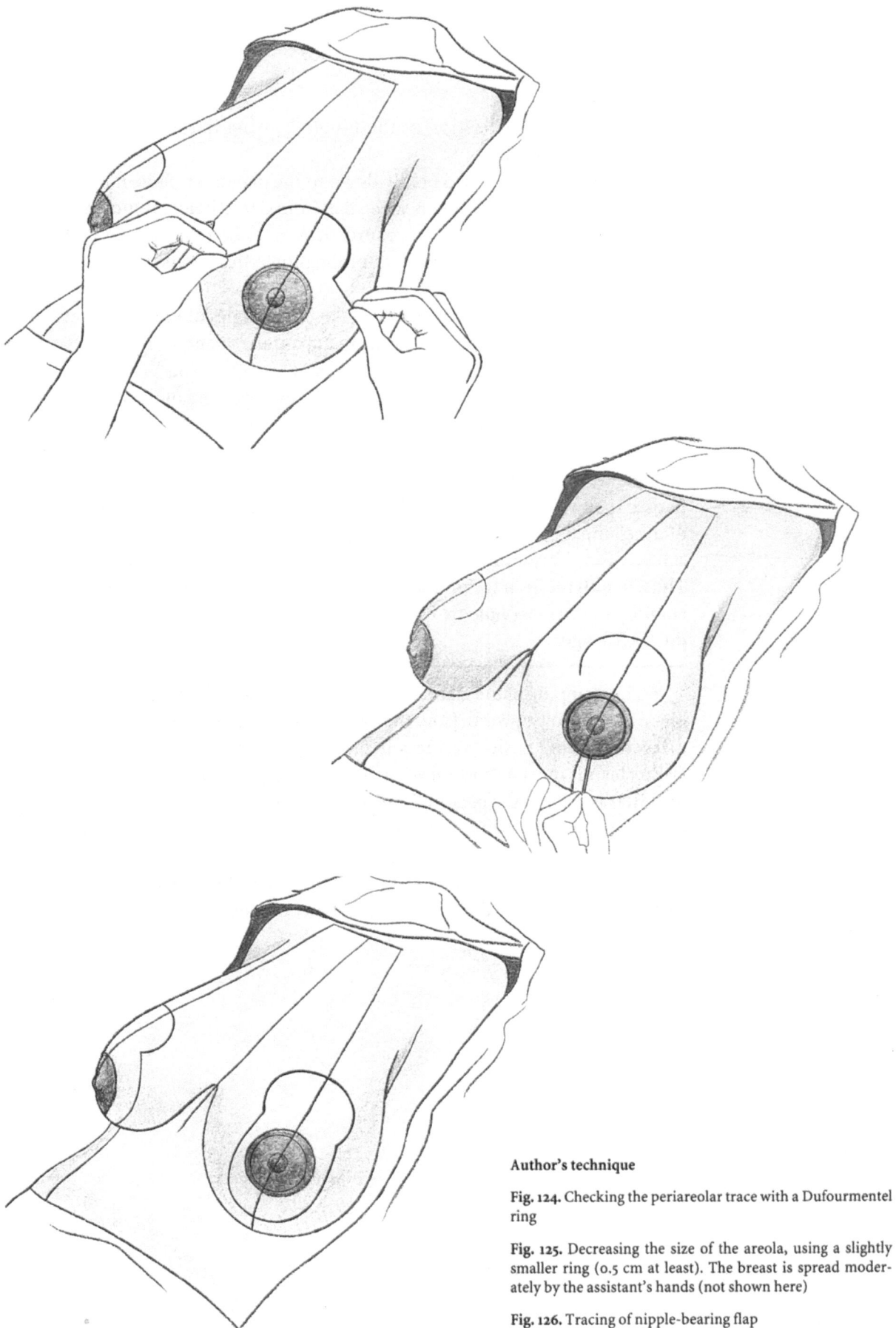

Author's technique

Fig. 124. Checking the periareolar trace with a Dufourmentel ring

Fig. 125. Decreasing the size of the areola, using a slightly smaller ring (0.5 cm at least). The breast is spread moderately by the assistant's hands (not shown here)

Fig. 126. Tracing of nipple-bearing flap

• the tracings of the two sides are made simultaneously at the start of the procedure in order to ensure their symmetry.

2) Dissection :

• The de-epithelialisation of the nipple-bearing flap is performed using a mammostat (fig. 127);

• the skin is then incised boldly down to the glandular plane for the length of the lower border of the nipple-bearing flap from C to D before removing the mammostat, which facilitates the procedure; then, after its removal, along the axis of the breast from the lower extremity of the nipple-bearing flap to the inframammary crease (fig. 128);

• two Kocher's forceps are placed at the inner angles of these incisions and the skin is freed vertically, passing from the glandular plane to the inframammary crease. This stripping extends laterally above to points C and D, but below it is not carried further than 5 cm from either side of the lower end of the vertical incision, ie from point B (fig. 129);

• at this stage there effectively exists a cutaneo-glandular cleavage intended to facilitate the subsequent dissection and the glandular resection; but these skin flaps actually correspond to the skin that will be resected at the time of application of the clamp.

Thus, like all modern techniques ensuring vascular security and the best possible stability of the morphologic result, this technique is devoid of any cutaneo-glandular cleavage.

• The stripping of the gland from the deep prethoracic and prepectoral plane is made from below upward, from the lower border of the gland to its upper pole, the dissection being easier and less hemorrhagic if the perimysium is respected. Hemostasis is most important at the zone of stripping situated betwen the fold and the lower border of the pectoralis major, as several vessels emerge from the depths at the lower border of this muscle. This dissection may be pursued without risk under the·medial and lateral quadrants of the gland as far as their peripheral limit, since, as with the dermal vault technique, this is a technique with a superior pedicle vascularised by the dermal and subcutaneous plexus.

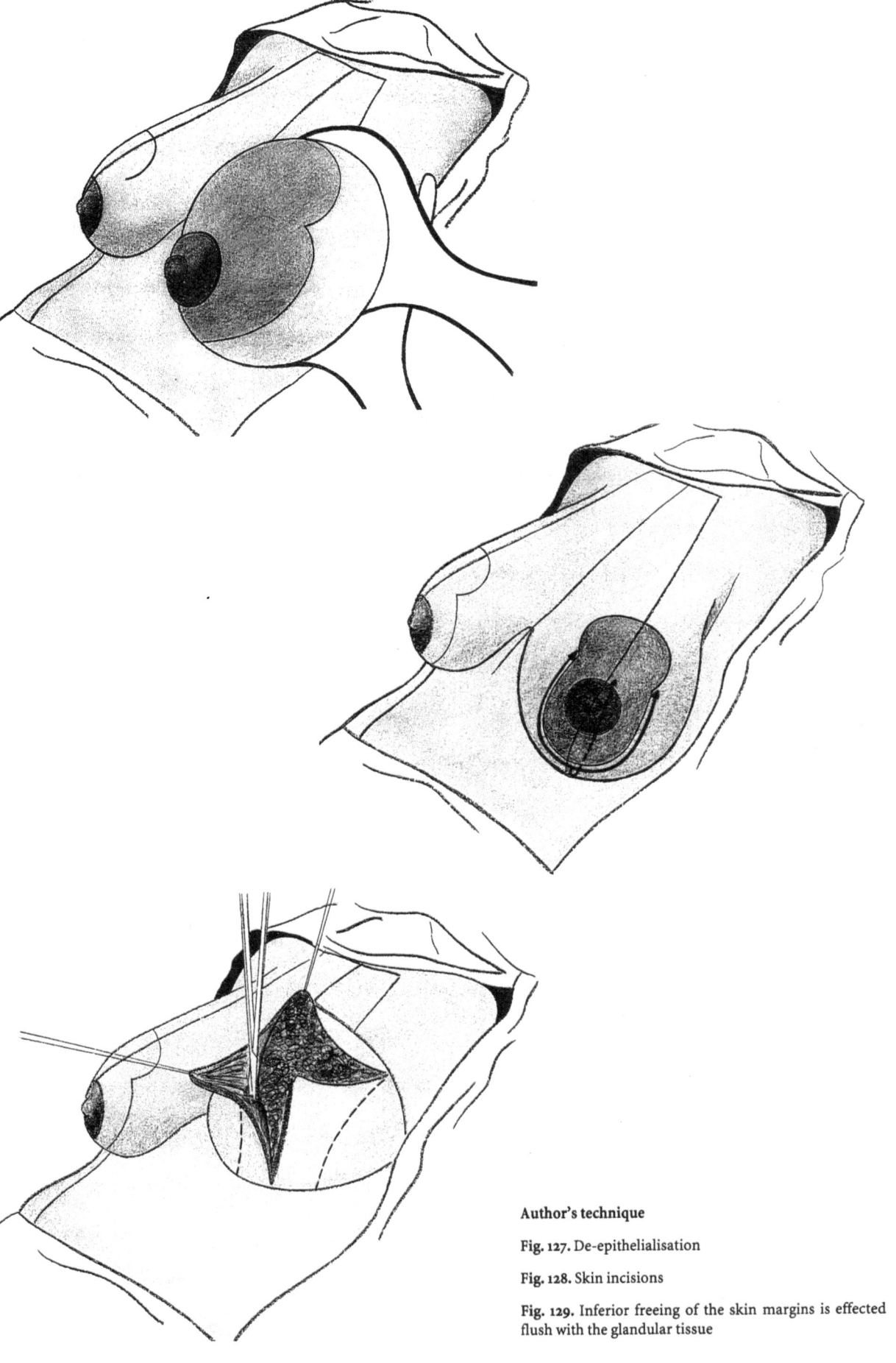

Author's technique

Fig. 127. De-epithelialisation

Fig. 128. Skin incisions

Fig. 129. Inferior freeing of the skin margins is effected flush with the glandular tissue

3) The glandular resection

• With the flat left hand under the gland, the glandular incision is begun at the lower border of the nipple-bearing flap, from C to D, creating a glandular slice 1 to 2 cm thick, this slice being thinner when the nipple-bearing flap is longer (fig. 130);

• two Kocher's forceps are clamped on the lower border of the nipple-bearing flap, seizing both dermis and gland, and held vertically by the assistant who lifts them in time with the progress of the dissection. The latter is performed from above downward, leaving a slice of constant thickness, the regularity of the section being constantly monitored by the flat left hand applied behind against the nipple-bearing flap (fig. 131);

• this uniform glandular resection is extended under the inner and outer quadrants; it can be pursued medially without risk as far as the inner limit of the gland since this technique no longer uses a dermo-glandular coiled flap (figs. 132 and 133);

• the resected mass is weighed (the operation has begun with the breast that appears smaller if there is asymmetry), and this weight serves as a reference standard for resection of the other side. Careful hemostasis is made; the important zones here are the lower border of the pectoralis major and the outer limits of the stripping, where the branches of the lateral thoracic artery ramify.

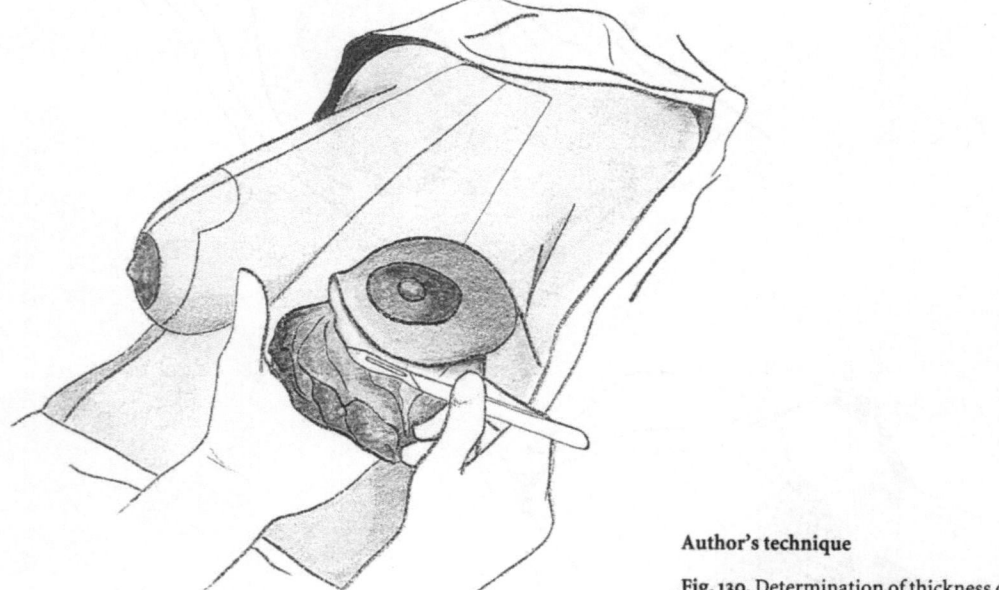

Author's technique

Fig. 130. Determination of thickness of the nipple-bearing flap

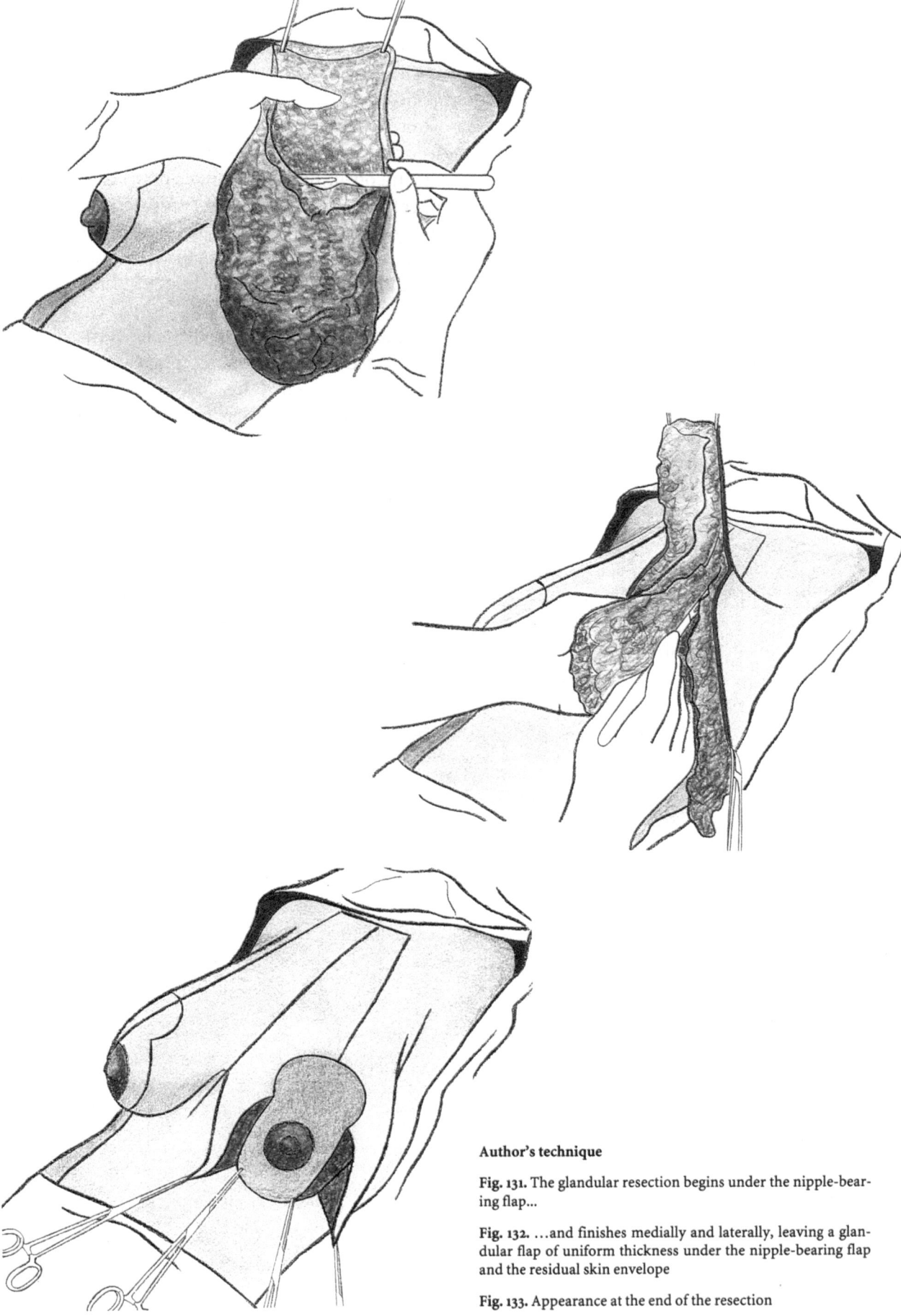

Author's technique

Fig. 131. The glandular resection begins under the nipple-bearing flap...

Fig. 132. ...and finishes medially and laterally, leaving a glandular flap of uniform thickness under the nipple-bearing flap and the residual skin envelope

Fig. 133. Appearance at the end of the resection

4) Reconstruction

• The areola. Point A is attached to the areola by a temporary nylon suture (fig. 134). C and D are also attached to each other by a stitch whose ends are left long so that traction may be applied by a Halsted forceps; this stitch grasps in passing the point of the areola diametrically opposite to A (fig. 135). The periareola thus closed does not assume a circular shape because of the weight of the residual gland on a skin envelope that is still open. To tack the areola down in a harmonious manner we slip a drape under it to spread it out, which facilitates the placing of six other stitches for the areolar construction; these are inverting dermal sutures passed simply on the inner areolar slope and in U form on the outer slope, so as to compensate for the inequality of the two circles (avoiding puckering as far as possible) (fig. 136);

• the drape is removed and the assistant holds the taut stitches vertically from the inferior areolar point by the Halsted forceps, two compresses aiding in grasping the inferior skin flaps, and the clamp is applied (fig. 137).

When we first started using this technique, and were still somewhat apprehensive about correct placement of the clamp, we continued to trace the margins of the ellipse in ink at the start of the operation to guide our procedure, but these corresponded so regularly to the limits of the flaps taken in the clamp that we soon abandoned this landmark.

We are in the habit of using two clamps of differing curvatures. When the breast is very spread out, with an almost horizontal inframammary crease and a very wide base, we use a clamp with a large curvature. When the breast has a narrower base and the crease is more curved, we use a clamp whose radius of curvature is smaller. In practice, while this technique necessarily reduces the base of breast implantation, this reduction nevertheless has its limits and depends partly on the initial breast base if it is desired to preserve harmony between the reduction of the breast base and the anterior projection of the diminished breast.

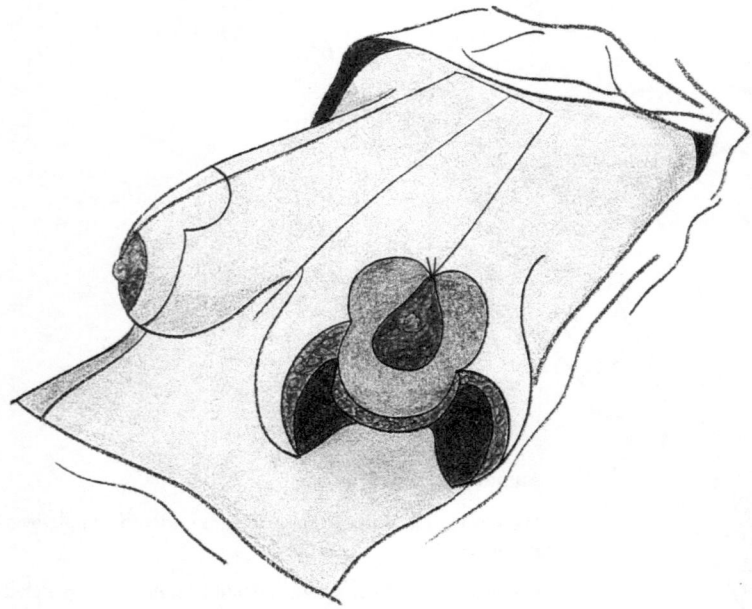

Author's technique

Fig. 134. Fixation of the upper areolar stitch

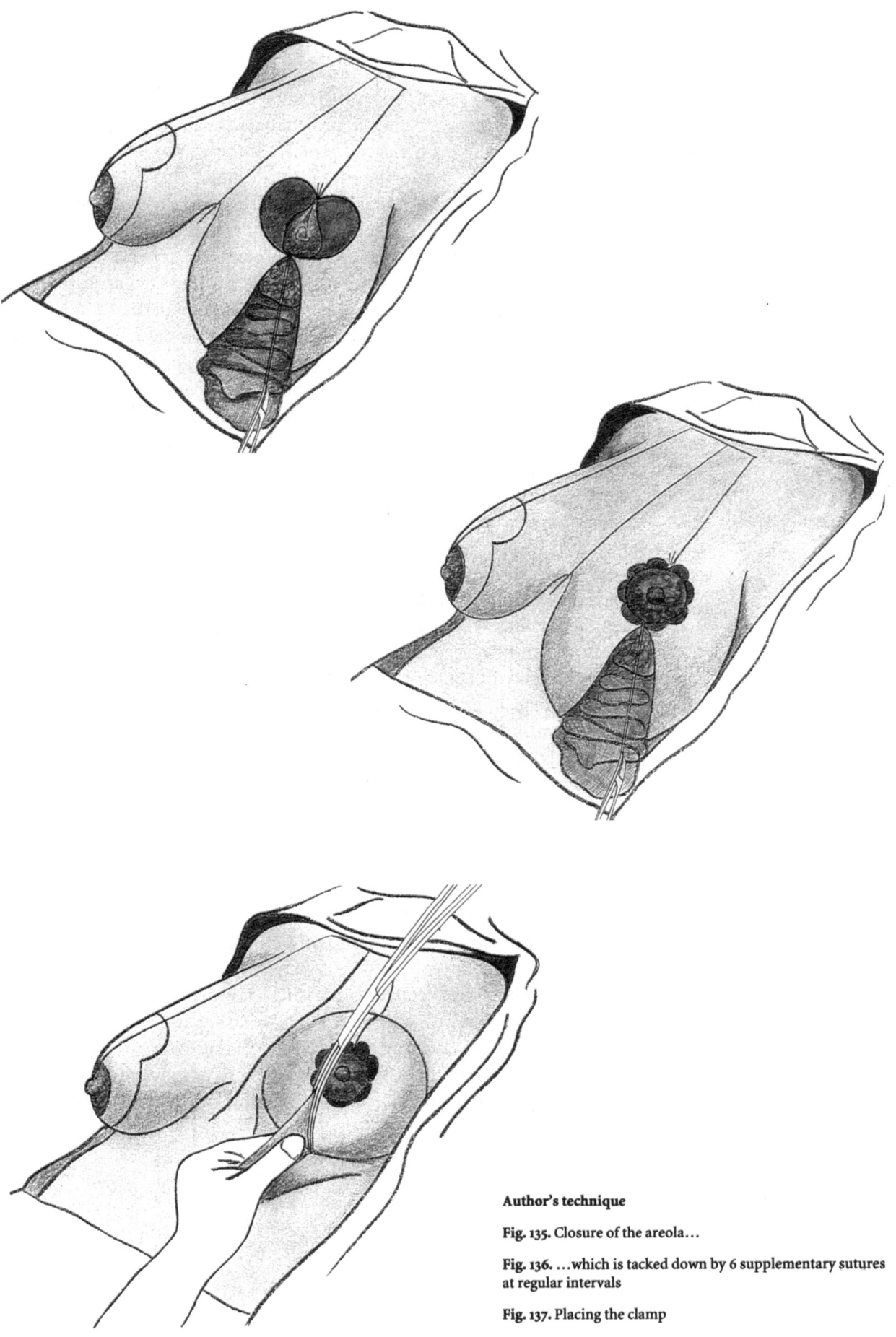

Author's technique

Fig. 135. Closure of the areola...

Fig. 136. ...which is tacked down by 6 supplementary sutures at regular intervals

Fig. 137. Placing the clamp

Care must be taken to ensure that the clamp is neither too vertical (base insufficiently reduced, areola situated too high and facing upward, segment III too long and risking uncoiling with glandular ptosis) nor too horizontal (base over-reduced in relation to an excessive anterior projection, with an areola tilted downward and segment III too short, risking ptosis), and always distributing the tension uniformly along the whole of the edges of the clamp.

• Once the clamp appears to be in satisfactory position, a line is drawn along its edges and it is removed (fig. 138). The skin incisions are made a little within these guidelines, about 0.5 cm from the lines, so as to prevent an excessive reduction leading to exaggerated tension on the margins of the vertical subareolar scar;

• the vertical subareolar scar is tacked down with inverting dermal stitches of fine slowly-absorbed material up to a height (without stretching) of 4.5 cm, and the lower end is tethered to the fold (fig. 139). If at this stage the areola faces upward and does not seem circular, with an inferior hemicircumference that is too flattened, the vertical suture is prolonged by 0.5 to 1 cm, its lower end is reattached to the crease, and a supplementary depithelialisation is made at the lower border of the areola allowing rounding-off and reorientation of its lower portion, and bringing the vertical subareolar scar to 4.5 cm in length (fig. 139, inset);

• after insertion of a suction drain, it remains to perform the lateral resection of the dog-ears. The upper tracing is marked in the inframammary crease, which spontaneously assumes its shape. The lower line must follow the limit of the former fold, an anatomic entity which corresponds to the transition from the superficial fascia of the subcutaneous plane to the retroglandular plane. Very often, after this resection, the lower margin of the resection appears longer than its upper margin. This inequality of length is compensated by a "lift" effect at the time of suture, by suturing the inner margins from within outward and the outer margins from without inward, ending the sutures under the vertical scar (fig. 140).

Here, too, the possibilities of compensating for the inequality of the margins depends on the skin elasticity. If the suture does leads to puckering, it is better to revise the resection of the upper margin and to lengthen it somewhat, rather than to run the risk of a hypertrophic scar by an excessive imbalance of tension between the two margins.

• The suturing is completed, with a continuous rapidly absorbed superficial intradermal suture for the limbs of the inverted T and a superficial continuous monofilament nylon suture for the areola or a slowly-absorbed intradermal suture;

• a moderately compressive modelling dressing is composed with tulle gras, absorbent pads and adhesive hypoallergenic adhesive strapping. This is removed with the drains after 3 to 4 days, and is replaced by adhesive strips across the suture line for two weeks and the wearing of a brassière day and night for two months. If made with nylon, the periareolar continuous suture is retained for four weeks.

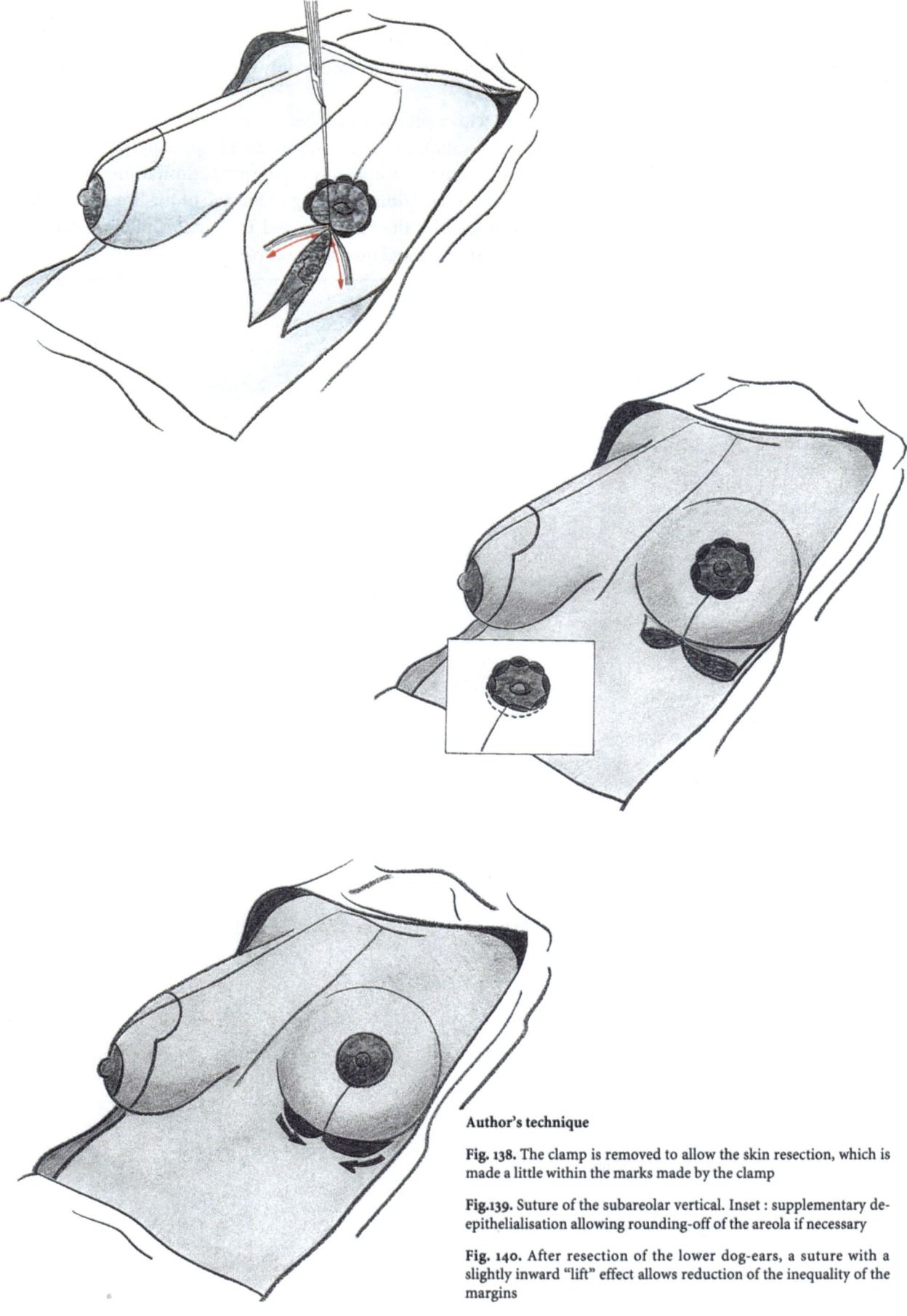

Author's technique

Fig. 138. The clamp is removed to allow the skin resection, which is made a little within the marks made by the clamp

Fig. 139. Suture of the subareolar vertical. Inset : supplementary de-epithelialisation allowing rounding-off of the areola if necessary

Fig. 140. After resection of the lower dog-ears, a suture with a slightly inward "lift" effect allows reduction of the inequality of the margins

This technique combines (figs. 142 and 143) :

    – a preoperative design which predetermines only the size and position of the areola,

    – a nipple-bearing flap with a superior pedicle,

    – extensive de-epithelialisation, helping to secure the blood-supply,

    – a uniform glandular resection without any topographic limitations,

    – clamp control of the skin resection, allowing reduction of the breast base as required, and which, together with the final inverted T resection, allows adaptation of the skin envelope to the residual breast size at will.

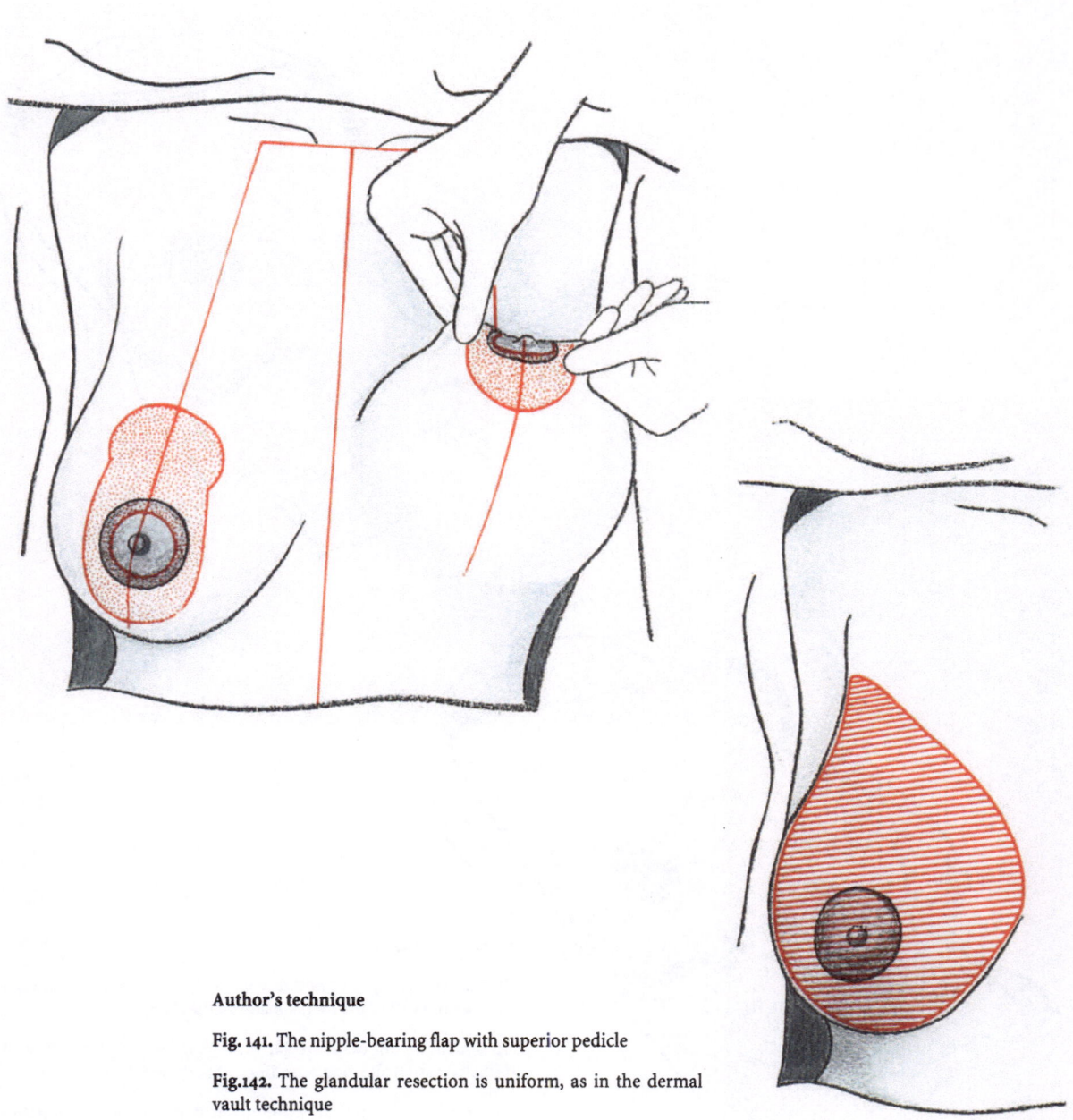

Author's technique

Fig. 141. The nipple-bearing flap with superior pedicle

Fig.142. The glandular resection is uniform, as in the dermal vault technique

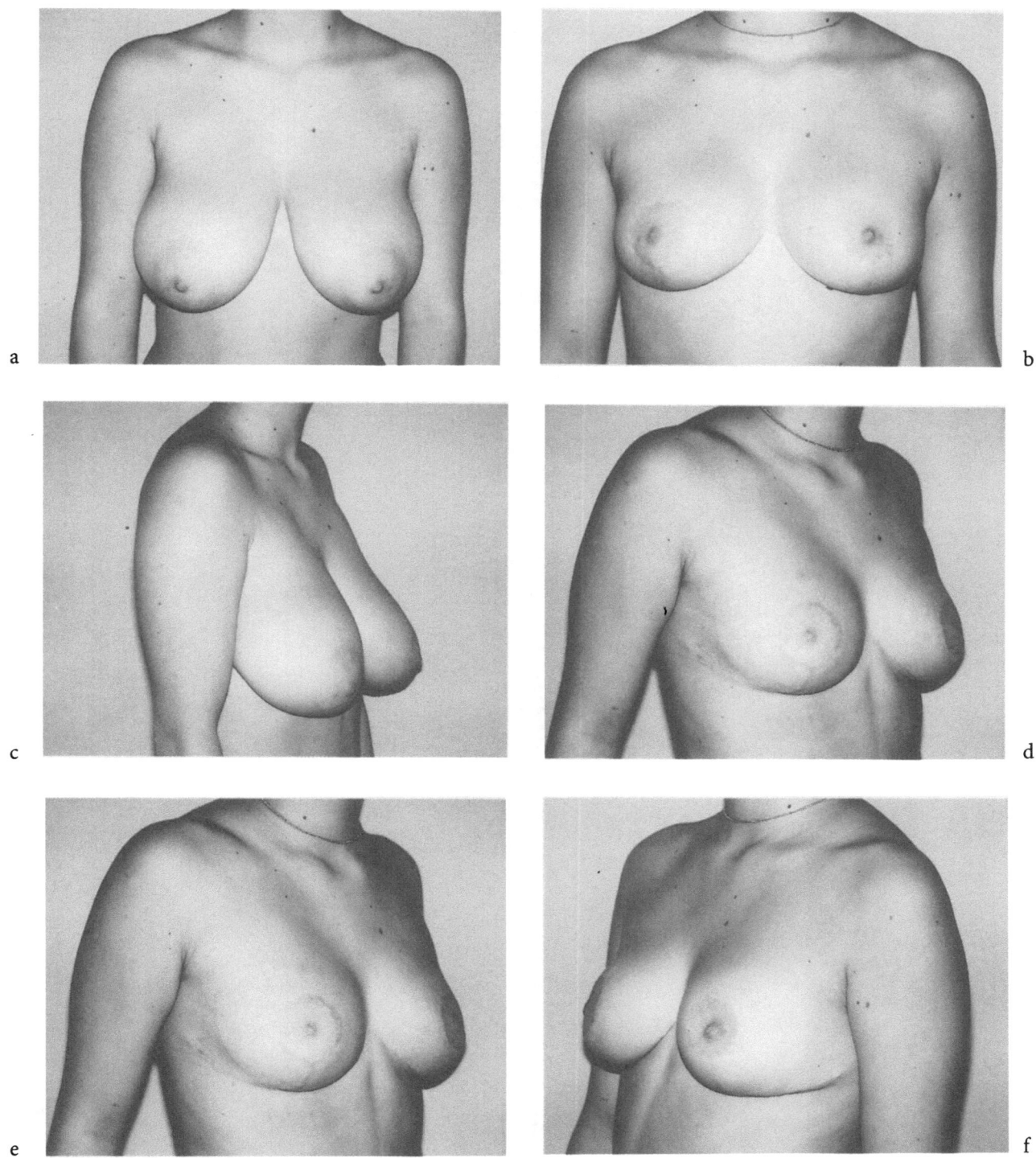

Fig. 143 a-f. 17-year-old : moderate hypertrophy, poor skin quality (striae). Resection of 480 g left, 450 g right. Defects : long horizontal scar (but breast base large initially, and inframammary crease extending to the mid-axillary line); residual areolar asymmetry

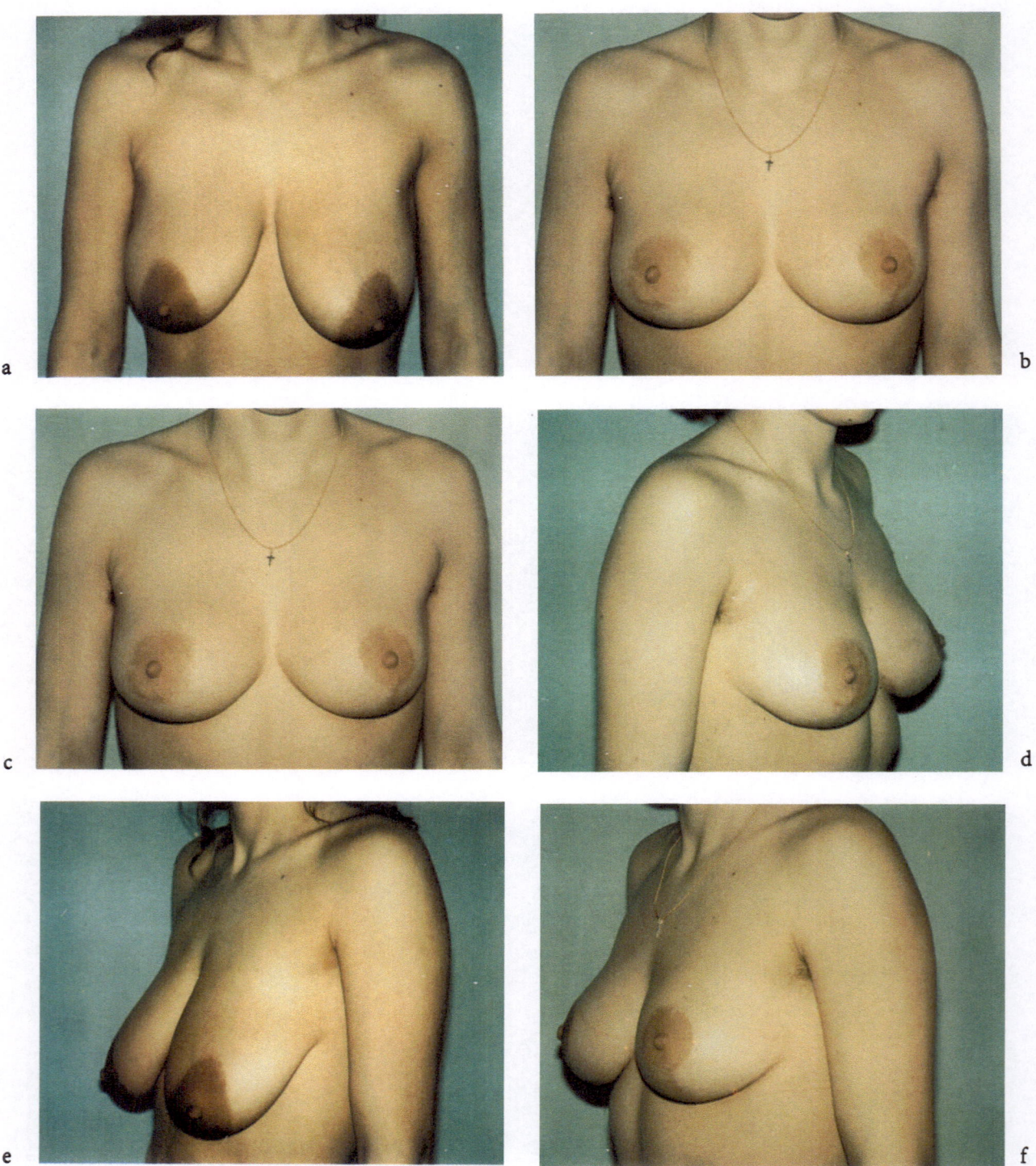

Fig. 144 a-f. 22-year-old : glandular shrinkage after pregnancy and lactation; good quality skin, ptosis exceeds degree of hypertrophy. Skin asymmetry greater than asymmetry of size. Resection of 210 g left and 170 g right (the difference in areolar color is due to the fact that the operation was performed 6 months after delivery and 4 months after weaning). Result at 2 years

Recent developments

Certain techniques or their recent modifications tend to lay special emphasis on a particular feature of the mammoplasty, whether this is a problem of the pedicle, or the position and especially the length of the scars.

Inferior pedicle techniques

These were described by Ribeiro (1975) and Robbins (1977). They are based on the principle of conservation of the subdermal vessels at the level of the inframammary crease, of the deep glandular branches emerging at the lower border of the pectoralis major, and also of the so-called artery of the nipple.

It is actually a technique of McKissock's, since it uses a vertical dermoglandular flap whose superior attachments have been severed (fig. 145).

The best indication is in cases of very great hypertrophy with ptosis, where the sterno-areolar distance is thought to be too great for survival of a nipple-bearing flap with a superior pedicle.

The width of the inferior pedicle must be at least 8 cm; the peripheral glandular resection, by which reduction of the breast base is achieved, is of horse-shoe shape (fig. 146).

After ascension and fixation of the nipple-areolar plaque, the skin envelope is adjusted to the residual breast size.

The inferior pedicle techniques combine:
  – an inferior nipple-bearing dermo-glandular flap,
  – a superior and lateral glandular resection,
  – a final T-shaped scar.

While the advantages of this technique are essentially represented by its security as regards blood-supply and secondarily by preservation of the deep innervation of the nipple (not that the sensitivity of the nipple is a minor matter, but we have seen that with a superior pedicle nipple sensation is nearly always preserved, which suggests that this innervation is not solely of deep origin), it has certain disadvantages:

– the principle is simple but its realisation is not always easy, either for a good choice of position of the nipple-areolar plaque or for readjustment of the skin envelope, dissociated from the residual breast size;

– the inferior scar is necessarily long because of the absence of major skin reduction opposite the vertical subareolar scar and the impossibility of mobilisation of the inframammary crease. In fact, while the crease is fixed to the skin for anatomic reasons (passage of the superficial fascia behind the glandular plane), it can be mobile relative to the thoracic plane, and therefore capable of ascending on the parietal plane, provided the glandular plane has been freed from this parietal plane, which is not the case here for fear of injury to the blood-supply;

– we criticise it particularly for its creation of a cleavage between the superior skin envelope and the dermo-glandular pedicle, which is more exposed to the effects of gravity than a superior pedicle; the risk is therefore that of secondary ptosis comparable with glandular ptosis, with uncoiling of segment III, which becomes exaggeratedly convex, and emptying of the glandular content of segment II.

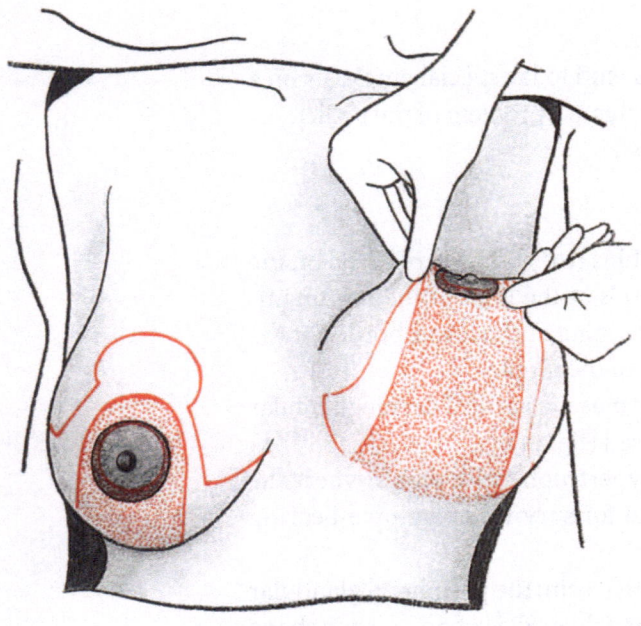

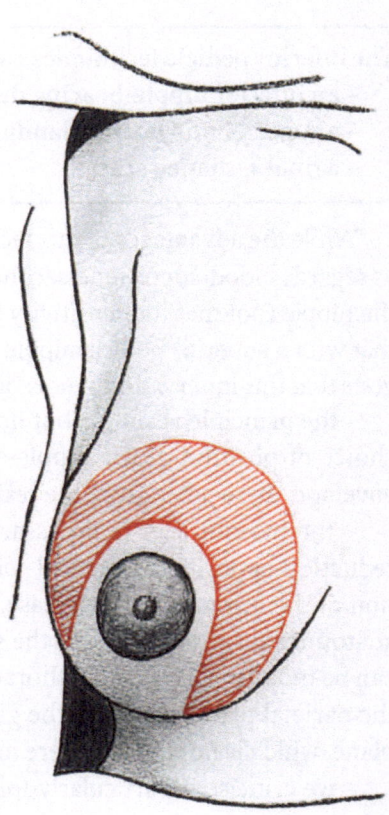

Inferior pedicle technique

Fig. 145. Design of dermo-glandular flap and skin incisions

Fig. 146. Horse-shoe glandular resection, above and laterally

Posterior pedicle techniques

Some authors postulate that, with an inferior pedicle, the essential part of the blood-supply does not come from the dermis but from preservation of the posterior glandular arteries, which has led them to describe a so-called central or posterior pedicle technique.

After the periareolar incision, with preservation of the nipple-areolar plaque by Schwartzmann's maneuver (which is imperative because there is again a cutaneo-glandular cleavage), the stripping of gland and skin and the glandular resection itself must be halted some cm from the muscle plane to be sure of preserving an adequate blood-supply, ie by respecting the cutaneous and glandular branches of the lateral and internal thoracic arteries

---

The posterior pedicle techniques are based on :
   – preservation for the gland and areola only of the posterior glandular vessels,
   – Schwarzmann's maneuver, and cutaneo-glandular cleavage.

The risks of these techniques are :

– an inadequate resection due to the fact that the need to preserve a thick peripheral cutaneo-glandular flap, separation of which from the deep plane must stop a few cm from the muscle plane, limits reduction of the breast base;

– secondary glandular ptosis with uncoiling of segment III for the same reasons as in the inferior pedicle technique;

– and above all a risk of damage, even amounting to necrosis, of the nipple-areolar plaque if the posterior vessels are not totally respected (their position may be difficult to assess in cases of ptosis).

To reintroduce into a modern technique the concept of cutaneo-glandular cleavage seems to us a retrograde step.

It cannot be over-emphasised that it is the techniques without cutaneo-glandular cleavage which have brought security of vascularity and that, among these, the superior pedicle techniques are those which ensure the best possible stability in morphologic terms.

Other techniques seek to reduce the length of the scars.

Peixoto's technique

The design of the skin resection is aimed at being as narrow as possible to minimise the horizontal limb. Depending on the degree of ptosis and hypertrophy, there may be a single vertical subareolar incision without a circular periareolar resection intended for glandular access, or a limited peri-areolar resection with a narrow vertical ellipse stopping 12 cm above the inframammary crease, or an hour-glass incision, wider and longer and reaching the crease (fig. 147).

The glandular resection is made at the deep aspect of the gland and eliminates a conical section of varying length, which reduces the breast base solely at its periphery (fig. 148).

A large part is accorded to "spontaneous" skin retraction, in the hope that the skin envelope will retract harmoniously on the residual breast volume.

In our view, this technique can only be satisfactorily applied to minor or moderate hypertrophy in the young woman with a highly placed areola, where the skin still retains excellent elastic quality. Its field of application is therefore limited, and it may also be remarked that in these situations the superior pedicle technique with skin reduction as required on the clamp also gives a horizontal scar which is very short or even absent.

When the areola is situated relatively low on the thorax, this type of design does not recenter it high enough; the breast remains badly centered and too spread out transversely with the areola too low, a concave segment II and an insufficiently

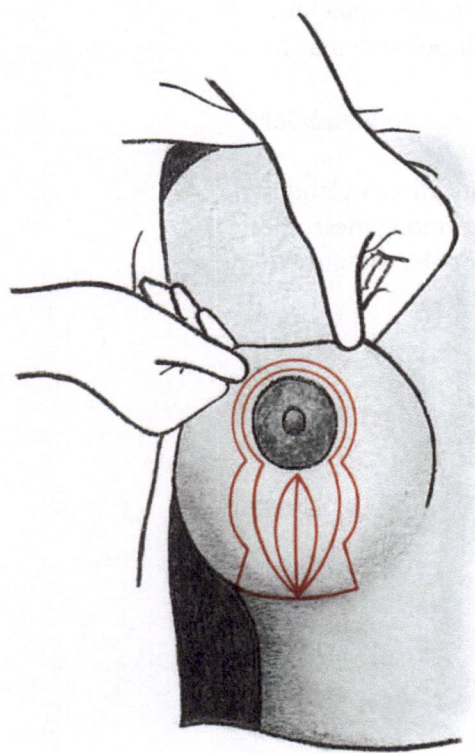

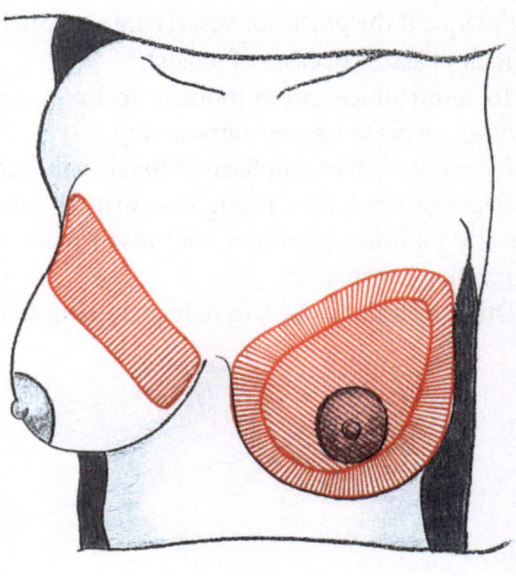

Peixoto's technique

Fig. 147. The different skin incisions

Fig. 148. The glandular resection involves a conic segment at the posterior part of the gland

reduced base, the ptosis being the more marked when the skin has been unable to retract adequately because of its poor elasticity.

Marchac's technique

The principle is the same: to minimise the horizontal inframammary limb of the T-shaped scar.

The "gateway" design of the skin resection is wider, but stops sharply higher up above the inframammary crease (fig. 149).

The glandular resection is made in central fashion, on the deep aspect of the gland, remembering to preserve sufficient tissue behind the areola to ensure its projection.

The skin between the lower extremity of the "carriage entrance",which is mammary skin, must be completely peeled from the residual gland as far as the anatomic fold, in front of the supplementary horizontal incision, to ensure that the horizontal scar does not reascend on the lower slope of the breast.

Here lies the real risk of this technique : one may not trifle deliberately with the inframammary crease. If this procedure is exaggerated, the horizontal scar is situated on the inferior slope of the breast; if it is even a little short, one may wonder whether the scar defect is not then more dis-pleasing than a scar that may be a little longer but which is perfectly situated in the inframammary crease and does not transgress at all on the base of the breast.

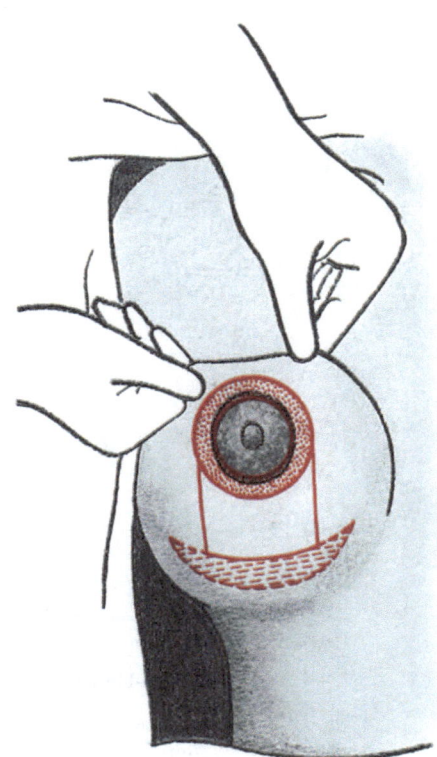

Marchac's technique

Fig. 149. The stippled zone corresponds to the de-epthelialised surface. The hatched zone corresponds to the supplementary skin resection (the upper part of the crescent is traced at 5 cm from the inframammary fold, the lower part at 2 cm)

The "round block"

The "round block' and the techniques describing it certainly constitute the extreme in the matter of skin economy, since the excision involves only the peri-areolar ring (fig. 150).

The skin reduction is confined to the periareolar region, without any possibility of reduction of the breast circumference and thus of any correction of the base of an asymmetry, which is so common (fig. 151)…

This means that its indications are few and it overlooks the fact that such incongruence between the outer and inner areolar circles, without the possibility of balancing and stabilisation by resection of a vertical or oblique lateral triangle with an areolar base and peripheral apex, necessarily risks broadening of the scar because of the radial tensions exerted throughout its extent, or a sprading of the areola and decrease of its anterior projection.

It also ignores the fact that the periareolar scar is invariably the most visible scar in a mammoplasty.

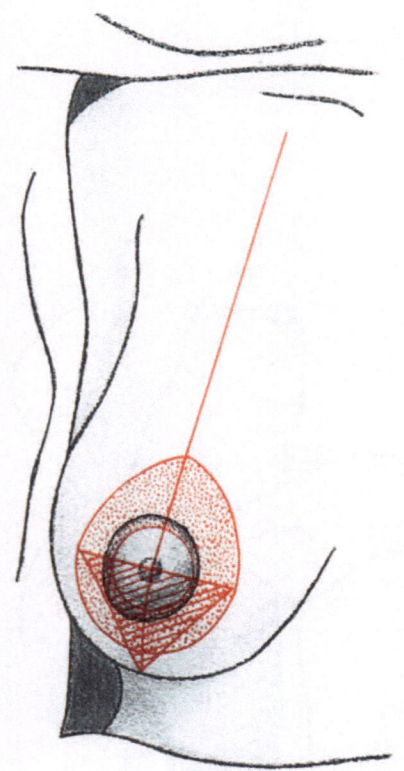
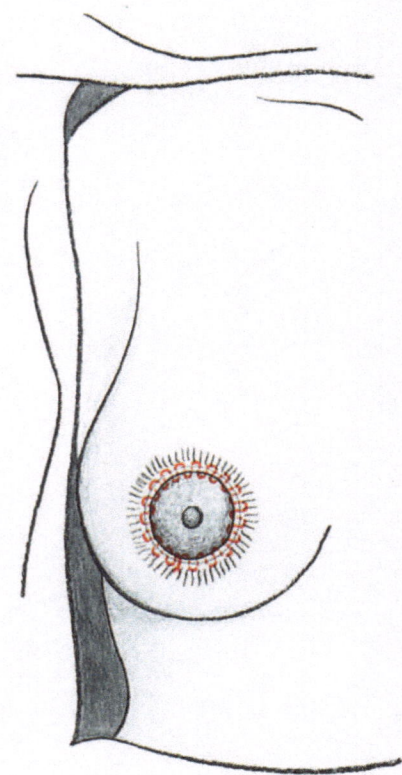

Round-block technique (of Benelli)

Fig. 150. The stippled area is the zone of periareolar de-epithelialisation; the triangular hatched area is the zone of glandular resection

Fig. 151. The incongruence of the two areolar tracings can be resolved only by creating major puckering post-operatively. Suture is made with nonabsorbable material left in place, the only way of avoiding excessive broadening of the scar or spreading of the areola. And what if the suture is extruded or breaks ?

Amputation of the breast with areolar graft (Thorek)

Whether this refers to Thorek's original technique (1939) or a derivative without a pre-established design, we must stress from the outset that this procedure, in our view, is to be reserved for a particular situation : gigantomasty in a woman in her fifties, often obese, in whom the skin, grossly stretched by the weight of the gland and the action of the years, has entirely lost its capacity to retract, and where the length of the nipple-bearing flap creates doubt as to the viability of the nipple-areolar plaque.

Therefore it concerns only those cases where the nipple is situated more than 40 cm from the suprasternal notch, on a skin of poor quality exhibiting numerous striae, and where the dermis is thinned: the dermal vascular plexus risks being defective at the end of such a pedicle, with damage to the areola.

Operative technique

The axis of the breast is drawn starting from a point situated 5 cm lateral to the suprasternal notch and ending at B in the middle of the inframammary crease (fig. 152).

A point A is located on this axis 18-19 cm from the apex of the axis (corresponding more or less to the final position of the nipple and not being placed too high to be included in the areola.

Two lines are drawn vertically joining A and B, with the breast moderately retracted laterally and then medially. It is confirmed that the tangent to the most medial part of the medial line is situated no less than 12 cm from the midline.

Two points C and D are located on these lines, projecting slightly below the inframmary crease. C and D are connected at the two ends of the fold to C' and D' (CC' + DD' = C'D'). The nipple-areolar plaque is removed and preserved in normal saline, after reduction of its size to 4.5 – 5 cm in diameter.

The incisions are made boldly, initially through skin and gland at right angles to the skin, down to the parietal plane (figs. 153 and 154).

The gland is apposed by several absorbable sutures after checking the hemostasis, and a suture is passed at point A and drawn upward to facilitate construction of the subareolar vertical. At this point a decision must be made as to whether a supplementary posterior glandular resection will be needed. Drainage is inserted and the horizontal scar is placed in the crease.

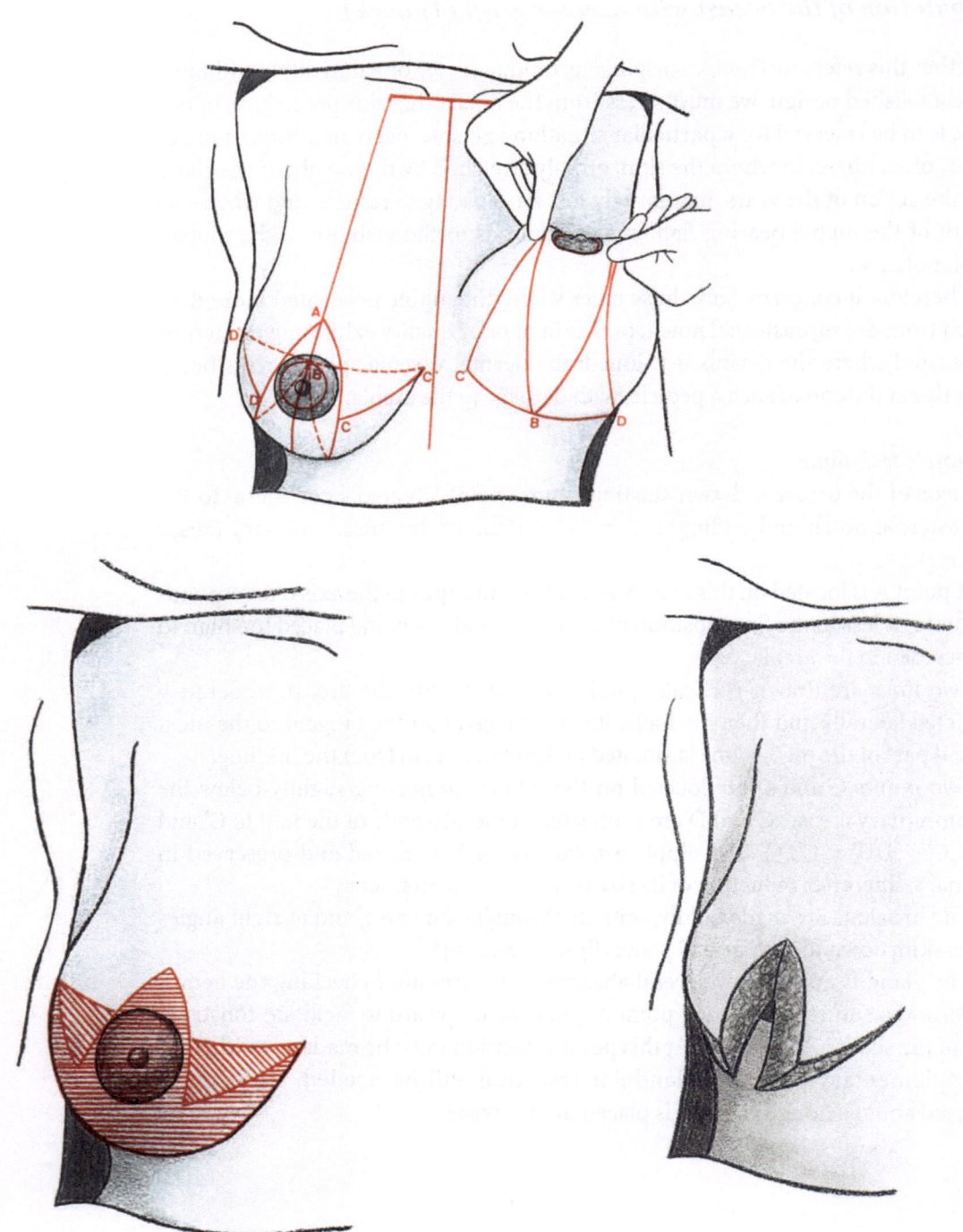

Thorek's technique

Fig. 152. Skin incisions

Fig. 153. Projection of the zone of glandular resection

Fig. 154. After the cutaneo-glandular resection

Finally, the areola is grafted in the de-epithelialised receptor site at the apex of the breast cone. The areola must face forward and slightly outward and the subareolar vertical must not exceed 5 cm in length.

The nipple-areolar graft, carefully thinned with fine scissors in its areolar zone and preserving a nipple 0.5 cm thick, is fixed under a tie-over bolus left in place for 6 days.

This technique is characterised by :
- **– an amputation-graft of the nipple-areolar plaque,**
- **– absence of cutaneo-glandular cleavage,**
- **– a preestablished design.**

While the morphologic results are satisfactory, there are disadvantages of the method that lead us to reserve it for the indication given above : the nipple-areolar plaque, because it is a free graft, is devoid of the sensitivity and erectile nature of the nipple; moreover, secondary flattening of the nipple is often seen, and the graft sometimes becomes discolored.

The scar defect

The responsibility for the scar defect of a mammoplasty, both in extent and quality, is shared between:
- the surgeon,
- the breast,
- the patient.

The surgeon's responsibility

The technique used

It is attributable primarily to the technique used, as regards both the glandular procedure and the management of the skin.

The glandular procedure

• The site of the resection plays a part since certain techniques allow only a resection limited in extent and site. This determines the site of the scars and also their length and quality. The scars may be relatively short, but sometimes at the expense of an inadequate resection. We prefer techniques permitting an "unlimited" resection, especially if uniform.

• The choice of position of the pedicle also affects the length of the scars. Only the superior pedicle techniques allow control of the length of the inframammary scar, since it is here that they achieve reduction of the breast base. For technical reasons, on the other hand, in the inferior pedicle methods it is inevitable that the inframmary scar is relatively long.

• In practice, the glandular procedure especially affects the degree of residual breast volume, which will affect both the length and quality of the scars.

• If residual breast volume is small — provided of course that the skin envelope is correctly adjusted to it — the scars will be relatively long but of good quality since skin tension will be minor.

• However, if the residual volume is excessive (due to inadequate resection), the scars will certainly be relatively short but of poor quality (due to excessive skin tension).

Moreover, for the same residual breast volume, the length of the scars is a function of the extent of the glandular resection :

– for a similar residual breast volume and glandular resection, the length of the scars is proportional to the extent of skin resection; this is a **content** *to which the* **container** *is adjusted. The scars will be longer after treatment of hypertrophy with ptosis than of an equivalent isolated hypertrophy.*

But here we become involved with the concept of skin quality.

Cutaneous procedure

If the glandular procedure predetermines the extent of the scar, it is the cutaneous procedure that is the culmination, since it:
- fixes the site and distributes the different segments of the scar;
- determines its length and skin tension (which must be as small as possible).

Scar sites

These are periareolar, radial and peripheral, at the circumference of the implantation base.

Techniques comprising only a periareolar circular scar lead inevitably to morphologic failure, with anteroposterior flattening of the shape of the breast, spreading of the areola and broadening of the scar.

Radial scars, whether vertical or lateral and oblique, must have the length of segment III since it is impermissible to deliberately interfere with the inframammary crease. In fact, the crease is determined anatomically, for it is at just this site that the superficial fascia departs from the subcutaneous plane to pass on the deep aspect of the gland. It is closely connected to the dermal plane by the crests of Duret.

Attempts to place the crease higher, in breast skin, are doomed to failure, and techniques that tend to transform the breast skin of segment III into thoracic skin, if there is marked hypertrophy run the risk of "the revenge of the breast, which retrieves its skin" (Lalardrie).

The crease inexorably regains its place, below the scar. Though it is fixed relative to the skin, it is relatively mobile relative to the costomuscular thoracic plane.

It is therefore impossible to vary the length of the radial scar for a given volume and fixed implantation base, whether this scar be vertical or lateral-oblique. It remains equal to the length of segment III. It is only possible to vary the periareolar scar in relation to the inframammary scar, in inversely proportional manner.

But all such maneuvering has its cost. The endeavour to reduce the inframammary scar too much carries the risk of periareolar puckering, or excessive broadening of this scar with spreading of the areola, this spreading not necessarily being uniform as it occurs along the radii of maximal tension.

Conversely, a periareola that is too small results in a poorly reduced breast and an inframammary scar that is too long and too horizontal. This defect is seen especially when the upper border of the future areola is positioned too high. The distance to the suprasternal notch is too long, for which the surgeon usually compensates by a shorter segment III. The course is marked by ptosis with horizontalisation of segment III, defective skin reduction, a conical breast and a horizontal inframammary fold.

An areola placed too high runs the opposite risk, which is even more difficult to make good : segment III is over-long and the course is towards glandular ptosis with unwinding of segment III, and a radial scar that is too exposed to view. The ideal position for the areola is actually at the apex of the bulk of the gland, which usually corresponds at the end of the operation to an areola situated very slightly below the apex of the gland and facing somewhat downward and slightly outward, this because of the ptosis — inevitable in the first few months — which will remain moderate if the technique is satisfactory.

An areola that is too medial is one of the most difficult defects to correct, while areolae that are too high are irreparable.

Suture techniques

The care given to suture technique also affects the quality of the scar.

Thus, the areola may be sutured in two layers : an inverting dermal suture of very fine (4/0) absorbable material and a continuous superficial intradermal (subcuticular) suture of slowly absorbed material or monofilament nylon (3/0 or 4/0) left in place for 3-4 weeks.

The radial and inframammary scars are also sutured in two layers: the deep dermal layer with interrupted absorbable stitches (20/100 mm or 3/) and a continuous intradermal suture of rapidly absorbed material (3/0) or monofilament nylon (25/100 mm = 2/0).

The dressing also plays a part since it exerts a constraint at the scars; adhesive strips or film are left at least until removal of the sutures, or even longer in some cases.

The breast factor

The quality of container and content are closely linked

Cutaneous factor

The greater the hypertrophy. the more it will act to stretch the skin, which loses its elasticity and exhibits striae, and the dermis becomes thinner. This factor worsens with time, so it is better to operate for hypertrophy while the patient is still young, when the skin envelope is less impaired and can readapt better to the glandular content. When the skin has retained its elasticity, the necessary resection will be less extensive and the scars will be shorter.

Glandular factor

• The breast of the young girl (of normal height-weight ratio) is firm but easy to model, since it contains essentially glandular substance; it is also white on section. This is the so-called idiopathic hypertrophy, the causes of which are unknown. On the other hand, the breast of an obese young girl is much softer and contains a great deal of fat, sometimes virtually no gland substance at all except in the retro-areolar region, especially if the overweight accompanies puberty. This indicates how harmful a sudden rapid gain in weight at this stage of reproductive life is for the shape of the breast. It is our impression that some of these "associated " hypertrophies might have been avoided by preservation of a normal height-weight ratio; how is one otherwise to explain the virtually total absence of gland substance specific to this type of breast, as confirmed by the histology ?

Some authors have even suggested treating these fatty hypertrophies by liposuction, but this ignores the fact that the skin envelope is simultaneously distended as evidenced by the presence of striae, and that simultaneous readaptation of the skin sac is necessary for a good morphologic result.

• With pregnancies glandular involution develops, with a greater proportion of fatty tissue; the skin is easy to reshape but with less "grip". The role of the skin in the quality of the morphologic result is more important; the skin resection will be greater than in a young girl, since the degree of ptosis due to the glandular involution is more exaggerated than the residual hypertrophy would suggest.

• Caution is called for with the hypertrophic breast in the woman of fifty, often very dystrophic, rigid and difficult to shape. It is necessary to resect more gland than in a younger woman, particularly at the level of the nipple-bearing flap, to reconstruct the breast satisfactorily without immediate excessive skin tension at the periareolar scar and at the angles of the T (fig.155).

Often, at the end of the operation, the breast exhibits a "tyre-like" appearance with a periareolar glandular rim and an areola that is too flat. If this appearance is due entirely to the rigidity of the gland it will correct itself spontaneously in a few weeks, being already considerably improved even at the first dressing. If, however, this appearance is associated with over-resection under the nipple-bearing flap, so that it is thinner than the rest of the skin envelope, it may persist. Hence the importance, once again, of a uniform glandular resection.

• The dystrophic breast can be dealt with by resection in a precise quadrant; preoperative mammography will form part of the assessment, whatever the age.

The morphology of the breast

This factor exerts its influence primarily through the extent of the breast base. Not all the techniques allow reduction of this base, hence the length of the scar will depend on the shape and length of the inframammary crease. It is preferable to use techniques that do allow its reduction.

• When the breasts are asymmetric — if the asymmetry of size is corrected — the scars will be longer on the side of the bulkier breast. If asymmetry is marked, and the skin still seems to be elastic, one should take care in making the preoperative design that the upper border of the future areola is positioned a little lower on the bulkier side, since the skin is more stressed on this side and this point will reascend spontaneously more after the glandular resection.

It is best to begin the operation with the smaller breast, the weight of resected gland tissue serving as a reference for the minimum to be removed from the other side.

• The areola is not always centered at the apex of the breast cone. If the areola is more medial, the design is centered on the axis of the breast, here passing lateral to the nipple. Otherwise, depending on the technique employed, there is a risk that the areola will be situated :

  – either at the apex of the breast cone, but the breasts will be convergent, the subareolar scar too medial and the breast volume badly distributed, being too great medially;

  – or medial to the breast cone, with too short a distance from the midline to the areolar scar.

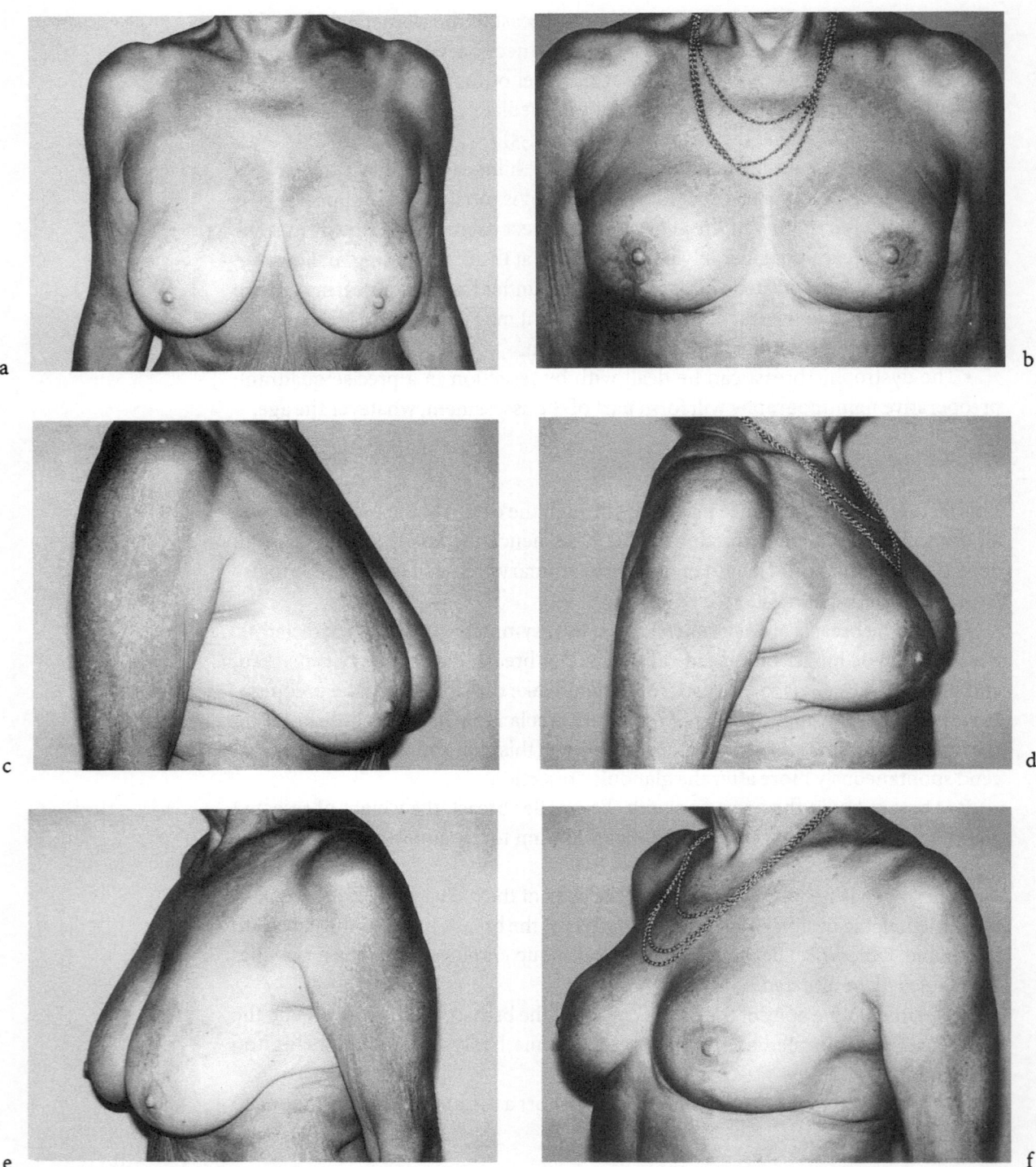

a

b

c

d

e

f

Fig. 155 a-f. 79-year-old : fatty involution of the gland, relative rigidity, ptosis, poor quality skin. Resection of 280 g left and 220 g right

Patient factors

Age

The younger the patient, the better the quality of the skin. The morphologic result is better and the breast more stable with time, but the dermis is thick and the scars are more likely to be hypertrophic.

If all the scars are uniformly hypertrophic, this is due to the skin quality. If they are hypertrophic only in some places, the fault lies with the surgeon, due to excessive and unequally distributed tension at this site, or poor apposition of the margins.

In older women, whose skin is atrophic, the dermis is thinner. The loss of cutaneous elasticity requires a more extensive resection and the scars will be longer but finer.

Life style

Tobacco, alcohol and sunlight have an injurious effect on skin quality as regards both its vascularity and elasticity.

Stage of reproductive life

This affects the scars by virtue of the degree of estrogenic activity.

This is one of the reasons why the scars are more likely to be red and hypertrophic in young women.

It is therefore best not to prescribe estrogenic contraceptives for at least 2 months, or even 6 months, after operation, and to caution against starting a pregnancy less than two years afterwards.

Further, oral contraceptives should be discontinued one month before operation, because of the risk of calf thromboembolism and of peroperative hemorrhage.

Obesity

If possible, it is better to have the patient lose weight before operation. This is more difficult in women of mature age and is more easily achieved in young girls, if care is taken to explain properly what is at stake. As breast size is adapted to general body build, it is preferable to lose the excess weight before operation, rather than to diet afterwards (this is a common "spontaneous" occurrence once the young girl is relieved of the physiologic and psychologic burden of her hypertrophy), which is combined with some degree of ptosis due to the decrease in residual breast size.

Dieting before the operation is both an advantage and a disadvantage for the surgeon. The disappearance of abdominal fat facilitates resection in the inframammary crease, but the amount of skin to be resected is somewhat more difficult to assess when loss of weight occurs, this problem varying with the quality of the skin, its degree of elasticity and its capacity for recovery.

The obese patient has a crease that is horizontalised by the excess of abdominal fat; the breast base is more difficult to reduce, and the horizontal scar is therefore longer but well hidden in the crease. The outer limb of the horizontal scar is often more difficult to position, and will be long because of the lateral thoracic rim.

Revision procedures

The problems posed by revision of mammoplasties , apart from the morphologic problems, are those of the scars : which should be revised, and why, when to revise them, and how ?

The scar problem is an isolated one

• The morphologic result is satisfactory, ie :
– the residual volume is adapted to the skin envelope and to the patient's build;
– the areola is properly placed, facing forward and slightly outward and situated at the apex of the projection of the breast;
– the breasts are symmetric in shape and size;
– secondary ptosis is absent or minor.
• However, the scars may be too evident because hypertrophied (between 2 and 6 months after the operation).

This hypertrophic reaction may be localised to one segment of the scar; this is due to an error of technique, the hypertrophy occurring precisely where the tension has been excessive.

If the scars are everywhere hypertrophic, this is due to the state of the skin.

At this interval after operation, whether the scar hypertrophy is isolated or diffuse, treatment is medical : by compression, and long-acting corticosteroids as cream or injected.

After 6 months, such treatment will be ineffective; only time will lessen the obviousness of the scars, they will remain broadened but become paler, though this may take two to three years. If surgical revision is envisaged, it should be delayed until the scars have paled, a sign of stabilisation and disappearance of the inflammatory reaction, and the operation should be followed by a course of corticosteroid treatment

There is an associated morphologic problem

There is a logical indication for surgical revision, but not before at least a year after the original operation, so that the result — and therefore the damage — has become stabilised.

An attempt should always be made to obtain the report of the first operation, so as to discover the technique used, of which the shape and position of the scars will in any case give some idea.

One should be wary of purely cutaneous techniques, since these have been associated with cleavage between skin and gland and the revision runs a not inconsiderable risk of glandular necrosis, a risk whose extent is difficult to predict and of which the patient should be informed.

The revision is a function of the residual breast size, the degree of ptosis and the position of the areolae. It should generally be done using a superior pedicle technique, the only absolutely reliable method of revising a breast previously operated by an inferior pedicle technique.

Care should be taken in evaluating the different basic distances: the position of the areola in relation to the suprasternal notch and to the midline, the size of the areola, the distance to the inframmmary crease, possible asymmetry.

Even more than at the first operation, one should beware the pitfalls of a pre-established design, which cannot assess the inequalities of skin tension at certain segments and whose importance may only become apparent during the procedure, after the incision. In these often difficult revisions we rely entirely on procedures using a clamp.

The revision is aimed primarily at restoration of satisfactory shape and the correction of any areolar malposition, but this is not always possible if the areolae are much too high and medial.

Thus, elimination of the anterior scars is not the primary objective; it may even be best to dispense with this and to take no account of them if they are completely outside the tracing used. To attempt to revise a mammoplasty at all costs by anterior scars, if these are badly placed, courts the risk of failure to correct the dysmorphism or even of worsening it.

Some scars will be eliminated because they are included in the skin incision of the revision procedure. Others will not; this is the case with high lateral horizontal scars, which are nearly always enlarged, and it is also the case with scars which are secondarily displaced on the breast contour, usually the result of a technical error.

The surgical indications for such revision procedures must therefore be very strict, and the patient should be warned of the possible persistence of part of the scar (and that others will be added). The postoperative surveillance must be very attentive because of the risk of glandular and sometimes even cutaneous necrosis.

Conclusion

The surgeon is responsible for the scars he creates on a given breast in a given patient.

The scar defect of a mammoplasty is never negligible, whatever the morphologic gain. It is acceptable only provided there is satisfactory morphologic correction, ie:

– a size adapted to the general build of the patient;

– an attractive shape, the breast being harmonious and the areola neither too high nor too low, but correctly situated at the apex of a well-concentrated glandular volume.

This means that one should not be satisfied with correction of the hypertrophy or ptosis alone, but that the shape and size obtained must conceal any secondary ptosis, whether cutaneous, due to inadequate readjustment of the envelope, or glandular, due to inadequate resection or inadequate measurements (particularly a subareolar distance that is too long).

We prefer techniques without cutaneo-glandular cleavage and with a superior pedicle, as a guarantee of vascular security and morphologic stability.

The best techniques, in our view, remain those which are not bound to a preestablished pattern, the adjustment of the container to the properly reduced content taking place as the operation proceeds, on a patient in the semi-seated position so that the level of the breast can be correctly assessed against the effect of gravity.

We repeat once again that a mammoplasty is a whole, that container and content are inseparable, that the main concern should be the shape, and that this must not be sacrificed to limit the length of the scars at all costs.

However, every effort should be made to limit the scar defect as much as possible in quantity and quality; therefore particular attention should be given to certain features:

– a fine periareolar scar (no exaggerated tension, no marked incongruence between the two circles);

– a fine vertical or oblique scar (no excess tension) and one that is relatively short (the subareolar distance must not exceed 4-5 cm at the end of the operation, so as to avoid derotation with secondary glandular ptosis);

– a horizontal scar sparing the intermammary crease medially and not transgressing on the base of the breast laterally, and above all remaining within the fold.

The operation must be proposed with discernment, with an eye to all these factors, and after carefully informing the patient. The morphologic gain must compensate for the scar defect, since experience teaches humility where mammoplasty scars are concerned.

References

Bricout N, Chavoin JP, Flageul G, Ohana J, Ricbourg B (1989) Hypertrophie mammaire. Rapport du XXXIVᵉ Congrès de la Société Française de Chirurgie Plastique, Reconstructrice et Esthétique, 21 October 1987

Goldwyn RM (1990) Reduction mammaplasty. Little, Brown and Company, Boston, Toronto, London

Lalardrie JP, J Jouglard JH (1974) Chirurgie plastique du sein. Masson, Paris

Bricout N, Lalardrie JP (21 October 1987) Cicatrices et plasties mammaires. Cours de la Société Française de Chirurgie Plastique, Reconstructrive et Esthétique

Breast augmentation

The surgery of breast augmentation is directed towards very different situations:

– minor anomalies or malformations such as hypoplasia,

– more serious disorders of differing degrees, ranging from aplasia to Poland's syndrome,

– and finally where the demand is purely cosmetic, the breast being of normal size but regarded as inadequate, or where it has decreased in size with age.

The operative indication and its technical performance should not view the problem as simply one of providing supplementary volume; once again, container and content are indissolubly linked, and it would be a mistake, penalised by an unsatisfactory result, to treat this aspect in isolation without incorporating it into the wider context of the state of the skin envelope, which may require an associated procedure, of thoracic morphology and general body build, and of course of the patient's wishes and motivations.

While in the past a number of techniques using fatty, dermo-fatty, omental or even glandular autotransplants have had their vogue, necessarily ephemeral because of the inconsistency of the results (inadequacy of the volume obtained being the least of the complications observed), today the sole valid method for augmentation of breast size is the use of prosthetic implants. Although these have made notable progress, we shall see that no implant is yet ideal, and that in this field of breast surgery the patient must be kept fully informed.

We shall first consider the problems posed by simple augmentation with a skin envelope of good quality. The particular problems posed by secondary hypertrophy associated with ptosis will be treated separately.

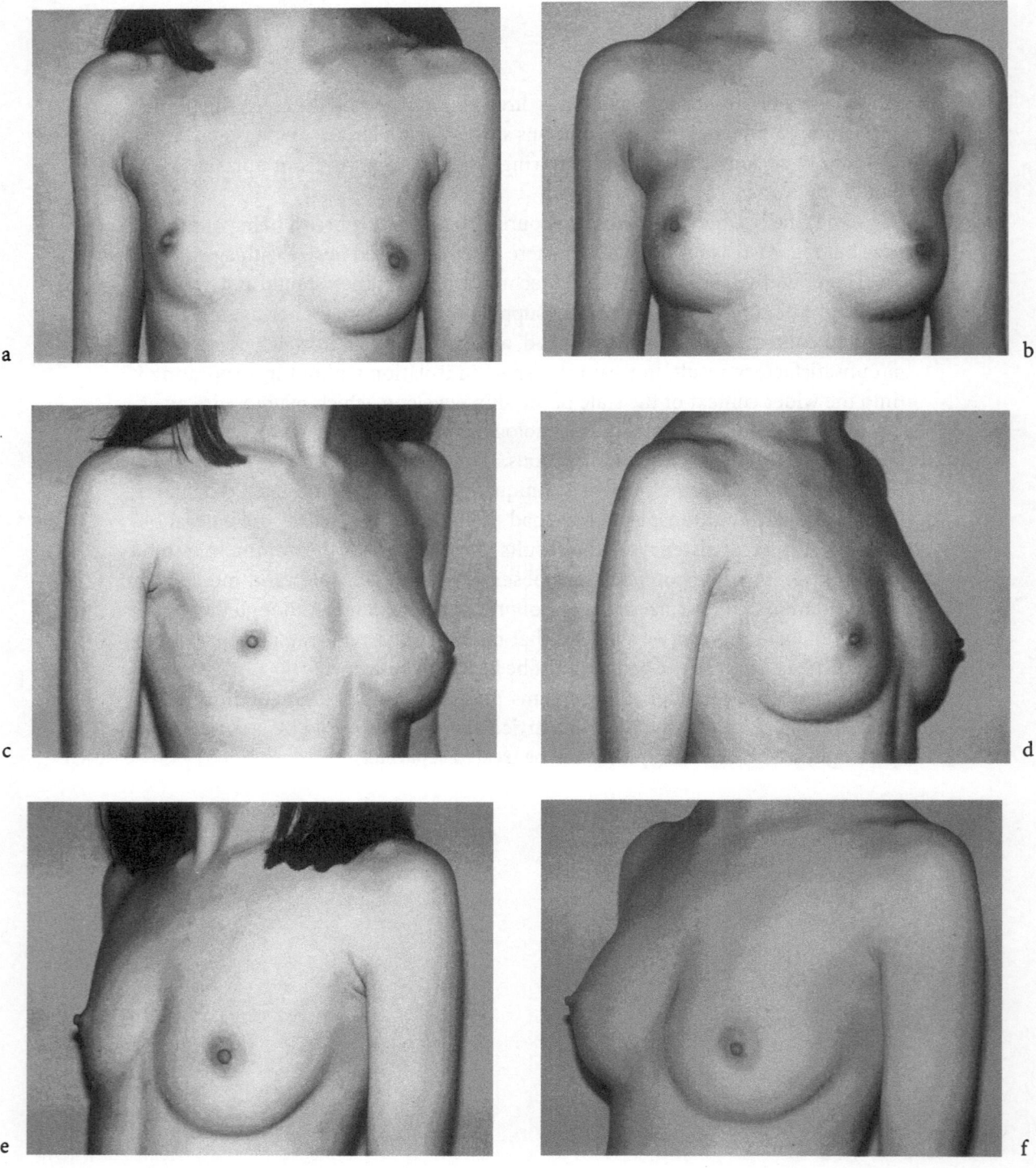

Fig. 156 a-f. Unilateral mammary hypoplasia verging on aplasia. Access: presumed level of inframammary crease in its inferolateral part, with tethering. Ist stage: insertion of a round Sigma Dow Corning expansion prosthesis with remote valve, diameter 12 cm, theoretic content 600 ml, initial filling 130 ml, final filling 250 ml. 2nd stage: replacement by a textured inflatable implant (Sebbin LS21) of 200 ml, filled with 230 ml (diameter identical with expansion prosthesis)

Definitions

Amazia

This is complete congenital absence of the breast, without any glandular component or a nipple-areolar plaque. The malformation is usually unilateral and is not accompanied by any anomaly of thoracic morphology.

Aplasia

Aplasia is characterised by absence of the mammary gland, but with the presence of a nipple-areolar plaque. However, this areola is often very small, of infantile type, smaller than that of the opposite breast which is normally developed. This malformation is actually more often also unilateral, and is unassociated with any regional malformation.

Hypoplasia

The mammary gland and areola are present, but the gland is inadequate in volume and the areola of variable size. The disorder is linked to insufficient development of the mammary gland at the time of puberty, glandular growth at this period occurring under the influence of estrogenic secretion (fig. 156). The mammary hypoplasia is usually bilateral, but may be asymmetrical.

Hypoplasia of congenital origin is to be distinguished from iatrogenic hypoplasia associated with a surgical or medical procedure in childhood, such as the drainage of an abscess or the irradiation of an angioma. The rudimentary breast is very vulnerabe, and even without having undergone obvious damage at the time the effects of injury will only become evident at puberty through absence of development of the breast.

The breast involvement in Poland's syndrome varies in extent, as do the associated lesions: hypoplasia, aplasia and even, more rarely, amazia. Agenesis of the sternocostal head of the pectoralis major is virtually constant, and the pectoralis minor is more or less involved as are the upper dentations of the serratus anterior. There may also be a thoracic depression due to hypoplasia or agenesis of one or more ribs between the 2nd and the 6th (fig. 157). Finally, malformations of the fingers (brachymesophalangy, syndactyly) are common, and may or may not be associated with other and more serious lesions of the hand: "mitten hand", club-hand, etc. The malformation is unilateral.

Atrophy

Whereas hypoplasia relates to inadequate development of an organ, atrophy in the strict sense of the term is the outcome of "defective nutrition of an organ, usually leading to its failure". In mastology, this term is therefore reserved for secondary decrease of the size of the breast. This is a consequence of changes in the mammary gland with age, and may be exacerbated by various factors such as weight-loss and especially by pregnancy and lactation, which are secondarily responsible for breast collapse of varying degree in different patients.

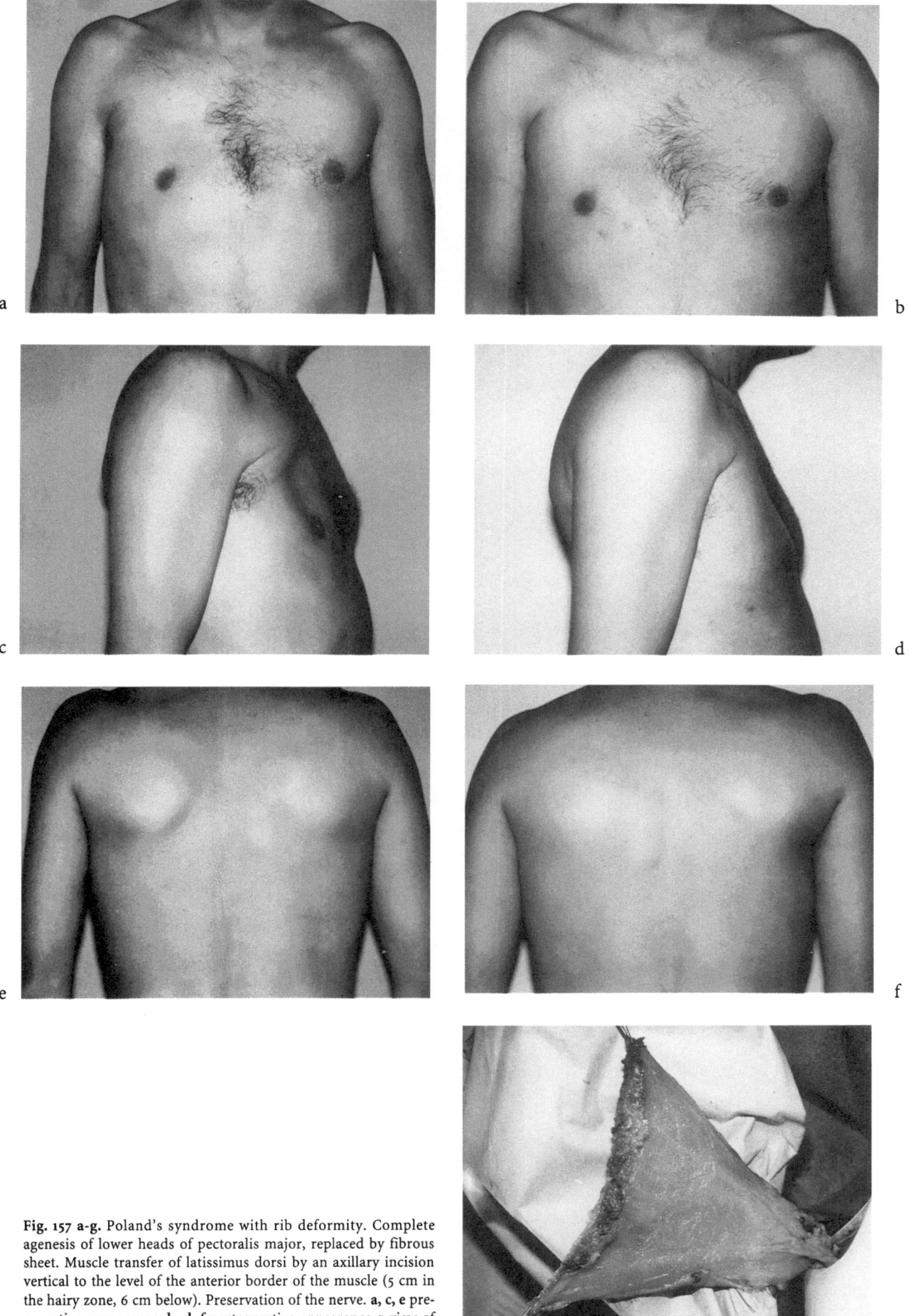

Fig. 157 a-g. Poland's syndrome with rib deformity. Complete agenesis of lower heads of pectoralis major, replaced by fibrous sheet. Muscle transfer of latissimus dorsi by an axillary incision vertical to the level of the anterior border of the muscle (5 cm in the hairy zone, 6 cm below). Preservation of the nerve. **a, c, e** preoperative appearance; **b, d, f** postoperative appearance **g** view of muscle and vascular pedicle

Physiopathology

Explanations of these malformations can be no more than hypotheses, supported by our knowledge of embryonic development:

To explain amazia, it may be supposed that the mammary ridge has developed normally, but that its regression has also involved the rudiments of the 4th pair, which would seem more likely than that the mammary ridge has not developed at all due to ectodermal agenesis.

In mammary aplasia, the rudiments of the 4th pair are normally persistent, but development is arrested at the time of proliferation of the lactiferous sinuses.

Hypoplasia could be due to an anomaly of development at various stages, either as arrested development during the third trimester of pregnancy, or as growth disturbance at the time of puberty; when puberty is otherwise normal, this suggests the idea of an abnormal tissue hormonal receptivity. But all this is only hypothetical, especially as a certain number of breast hypoplasias are seen in tall slender women of rather masculine build, in whom pubertal hormonal secretion may have been disturbed.

In Poland's syndrome, for lack of an etiologic hypothesis, there is a more precise idea of the time of appearance of the anomaly, since it is known that the middle phalanges and the pectoralis major differentiate at the 46th day of embryonic development, which also corresponds to the period of development of the mammary ridges, which appear at the 6th week. Development of the sternocostal head of the pectoralis major, the pectoralis minor and most of the intrinsic muscles of the hand depends on the metamere D1, which explains why the anomalies are associated, whereas the clavicular head of the pectoralis major, like the latissimus dorsi muscle, depends on metamere C6 and is therefore spared.

Clinical examination

Analysis of breast size

Rather than measurement of volume alone, which is insufficient or may be considered as such, study should be devoted to the distribution and thus the shape of the breast, study of shape being inseparable from that of content.

The volume may be at the lower limit of normal, obviously hypoplastic, or even completely absent.

The shape of the breast may be slightly conical, with a very reduced base of implantation, or may correspond, when the gland is more spread out, to part of the circumference of a sphere. The breast may be reduced to a retroareolar disc, leading in the worst case to areolar prolapse. In this particular malformation the areola, whose size is disproportionate in relation to the rest of the skin envelope, is as if "blown up" by the gland, which exists virtually only immediately behind it. The skin envelope seems to retract to the periphery of the areola, segments II and III being short and concave.

This malformation further poses difficult problems in treatment, since it is necessary to consider both enlargement of the breast base and global augmentation of breast size, the latter being the easier to resolve by means of an implant, and especially to reduce the size of the areola and its prolapse by a periareolar reduction procedure involving skin and gland. The principle of this is simple enough, but in practice permanent stabilisation of the shape and size of the new areola is a difficult matter (fig. 158).

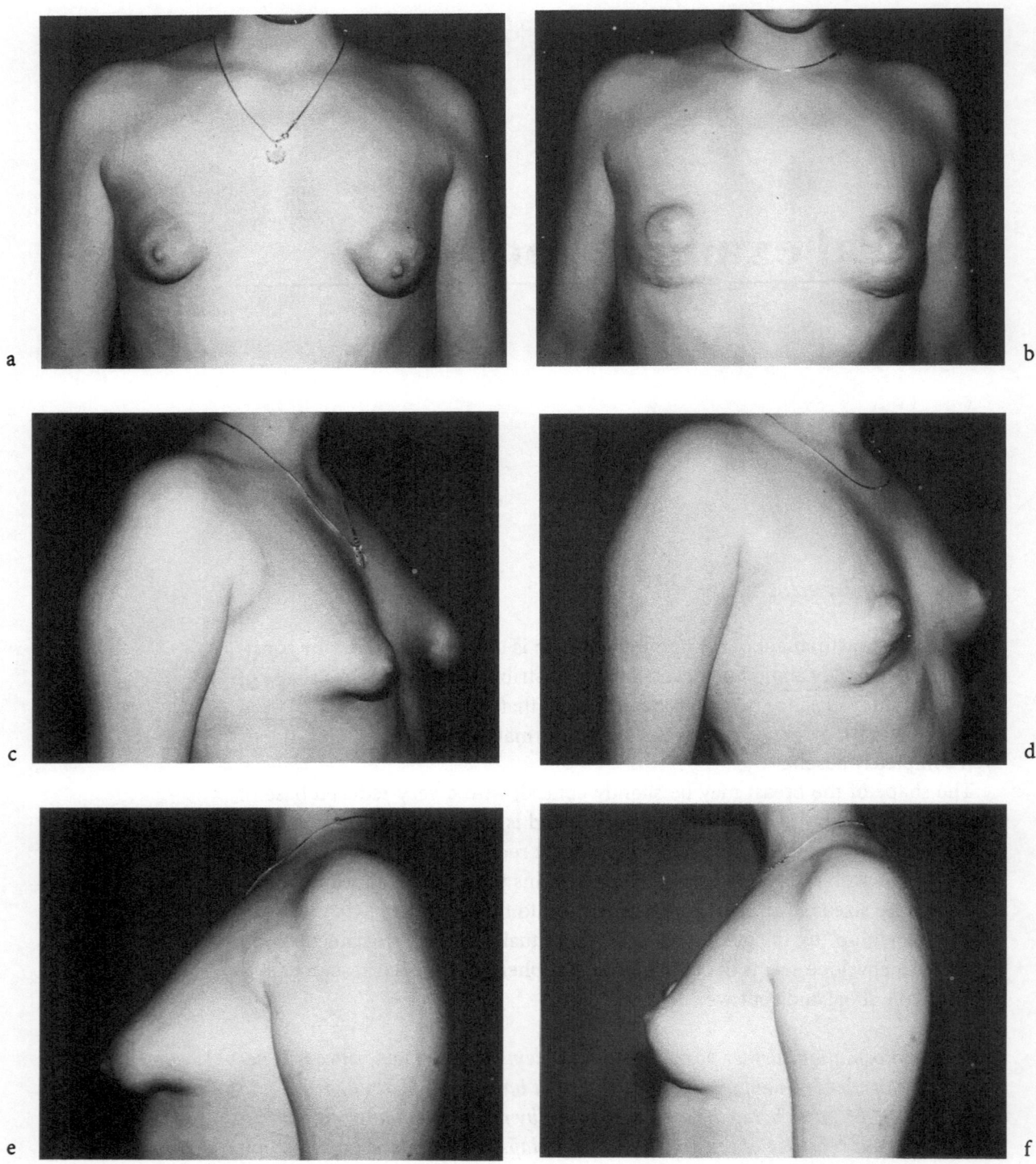

Fig. 158 a-f. Areolar prolapse: correction by periareolar embedding, the balance between the two circles being restored by a vertical triangular excision at the lower apex ending in the inframammary crease. Breast volume somewhat inadequate (patient declined an implant)

Analysis of content

In simple hypoplasias and atrophies, without ptosis, the skin is supple and of good quality and uniform thickness since it has not undergone previous stretching.

In aplasia and in Poland's syndrome, the skin may be tautly stretched on the thorax and not very mobile on the subjacent plane.

This factor must be properly assessed, since if the skin cover is not supple enough it will not allow stretching at a single stage, and will require resort to a procedure of cutaneous expansion. When associated with a muscular deficit, the lack of thickness will raise the supplementary indication for lining by a muscle layer, the better to isolate the implant from the superficial layers.

Certain measurements must be made starting from the areola, since they will determine the choice of implant (volume and diameter) and the route of access (fig. 159).

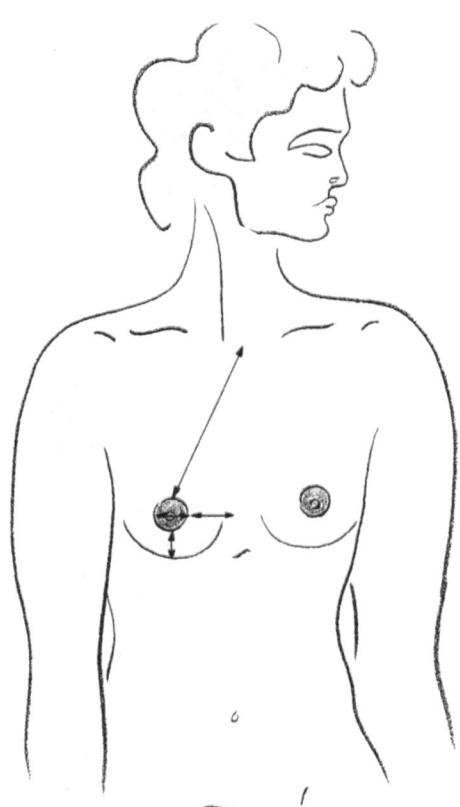

Fig. 159. Analysis of envelope: measurements

These are:
- the diameter of the areola, and
- its distance from:
  - the suprasternal notch,
  - the midline,
  - and the inframammary crease, which should also be noted as well-defined or not (fig. 160).

The choice of diameter of implant, which will in great part determine the breast volume, depends on these measurements. For the result of a mammary implant to be cosmetically satisfactory, the implant must recreate the normal breast base and must be centered in relation to the areola. If the areolae are divergent, which usually corresponds to a rib cage facing outward on a conically shaped thorax, the breasts will also be divergent (fig. 161). The patient should be forewarned, as it is not permissibve to try to juggle with the position of the implant relative to the areola. Nothing is uglier than an implant which is eccentric in relation to the areola because it is badly placed and too small in diameter.

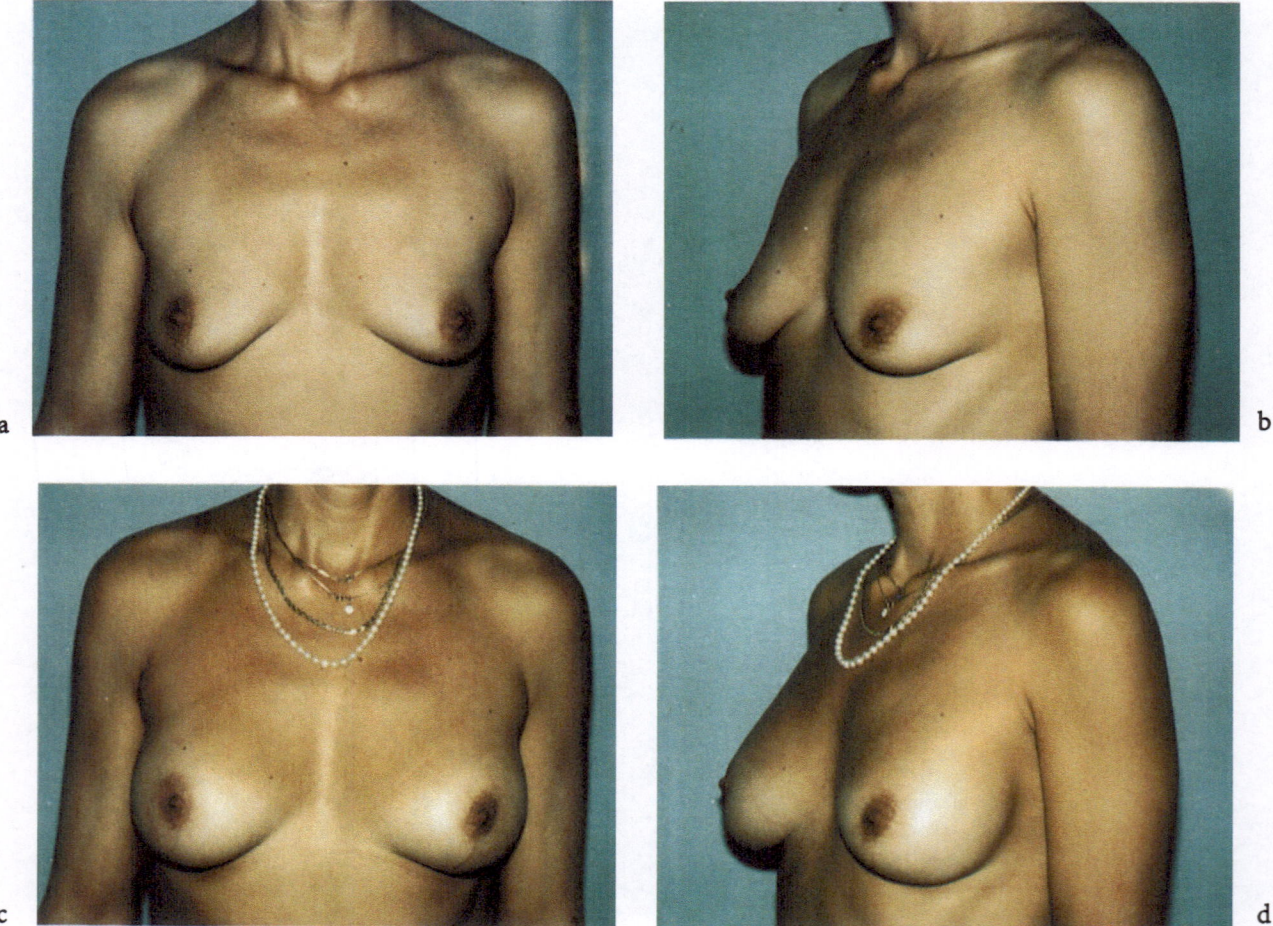

a b c d

Fig. 160 a-d. Mammary atrophy: inframammary creases at same level but distance between the lower border of the areola and the crease 5.5 cm left and 6.5 cm right. Insertion of textured inflatable implants (Sebbin LS21) of 175 ml, filled to 200 ml, by the inframmmary route with skin resection in horizontal crescent of 1 cm on the right to restore the balance of the subareolar distance

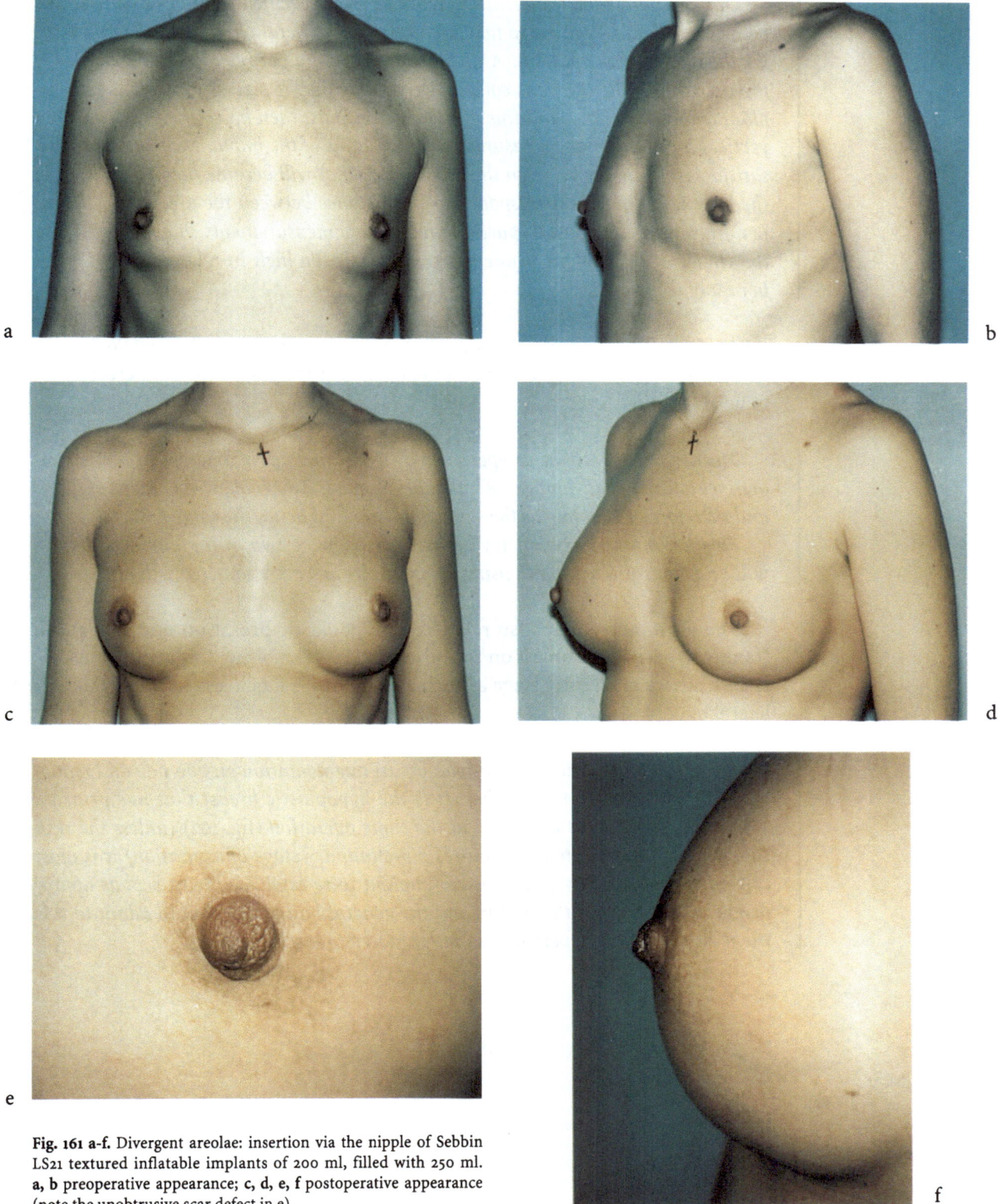

Fig. 161 a-f. Divergent areolae: insertion via the nipple of Sebbin LS21 textured inflatable implants of 200 ml, filled with 250 ml. **a, b** preoperative appearance; **c, d, e, f** postoperative appearance (note the unobtrusive scar defect in e)

One should rely on the measurements we have specified for the "ideal operated breast", without forgetting to take account of the general physique and in particular the height of the patient. A distance of 4 to 5 cm between the lower border of the areola and the crease is correct. Depending on the size of the areola, the implant chosen will have a radius of 5 to 7 cm. It must then be verified that this first vertical inframammary measurement (the radius of the implant) corresponds to a satisfactory distance between the areola and what will become the medial limit of the breast, ie that this corresponds to the distance between the areola and the inner ends of the intercostal spaces. Finally, these measurements should not lead to the choice of an implant whose upper border is too high in relation to the lower border of the clavicle.

Any asymmetry of size between the two breasts should be checked. When such asymmetry is related to bilateral hypoplasia, it is not rare for both creases not to be at the same level.

The asymmetry will be compensated by using implants of different sizes. This underlines one of the advantages of inflatable implants, which allow variations of filling and therefore of volume, for the same diameter and hence the same breast base.
Further, marked asymmetry of level between the two inframammary creases will be a contraindication to using the crease as an access route, as will be seen.

The asymmetry may also relate to a hypoplastic breast on one side and a frankly hypertrophic breast on the other. Patients exhibiting this anomaly usually seek advice at an early stage as such asymmetry is much less tolerable than bilateral hypoplasia.

The surgical procedure is two-fold: breast augmentation on one side and reduction of hypertrophy on the other. It is the hypoplastic breast that has priority. When both procedures are made at the same operation (fig. 162) (unless the skin substance is inadequate and requires a preliminary stage of expansion) it is most convenient to begin by inserting the implant to re-establish breast size as appropriate to the shape of the thorax and the general build, and then to adapt to this the reduction of the hypertrophic and/or ptosed breast.

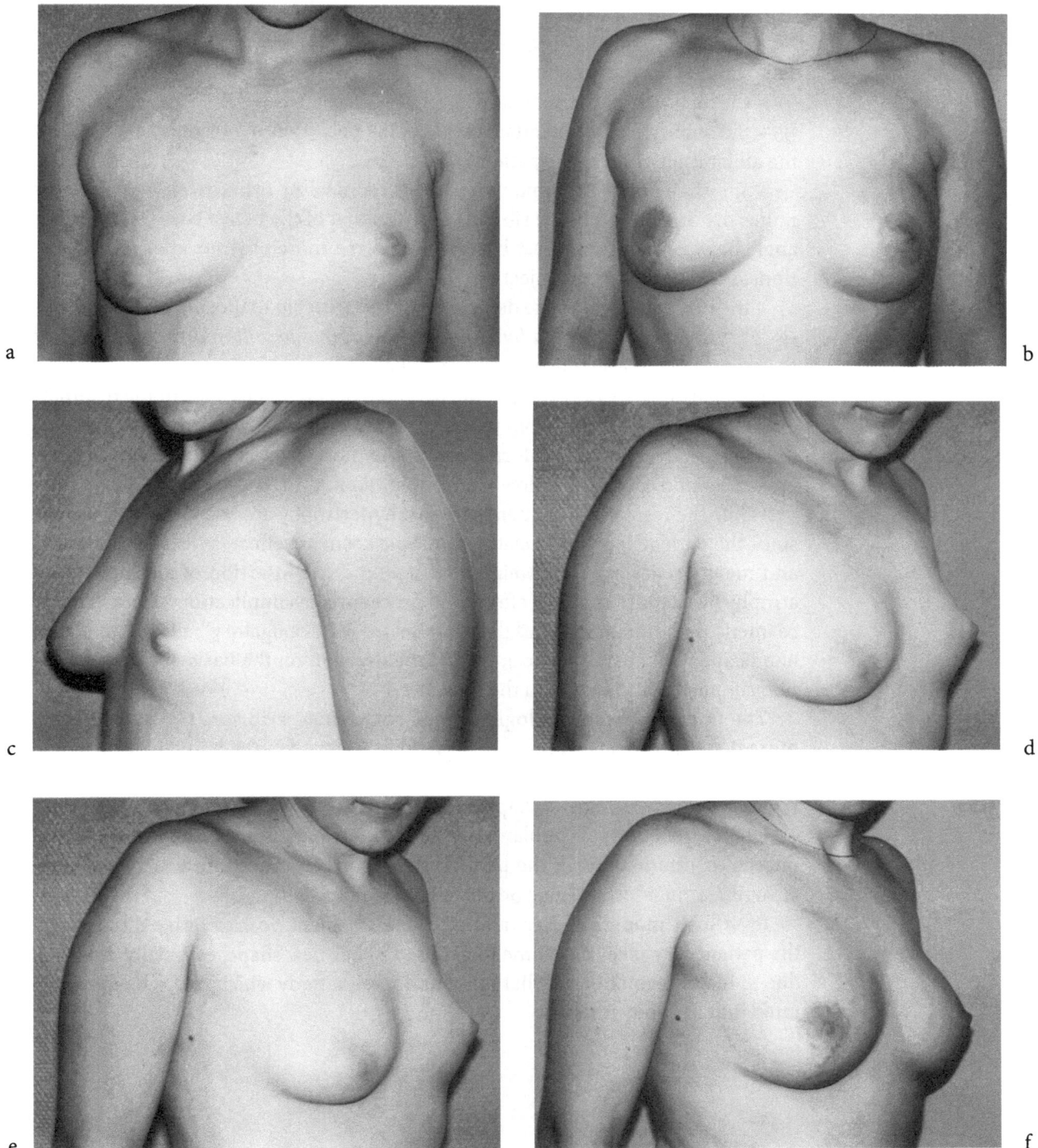

Fig. 162 a-f. Breast asymmetry: right, insertion by inframammary route, after preliminary expansion, of an inflatable implant of 150 ml filled with 170 ml of normal saline; left, mammoplasty with skin reduction. Size of left areola increased by tattooing

Overall analysis

This should take account of:
- the thickness of the subcutaneous fatty layer;
- the quality, shape and attachments of the pectoralis major muscle (as well as the athletic activities of the patient);
- the shape of the thorax, whether flat, conical or cylindrical, which determines the orientation of the rib cage and also that of the breast base. The varying angle between the two breast bases will become more obvious after augmentation, as will the anterior projection;
- the presence of thoracic deformity, linked with rib malformations or agenesis, *as this may necessitate a bulking-out procedure and will in any case influence the orientation or even the positioning of the implant.*

It will also assess the extent of the psychological repercussions of the disorder, as the patient will require from the surgeon not only, as always, the most complete and objective available information in the most accessible language, but also great attention especially following the operation.

While the results of treatment of breast hypertrophy are usually well accepted, since the patient soon appreciates, if not the cosmetic effect, at least the physical and mental relief from the weight and ugliness, the insertion of an implant for atrophy has a more complex effect. The procedure has implications that are more cosmetic than functional, and therefore seems less "obligatory"; the preoperative handicap is only psychological, so that the decision on the basis of the information supplied rests more with the patient.

The immediate morphologic change sometimes surprises the patient even more than she expected, and is not as readily accepted in the immediate postoperative period as one might have expected, even if the result is considered to be very satisfactory as regards shape and size.

One of the effects of implant insertion for atrophy may be the emergence of internal contradictions in the patient, since this is a procedure which produces an artifical "plus" which may be perceived as unwanted.

Even with moderate sizes, and after the transient postoperative discomfort, the patient may take some time to get used to her new shape, especially as this is due to the implantation of what remains a foreign body which has to be incorporated into the body image.

Supplementary investigations

The preoperative assessment is that of any surgical procedure: biochemical work-up, thrombo-elastogram, chest radiography, ECG, etc.

The clinical study of the breast is supplemented by mammography, which is sometimes difficult to perform in major hypoplasia and may then advantageously be replaced by ultrasonography.

Breast implants

The implants currently used consist of two parts: an outer wall made of an elastomere of silicone, of varying texture, sometimes covered with other materials, and a content of silicone gel, normal saline or some other substance.

Smooth-walled implants prefilled with silicone gel

This type of implant has been in existence since the beginning of the 1960s. Current implants are characterised by an outer wall made of one or more layers of an elastomere of silicone, filled with a viscous gel comprising many short-chain molecules.

The multiplicity and varying nature of the layers of the wall (with vinyl, phenyl and fluoride chains) is directed against transudation of the gel, which is the great drawback of prefilled implants, since this leads to a more severe inflammatory reaction and may have other consequences, as will be seen.

Models vary from one manufacturer to another as regards dimensions (degree of anterior projection in relation to the base) and shape: part of the circumference of a sphere with a variable radius of curvature, or the "tear-drop", theoretically of a more natural shape but one that seems incapable of giving better morphologic results because the quality of the result remains essentially linked to the degree of periprosthetic contracture.

The incidence of such contracture is such that means of obtaining better results have been sought. These studies have taken two main directions, concerning both the content but also the container. After the rapid recognition that factors favoring transudation of the gel (thinness of the wall and fluidity of the gel) resulted in a higher incidence of periprosthetic contracture, attention was directed to making implants with thicker walls and more viscous gel.

Another stage was reached some ten years later by modification of the texture of the outer wall of the implant, as will be shown.

Smooth inflatable implants

The first model of inflatable implant, Arion's prosthesis, was developed in 1965. Currently, the outer envelope is made of a relatively thick layer of an elastomere of silicone, thicker than that of most prefilled implants, and has a device allowing refilling which is usually a valve with a diaphragm situated at the middle of its anterior aspect (fig. 163).

These inflatable implants were initially smooth but are now available in a rough or textured version; these last forms are of recent development and seem to have markedly decreased the incidence of periprosthetic contracture.

Models vary between manufacturers, their bases being of differing extent for the same volume. For this reason we have criticised many models for having a base insufficiently extensive in proportion to their anterior projection, the shape being too approximate to a hemisphere, and this is a particularly sensitive problem in the context of breast reconstruction and in major hypoplasia. Our own preference, among the implants studied, is accorded to those whose base is relatively spread out in relation to their anterior projection, without being unduly flattened, and in which the suppleness of the elastomere of the wall allows some degree of freedom in filling.

The advantages of inflatable implants are based on the possibility of using a small surgical approach, so decreasing the scar defect in the cosmetic context, since the implant is inserted deflated, and with some degree of freedom as regards the filling, and therefore the global volume and anterior projection for a given diameter (facilitating the compensation of an asymmetry for the same diameter); also there is the assurance that the content is perfectly harmless.

However, care must be taken never to under-inflate an inflatable implant, since insufficient filling increases the risk of leakage from the valve and the development of creases, which give a palpable wavy sensation if the pre-implant tissues are not thick enough and at which the wall will suffer wear and risk perforation in the more or less long term.

The chief disadvantage of inflatable implants is precisely this risk of deflation, which may have several causes, and whose incidence is on average 2.5% per year depending on the series reported.

Deflation of an implant is certainly a very unpleasant event for both patient and surgeon, but is not serious apart from its psychological effect and the need to reaccess its compartment to replace it, which can often be done via a short incision under neuroleptic analgesia. We consider this risk as not comparable with that which may attach to prefilled implants as regards both complications and the

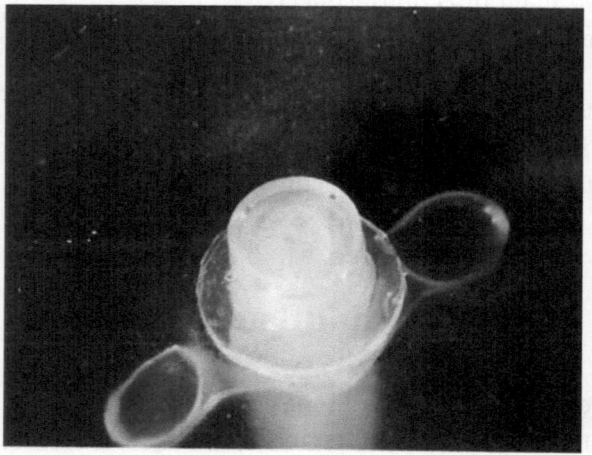
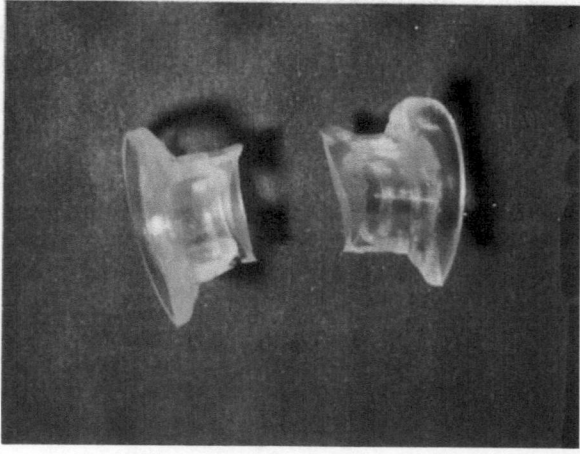

a   b

Fig. 163 a, b. Valve with diaphragm of Sebbin inflatable implant, seen from within and in section

risks associated with their content. Normal saline is immediately absorbed and eliminated, the more so since the problem is rapidly recognised. On the contrary, silicone gel can rapidly provoke a serious local inflammatory reaction, which is more damaging, especially if rupture of the implant is not recognised until changes in its shape occur as the gel starts to migrate. And this is only the beginning of the problem, since it is extremely difficult, or even impossible, to get rid of all the gel thus disseminated, and the tissues retain some inflammatory "memory" of the occurrence, which complicates and limits any reshaping procedure.

Deflation may be due to a problem with the valve, ie malfunction due to defective centering or poor closure of the valve by the plug of the protective tongue. This plug, which the surgeon must ensure is put in place after removal of the filling catheter, has no other function than to prevent the entry of connective tissue into the well of the valve and, by its proliferation, pressing on the diaphragm and promoting leakage.

Other causes of deflation relate to the envelope. Perforation of the wall may be due to damage to the implant during its insertion or, more rarely, to a manufacturing fault, so that the surgeon must check the implant by preliminary filling before its insertion into the body, a procedure that also serves to expel the air contained in the prosthesis.

Causes of perforation that may be regarded as iatrogenic are very uncommon: inopportune puncture to evacuate an effusion (a procedure obviously contraindicated), even perforation inflicted by the patient herself. We have personal knowledge of a case, in a patient who wanted breast augmentation but did not accept the result (though the size was only moderate). She had decided to decrease the size of her implants herself by puncturing them with a syringe and needle; what is astonishing is not that the implants evidently continued to diminish in size after the initial puncture, but that this decrease became stabilised after a few weeks!

Damage to the envelope (careless stretching during insertion, scratching by an instrument or the butt of a needle) may result in partial lesions that are not evidenced by perforation or tearing until after some weeks or months. This mechanism is certainly not specific to inflatable implants, but it is with these that the loss in size is seen most rapidly because of the rapid absorption of the normal saline, unlike the gel which remains in place (in the absence of secondary distal migration) and which poses other problems, as will be seen.

It is therefore important to be particularly careful to insert the implant in an atraumatic manner, without contact with an instrument (forceps, retractor, etc.) and to pay close attention at the stage of suture of the compartment.

There remain perforations of the envelope due to wear and tear, which are much the commonest. These are associated with the presence of creases, due to insufficient filling, or to periprosthetic contracture, or to wear of the prosthesis at its margins. These last causes should be eliminated with advances made by the manufacturers: the use of elastomeres more resistant to mechanical wear, reinforcement of thickness at the margins, increased security of the valve.

There is a final cause of deflation, often only partial, for which there is currently no satisfactory solution. The silicone elastomere that constitutes the wall of the implant may be to some extent considered as a semipermeable membrane, allowing the passage of substances with a molecular weight of less than 15,000. Evidently, water and salt traverse this barrier. Any excess pressure within the implant in relation to the external environment constituted by the body (due to over-filling or especially to increased pressure from periprosthetic contracture) will lead to an escape of fluid towards the exterior until a pressure equilbrium has been reestablished. Therefore a search has been made for substances to replace normal saline, with a molecular weight high enough not to traverse the wall. None of these agents has so far proved really satisfactory since, while their molecular weight for all its constituent molecules must exceed 15,000 not to pass the barrier, it must also be perfectly biocompatible and biodegradable (in case of accidental rupture), nontoxic, and yet have a molecular weight less than 40,000 so that it may be excreted if need be by the kidney to prevent its accumulation at various sites. Substances that have been tried and abandoned include macromolecules of glycide type, such as dextran, and the polyvinylpyrrolidones of a molecular weight above 40,000.

The future of inflatable implants certainly depends on the search for such a substance, which must satisfy the following requirements:

– nontoxicity, absence of provocation of an inflammatory reaction on tissue contact with the substance,

– biodegradability,

– possible excretion in the event of implant rupture or leakage,

– chemical purity,

– molecules of identical weight,

– negligible or no leakage

– a viscosity sufficient to guarantee the implant an agreeable consistency,

– and possibly the prevention of perforations of the envelope by lessening the formation of creases.

Prefilled implants covered with polyurethane

The first of this new generation of implants appeared at the beginning of the 1970s, the aim as initially stated being to diminish the risk of displacement of the implant on the thoracic wall by virtue of the adhesions provoked by its rough surface. But it was not until the 80s that they became widely used, following the publication of a series of reports giving a very large reduction in the incidence of periprosthetic contracture; this seemed due to the irregular outer structure of the implant, which disorganised the fibroblastic reaction and the orientation of collagen fibers. These implants remained however very controversial, as in some cases they led to an initial inflammatory reaction so intense that removal of the implant was necessary. Moreover, the insertion of this type of implant is awkward because it is very difficult to move it around; it is necessary to employ a technical artifice by inserting it in a plastic sac which is withdrawn once the implant is placed in good position. Finally, if it becomes necessary to remove such an implant, and as the periprosthetic tissue is extremely adherent to the implant because of the structure of the microthane, the dissection is very difficult and fairly hemorrhagic as it is calls for removal of the entire periprosthetic tissue.

Current debate on polyurethane relates to its fate, and that of the implant, after some years, since it seems that the polyurethane layer disintegrates with the passage of time, and it may be wondered what has then become of the periprosthetic membrane, whether it is stabilised, or whether there is any risk of secondary development of a contracture.

The questions posed also concern the degradation products of polyurethane, which can be carcinogenic in animal experiments, though these conditions seem remote from its use in clinical conditions. At the time of writing, the American Food and Drug Administration has suspended its wider use pending further information on the harmlessness of this product.

It may be said in conclusion that the greatest importance of implants covered with polyurethane has been to stress the advantage of roughened irregular walls compared to smooth walls in relation to the decreased incidence of periprosthetic contracture.

Prefilled implants with textured walls

The walls of these implants are made solely of silicone, but exhibit surface irregularities intended to disorganise the fibroblastic reaction by inducing a multidirectional orientation of the collagen fibers of the capsule.

The manner of treating the implant surface varies with the manufacturer, and it is too soon to say if any one procedure or type of roughness is more effective than another.

This process seems more stable with time than the addition of polyurethane, since the irregularities produced form part of the very surface of the implant and are not therefore a priori subject to disintegration and disappearance.

It will take some years, however, to confirm their superiority although the first results are encouraging; every new product usually profits from a certain indulgence and from results that are often more favorable than those shown by later studies.

Textured inflatable implants (fig. 164)

These have been developed since the improved results in the incidence of periprosthetic contracture observed with the textured prefilled implants which preceded them.

The results seem equally promising, and this is the type of implant we currently prefer.

In contrast with smooth implants, it is convenient to stress a particular technique. An implant whose surface is textured is somewhat more difficult to insert in its compartment because of the roughness of its wall, which tends to cling to the adjacent tissues, though this phenomenon is not at all comparable with what is observed with polyurethane-covered implants. Therefore more attention should be devoted than with a smooth implant to ensuring that, once the implant is inserted and filled, its base is perfectly spread out on the deep aspect of the stripping, and that there are no folds or creases on its edges or anterior surface.

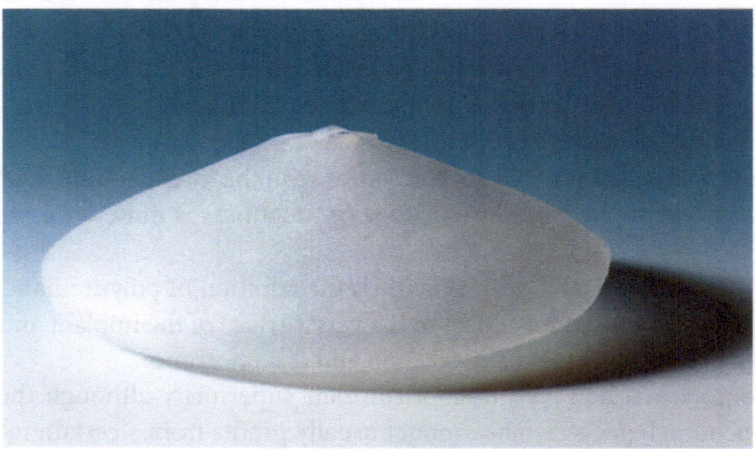

Fig. 164. Textured inflatable implant (Sebbin LS21)

Double-lumen implants

We need only say that these combine two compartments: an inner compartment made of a nucleus of silicone gel and an outer inflatable compartment furnished with a valve, or the converse arrangement: an outer layer of gel and an inner inflatable compartment. These implants seem to us to combine the disadvantages of both prefilled and inflatable implants.

Advantages and disadvantages of silicones

The particular properties of the silicones, especially their great physical and chemical stability, have long made them a material of choice in the biomedical field, a usage justified by the inertia of this class of substances. They are resistant to heat, oxidation, humidity and light.

But physical stability and chemical inertia are not synonymous with biological inertia and it is these very qualities of the silicones that are also their defects; though clinically inert, they are not biodegradable and cannot be excreted by the organism in which they are stored if there is accidental migration, unless there is a breach of the skin.

This migration of the gel if the outer wall of the implant is ruptured may be asymptomatic, but may also provoke very serious inflammatory reactions creating difficult therapeutic problems, while the accumulation of silicone particles is currently incriminated in the development of systemic reactions.

The different problems raised by the introduction of silicones into a living organism are better understood with some knowledge of their chemical nature.

Structure of the silicones

The basic structure of the silicones used in the biomedical field consists of atoms of silicon connected by oxygen bonds, and saturated usually by methyl radicals. This structure corresponds to polydimethylsiloxane, which repeats the primary

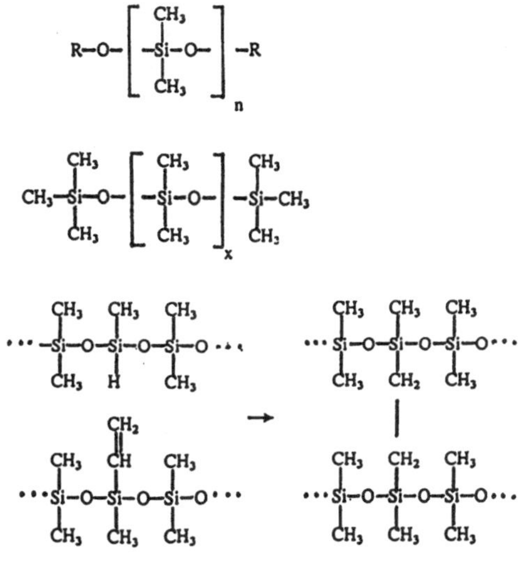

Fig. 165. Molecular structure of the silicones: above: general structure of silicone polymers most currently used; middle: structure of dimethylpolysiloxane, Dow Corning 360; below: the presence of a vinyl radical $C_2 = CH-$ allows the formation of a bond between two polymer chains

dimethypolysiloxane unit N times, where N may amount to several thousands, creating chains of varying length.

This yields the silicone oils, whose fluidity varies with the length of the chain. Chiefly used as lubricants, they have also been used by direct injection to augment breast volume. The gravity of the complications encountered has led to prohibition of such usage, but it is still used by some as injections to smooth out wrinkles.

The risk is connected with the way these oils are made, which does not secure chains of a single length; in particular, short chains persist, whose tissue toxicity is wellknown.

Polydimethylsiloxane is the basic polymer easiest to produce and the one most widely used in the construction of elastomeres of silicone. The insertion of other radicals, such as vinyl radicals, allows the creation of bonds within and between the chains in the presence of catalysts at a high temperature. These bonds give the polymer a three-dimensional structure and also its visco-elastic properties. This is how the gels such as those used in breast implants are obtained.

The more complex the bonds and the more the chains are intertwined among themselves, the greater the viscosity of the product, but the bonds between the polymers constitute only 10 to 20% of the gel as a whole, which may be considered as a network enclosing in its meshes shorter chains which are capable of migration. This tendency to migrate across the walls of prostheses may be lessened by lining their inner surface with other silicones of different solubilities.

By increasing the number of bonds between tand within the chains, complex products of increasing molecular weight are obtained which are formed by vulcanisation of elastomeres of silicone, used particularly in the manufacture of the envelopes of breast implants.

An implant is made by plunging a mold held by a mandrel into the basic silicone dissolved in a solvent. This soaking is repeated after evaporation of the solvent so as to superimpose several layers. The vulcanisation of the elastomere is performed either at a high temperature in an oven or at room temperature. The envelope thus obtained is removed from the mold, but it has a break of continuity at the junction of mold and mandrel, which is occluded by means of a lozenge of the same elastomere brazed on under heat or cold.

Finally, the silicones intended for biomedical use must not contain impurities such as antoxidants, colorants, plastifiers or catalyst residues. The final viscosity of the product depends on its molecular weight and the number of bonds: the less the viscosity, the more fluid the silicone will be and more capable of migration.

Reactions of the organism to silicones

When introduced into a living organism, the structure of the silicones is not modified because of their physical and chemical inertia. It was this absence of degradation that led to their being considered as eminently biocompatible and they have found numerous applications in the biomedical field, such as the Holter shunt used from 1955 in the treatment of hydrocephalus, various catheters for drainage of the lacrimal ducts, the restoration of patency to the urinary tact, the articular prostheses of Swanson, the outer envelope of testicular implants and breast prostheses. These implants of solid silicone may certainly fragment if subjected to mechanical constraints and repetitive movement (like Swanson's prostheses) but pose no problem of migration of the short chains contained in the silicone oils and the gel networks.

The idea of biocompatibility of the silicones must be reconsidered precisely because of what was considered as a good quality, their inertia, for it is this that renders them not biodegradable. As the organism cannot excrete them it reacts initially with a foreign-body reaction, whose consequences vary with the type of silicone present (fluid or viscous — though all viscous silicones contain some fluid — or solid silicone), exciting local, regional and even systemic reactions.

Local (foreign body) reactions

The introduction of a foreign body into the organism, of whatever nature, provokes an inflammatory response, the so-called elimination reaction to a foreign body, and this phenomenon is not, of course, specific to the silicones.

This reaction is evidenced locally, after an immediate phase of platelet aggregation, by vasomotor phenomena which promote the afflux of monocytes, macrophages and fibroblasts. The monocytes and macrophages are transformed in time into histiocytes, while the fibroblasts synthesise collagen, which becomes organised in fibers, and finally the foreign body will be completely surrounded by a fibrous membrane of varying thickness depending on the intensity of the reaction.

The periprosthetic capsule which forms around every breast implant is one example. Histologically, it has a twofold structure, which is recognisable clinically. In contact with the implant there is a fine, virtually avascular, membrane, with abundant collagen fibers oriented parallel to the surface of the implant. The second, outer, part of the membrane is richer in cells and vessels and the collagen fibers are not so oriented.

The intensity of the foreign body reaction is responsible for the morphologic fate of the implant, and hence the quality of the result. If the inflammatory reaction is low-grade, the periprosthetic membrane remains thin and supple, as it consists almost entirely of the inner layer, and the implant retains its spread-out shape and supple consistency, so that the breast has a natural shape and consistency whether there has been an augmentation for atrophy or a post-mastectomy reconstruction.

If there is a major inflammatory reaction, the periprosthetic membrane becomes thick by increase in the outer layer and tends to restrict the space available to the implant. At worst, it may become calcified.

As the volume of the implant is constant, and as the surface offered to it decreases, the breast becomes misshapen and tends to assume a spherical form, which is mathematically to be expected since a sphere has the smallest surface for a given volume; and as the content of the prosthesis, being fluid, is incompressible, this surface reduction is accompanied by an increase in pressure and the breast becomes firmer, even indurated.

Deformation and induration constitute what is, improperly, termed the "shell" phenomenon, ending in the irritating problem of the "hard breast". Though formation of a capsule is not a phenomenon specific to breast implants, since it is a general reaction directed against all foreign bodies, periprosthetic contracture is seen exclusively with these, since they are supple implants and it is desirable that they should retain this suppleness under all circumstances.

However, the problem of periprosthetic contracture is still not very well understood as not all the factors involved are known. Apart from a postoperative hematoma or an infection, these factors include the nature of the content of the prosthesis and the texture of its outer wall.

No prosthesis is perfectly impermeable because of the nature of the silicone elastomere composing its wall, even with the inner lining devices now employed.

This is verifiable by observing what happens in the open air. An inflatable implant will have its aqueous content evaporate in a few months, at a varying rate depending on the ambient humidity, and ends by containing only crystals of sodium chloride. A comparable phenomenon occurs with implants prefilled with silicone gel. Placed on a blotter, and after a variable period related to the quality and thickness of their wall, they leave a clearly visible imprint due to the "perspiration" of the gel.

Exchanges take place between the organism and the content of the implant through the meshes of the network of the elastomere which constitutes its wall and which acts rather like a semipermeable membrane. When the content consists of normal saline, the exchanges relate to substances normally present in the body and do not give rise to secondary inflammation. This is not the case with prefilled silicone gel implants, where the short chain molecules migrate and are themselves considered as foreign bodies since they are not biodegradable. It has to be borne in mind that it is these short chains which induce the most severe inflammatory reactions.

It has been shown that inflatable implants induce significantly less periprosthetic contracture than do standard implants prefilled with gel, a study made with adequate follow-up but at a time when prostheses with "anti-leak" layers did not yet exist. Moreover, in the periprosthetic membrane there can be found optically empty droplets (because of the solvents usually employed), surrounded by histiocytes and giant cells, and it can be shown by using other fixation techniques that these correspond to particles of silicone liquid or gel.

The diffusion of the gel is promoted by two features of the implant: the thinness of its wall (if there are one or more layers whose nature has been slightly altered by the introduction of other radicals, this decreases the transudation of the gel) and the viscosity of the gel itself. The prostheses with a fine wall and very fluid gel which have been fashionable for some years exhibit the phenomenon of transudation most markedly, and it does seem that the incidence of periprosthetic contracture is greater when the wall is thinner, since contact between gel and organism is responsible for an enhanced inflammatory reaction (fig. 166) with formation of a thicker periprosthetic membrane.

Thus, after having at one time proposed, for rather theoretical reasons, thin-walled and therefore more fragile implants, which risked not only the problem of leakage but also a greater risk of tearing, and a very fluid gel, the combination of both factors favoring increased transudation of the content, the manufacturers have reversed their stance and now suggest implants with thicker and double or even triple walls, and a more viscous gel. Recent studies, in need of confirmation by proper follow-up, seem to show a lower incidence of contracture with the new prefilled implants with little leakage, an incidence approximating that observed with prefilled saline implants. But it remains the case that, by its very nature, the silicone of the outer wall retains a certain porosity, and that, though the problem of oozing of the silicone may certainly be diminished, it cannot be guaranteed that an implant will be completely impermeable.

The texture of the outer surface of the implant wall is also involved in the development of periprosthetic contracture. Until relatively recently, every implant had a smooth outer surface. The use since 1981 of implants with a roughened outer surface, made irregular by the addition of a layer of polyurethane, has given rise to a number of publications reporting an incidence of contracture much lower than the previous average. Since, as we have seen, there is by no means unanimity on the use of polyurethane for other reasons, the manufacturers have suggested implants with a so-called textured wall, derived from the surface irregularity of polyurethane-covered prostheses (though microscopically the two appearances are not comparable). This new type of implant, which exists in both an inflatable and a prefilled version, also seems to give much more satisfacory results with a fall in the incidence of periprosthetic contracture.

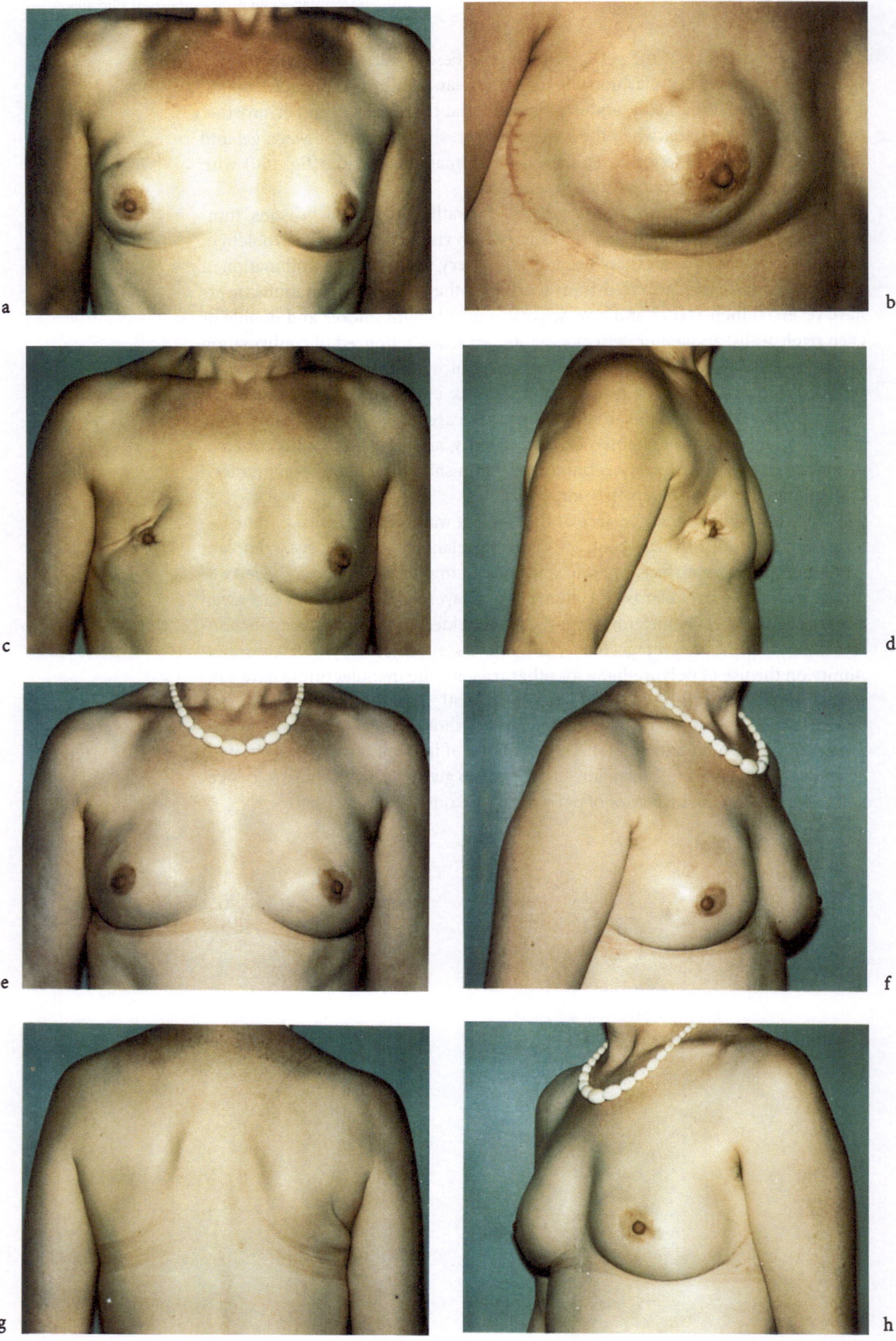

Other local problems

Besides the problems associated with transudation of the gel, other problems may arise in the event of accidental rupture of the implant, whether due to over-energetic external manipulation of the capsule intended to overcome periprosthetic contracture, or to wear of the wall at a crease.

Tearing of the envelope brings the tissues into direct contact with the gel and the outcome varies. In some cases there is an immediate and major response: a local inflammatory reaction accompanied by a painful increase in the volume of the breast, with fever and axillary lymphadenopathy. Radiologic or ultrasonic study may have already suggested the possibility of rupture of the implant and demonstrated the presence of a fluid effusion, usually sero-sanguineous, a diagnosis confirmed by surgical exposure. Surgery is of course the sole treatment applicable, with careful cleansing of the compartment as completely as possible to remove the residues of the gel. This procedure is difficult because of the tendency of the silicone gel to spread remotely and to form multiple loculations; and this usually makes it necessary, if all the residues are to be removed, to excise the periprosthetic membrane, which may be quite a hemorrhagic procedure. One can never be sure of having removed the diffused gel in its entirety, and mammography is required several weeks after the operation to check whether or not macroscopically identifiable residues have been left.

◄ **Fig. 166 a-h. a** Patient having undergone "subcutaneous mastectomy" with irradiation and insertion of implants prefilled with silicone gel; **b** appearance of inflammatory changes on right side. On exposure, the prosthesis appeared intact but its content had become yellow. Presence of a viscous periprosthetic effusion. Ablation of gel spindles and capsule difficult, with reoperation for hematoma after 24 h; **c, d** postoperative appearance: correction by transfer of latissimus dorsi muscle to isolate the implant from the superficial pectoral layer (pectoral thinned and damaged); **e, f, g, h** insertion on each side of a smooth inflatable Sebbin implant of 175 ml, filled with normal saline 300 ml right and 275 ml left. Note that the inflammatory reaction had extended to the axillary fossa, with presence of fibrous tissue impeding dissection of the subscapular pedicle

In other cases, rupture of the implant is not associated with a marked initial episode but remains completely asymptomatic until the patient or her doctor becomes worried by changes in shape or consistency, or even an abnormal radiologic appearance (multilocular appearance of the implant, double contour of the membrane, development of a periprosthetic effusion of differing density from the implant) (fig. 167). We have even once observed the development of calcification within the lactiferous sinuses, which was highly suspicious and was feared to be evidence of a malignant tumor. The diagnosis was only rectified by histologic study of the operative specimen.

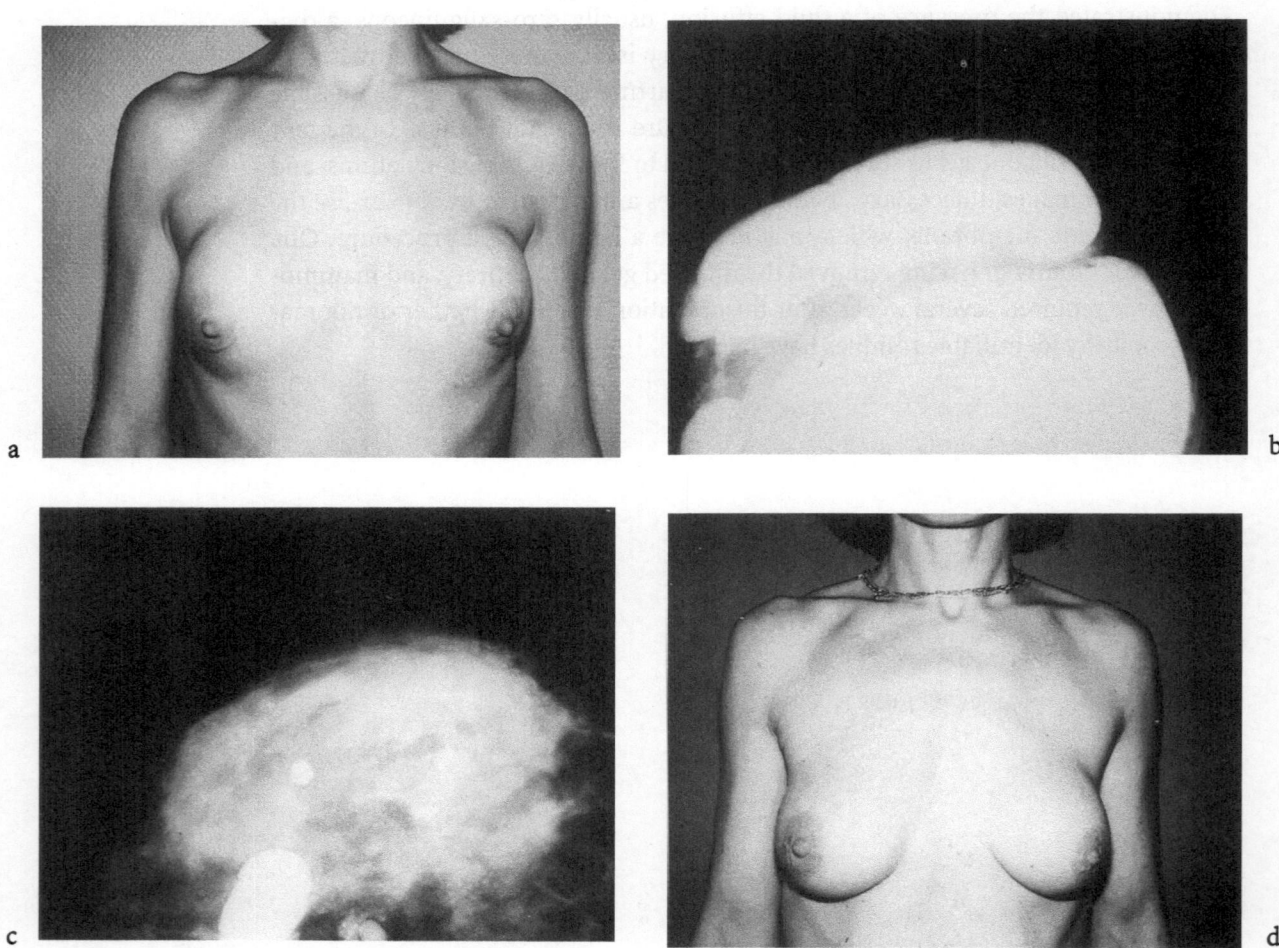

Fig. 167 a-d. a Patient had prefilled gel silicone implants 6 years ago. For two years, progressive modification of shape of left breast and deterioration of existing periprosthetic contracture; **b** preoperative mammogram identifying rupture; at exposure the implant was completely ruptured and its membrane was difficult to identify amidst the mass of gel, ablation of which was particularly difficult; **c** control mammogram at 2 months: persistence of nodules of gel; **d** after second cleansing and insertion of inflatable implants; on the side of the rupture the breast, though supple again, remains misshapen.

Regional and remote phenomena

In other cases it is not the local changes that attract attention but the development of swellings due to migration of the gel, more or less inflammatory and sometimes very remote from the implant. Such siliconomas have been noted at the sternum, the abdominal wall, the axillary fossa, the arm, and even at the elbow. A case of acute pleurisy was authenticated by aspiration, which withdrew a large amount of fluid on the surface of which there floated a fine oily layer of silicone! In some cases evident migration of the gel has occurred without actual rupture of the implant. Here again we have the phenomenon of transudation of the gel across its envelope and have to consider the problem of the fate of the silicone in the organism. The initial phase of inflammatory reaction unleashes an influx of macrophages, giant cells and histiocytes which devour the silicone particles, and these particles are then transported by these same cells into the structures of the reticuloendothelial system, where they remain permanently stored, ie in the lymph nodes but also in the liver, spleen and pancreas. This has led to the idea of a systemic pathology related to silicones, now the subject of much discussion.

Systemic problems associated with silicones

The first systemic problems were reported after massive direct injections of silicone in patients desirous of breast augmentation, or in transsexuals who had received injections into their breasts or hips. These injections have been proscribed by the FDA, but the material is still available and is widely used, even in France, in the treatment of wrinkles, admittedly in small amount but nevertheless involving direct subcutaneous injection.

Hepatic dysfunction has been reported in patients having received such injections into the breast, with silicone infiltration found at liver biopsy. One patient died suddenly after an injection of this kind, with acute pulmonary edema. The histologic studies made in a similar case showed particles of silicone in the lungs, liver, brain, kidneys, spleen and pancreas. The inflammatory reaction may result in the formation of chronic inflammatory granulomata around deposits of silicone, leading to a syndrome of hypercalcemia. This syndrome of hypercalcemia-hypercalciuria has led to the development of calcium urolithiasis in a transsexual patient who had been given silicone injections into the hips and breasts.

However, it has to be remembered that such very serious and acute accidents relate to direct injection of silicone into the organism, which is suddenly exposed to the presence of a large amount of silicone, and this should no longer occur after abandoning these techniques.

There is another pathology worthy of note, described after both direct injection and the insertion of implants, whether secondary rupture has been diagnosed or not.

These observations relate to the development of autoimmune disorders involving, in a way still poorly understood, factors of the HLA system. The first cases were described in Japan, then in the USA. These studies group pathologies related to different problems, observed not only after injections of paraffin, or of silicone of varying fluidity, but also after the insertion of implants prefilled with gel. The pathology reported is that of different collagen disorders: rheumatoid polyarthritis, systemic lupus, polymyosits, Hashimoto's thyroiditis, Gougerot-Sjö-gren's syndrome, morphea, less well-defined connective tissue inflammations and finally scleroderma. The physiopathologic hypotheses accord to silicones a role comparable to that of Freund's adjuvant (a suspension of tubercle bacilli in mineral oil), a wellknown experimental model used in the rat to provoke the de-velopment of arthritis. The latent period before development of the disease may be very long, a few months to 20 years. This syndrome has been called the "hu-man adjuvant disease:" by Japanese authors.

Since these initial studies, other observations have been reported associated solely with prefilled implants, the changes most often found being those of scle-roderma, with serologic anomalies such as the presence of antibodies. A causal relationship is difficult to prove, but it has been noted in certain cases that remo-val of the foreign material, even in one case by replacement with an inflatable im-plant, is accompanied by regression of the disease. The precise mechanism of the disorder, probably autoimmune, is still unknown but another physiopathologic hypothesis suggests involvement of degradation of silicone into silicon dioxide (SiO_2) during phagocytosis by the macrophages, the oxide itself being very anti-genic (the Erasmus syndrome). The macrophages which have absorbed the dioxide produce factors increasing the biosynthesis of collagen by the fibroblasts, which may perhaps account for the pathogenesis of the scleroderma apart from their role in producing thickening of the periprosthetic membrane.

In conclusion, there currently exist two main types of breast prosthesis: those not containing any silicone gel, ie prostheses inflatable with normal saline, and those which enclose a varying amount of silicone, ie filled prostheses with a va-ryingly thick envelope, "mixed' prostheses with an inflatable peripheral com-partment and a central nucleus of gel, or the other way round, and finally pre-filled prostheses with a polyurethane capsule. None of these prostheses, by the very nature of their envelope, can be considered as perfectly impermeable. The-refore, sooner or later they carry a risk of varying degrees of exchange of their contents with the organism, quite apart from problems of gross perforation or tearing.

In the case of inflatable prostheses, only substances normally participating in the homeostasis of the internal environment are concerned.

This is not the case for silicone gel, as we have seen. This is why, despite the criticisms that can be made of inflatable prostheses, ie the risk of deflation (less than 3% in our series), we remain faithful to such prostheses in both augmenta-tion surgery and breast reconstruction, since we are unwilling to let our patients incur the local and systemic risks of diffusion of the gel.

The different surgical approaches

The insertion of a breast implant and the creation of a compartment or pocket designed to receive it can be made through different incisions (fig. 168).

Each has its advantages and disadvantages, the aim being to perform the most atraumatic dissection possible (to eliminate one of the known factors in periprosthetic contracture), to carry out scrupulous hemostasis (hematoma formation is another cause of contracture), while allowing the introduction of an implant at the cost of minimal scar defect and without manipulation conducive to its rupture. There is a distinction here between inflatable and prefilled implants, the former being capable of insertion through a smaller access route than the latter.

In cosmetic surgery, while the surgeon's preference is fundamental, since it is based on technical arguments, attention should also be accorded within reasonable bounds to the wishes of the patient after having explained to her the advantages and disadvantages connected with each type of implant.

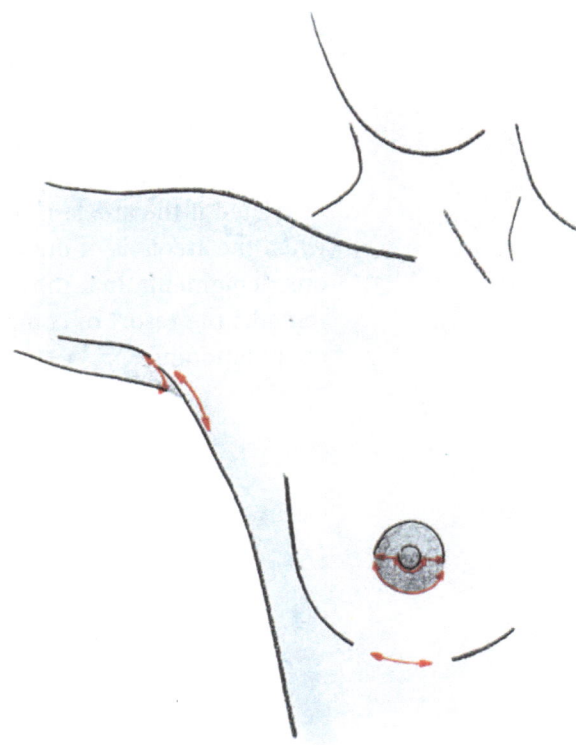

Fig. 168. The different routes of approach

Areolar approaches

These may be by an inferior alveolar route (fig. 169) or a transareolar route.

The inferior hemiareolar route is preferable to the horizontal transareolar approach when the nipple and areola are small, as it is a little longer than the corresponding transverse incision and gives a rather better exposure, facilitating dissection of the compartment, hemostasis and insertion of the implant. It is better to place the incision very slightly beyond the visible boundary between areola and mammary skin, to render the scar less obvious.

The horizontal transareolar route may either split the nipple transversely or skirt its lower half-circumference. In the first case, it is important to reappose the two halves of the nipple at their base carefully to prevent retraction and secondary deformity. For this reason, we prefer to skirt the base of the nipple, which eliminates any risk of deforming the nipple and leaves virtually no scar defect in this part of the incision.

The chief advantage of the areolar approaches is that they permit radial dissection, starting from what will correspond to the geometric center of the implant.

Via this route, the implant can be placed equally well in front of or behind the pectoral muscles. The simplest and least hemorrhagic procedure to reach the muscle after the skin incision is to traverse the gland directly down to the pectoral plane, and then to strip the upper part of the deep aspect of the gland from the muscle plane with the finger if a retropectoral position has been chosen, before the inferior inframuscular stripping which is always rather more difficult and more hemorrhagic.

If it has been decided to place the implant behind the muscle after having traversed it, it is also easier to begin the stripping with the finger behind the muscle in the upper and medial part of the compartment, as this plane is virtually avascular and easy to strip. However, care should be taken not to take the stripping too far medially, opposite the medial origins of the pectoralis, because of the presence here of intercostal perforating vessels whose hemostasis may be difficult since they retract into the muscle. The stripping is then continued downward and outward as before. It may be convenient to detach the lowest and innermost fibers of the pectoralis major to facilitate spreading of the prosthesis below and medially, which is equally easy by this approach.

The disadvantages of the areolar routes are two in number: first, access is restricted if the areola is very small, of infantile type as in the aplasias. Second, when the areola is of uniform color, both types of incision may leave very obvious depigmentation, the extent of which is difficult to predict. However, there remains the resort of compensating for such a defect in pigmentation by subsequent tattooing.

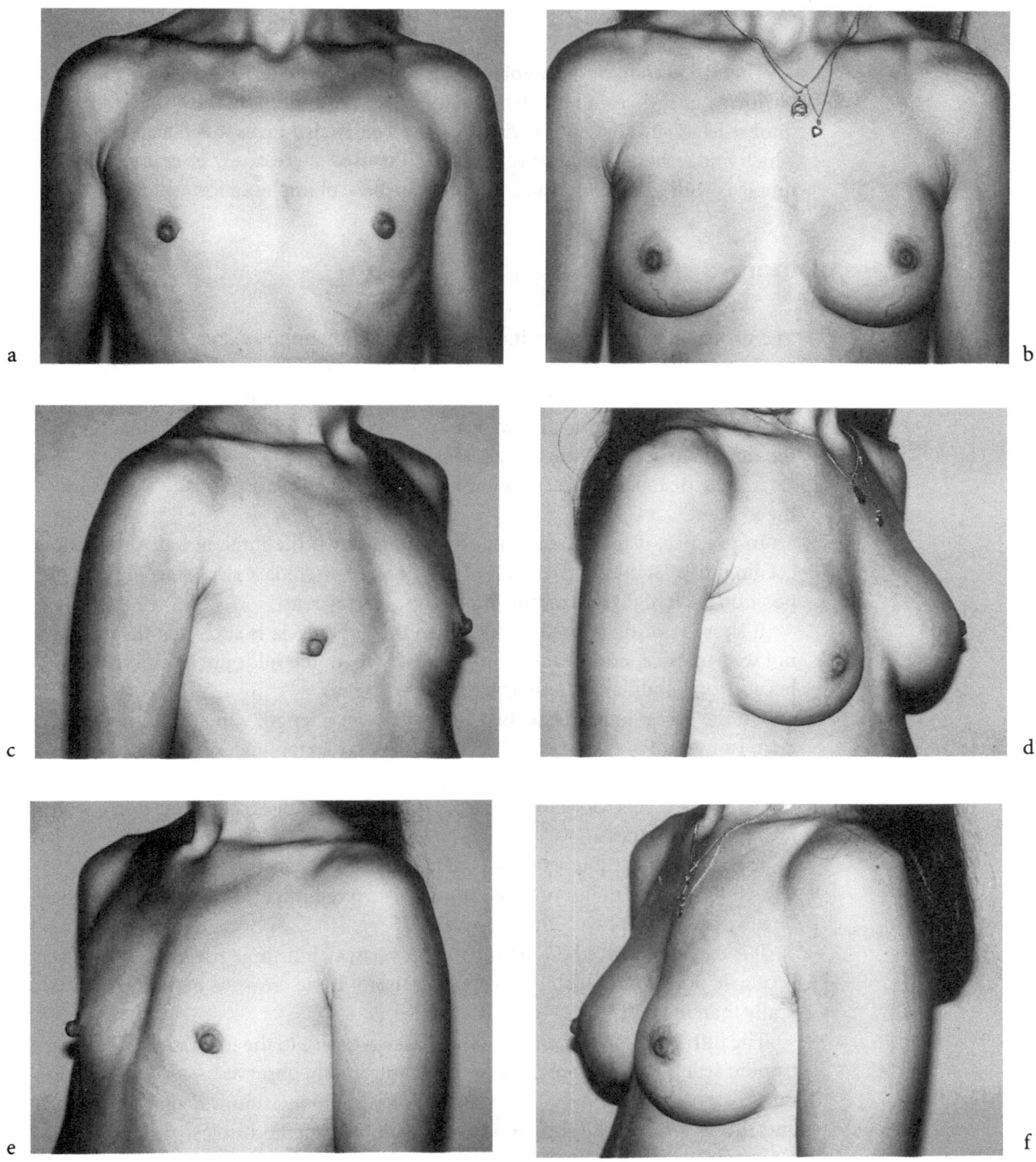

Fig. 169 a-f. Inferior hemiareolar approach. Insertion in retroglandular and prepectoral position of Sebbin LS20 implants of 200 ml filled with 295 ml. The appearance is acceptable because the skin envelope was of good thickness in the upper quadrants, but we now prefer to use the retropectoral position in cases of hypoplasia

The nipple approach (fig. 161)

This is a variant of the areolar route, but reduced to a single inferior periareolar incision. It gives a scar defect reduced to the minimum, and therefore very unobtrusive and virtually invisible. However, it also gives a reduced exposure, which makes hemostasis more difficult. It is used successfully in cases where the nipple is wide with a large and well-defined base of implantation.

The inframammary approach

The principle is to place the incision in the inframammary crease. It gives a very unobtrusive scar defect and is acceptable only provided it is placed very precisely in the crease. Therefore, in our opinion, it is to be used only:

– if the crease is fine and well-marked, but also circumscribed (this is often the case in atrophy but not in hypoplasia) (fig. 170);

– if the distance between the nipple and the fold corresponds to the radius of the implant.

In practice, if the crease is poorly defined, or if the implant has a radius exceeding the distance between areola and crease, there is a risk of seeing the scar position itself higher up on the lower slope of the breast.

It should not therefore be used when the hypoplasia is such that the crease is not well-marked, and certainly not in cases where the folds are at different levels because of glandular asymmetry.

On the other hand, it has the advantage, over a length which need not exceed 4 cm (for an inflatable implant), of allowing easy stripping, especially for the retropectoral route, and easy detachment of the innermost and lowest muscle fibers since these are very close to the access route. It gives an excellent exposure which facilitates hemostasis.

It is also serviceable when a wider approach is necessary and when it is intended to insert a bulky prefilled implant, or one difficult to manipulate as may be the case with a polyurethane implant.

It is usually centered on the subareolar vertical, but some prefer it to be a little eccentric outwards, which is particularly useful if the crease is better defined laterally than medially.

The inframammary incision sometimes gives rise to the formation of a hypertrophic scar — a phenomenon we have only rarely observed — in cases where the crease was ill-defined. This may be because the incision was not well placed, and this is a further argument for not using this method unless the inframammary crease is well-defined.

There is one precaution to be taken when starting the dissection: not to work behind the intercostal aponeurosis. Further, one must take care not to scratch the implant, which is quite close because of gravity, at the stage of closure of the compartment. If there is any doubt as to the stability of the crease, with a fear that the prosthesis may migrate downward, and in particular if one has the impression of having taken the stripping a little lower than the crease, it is possible

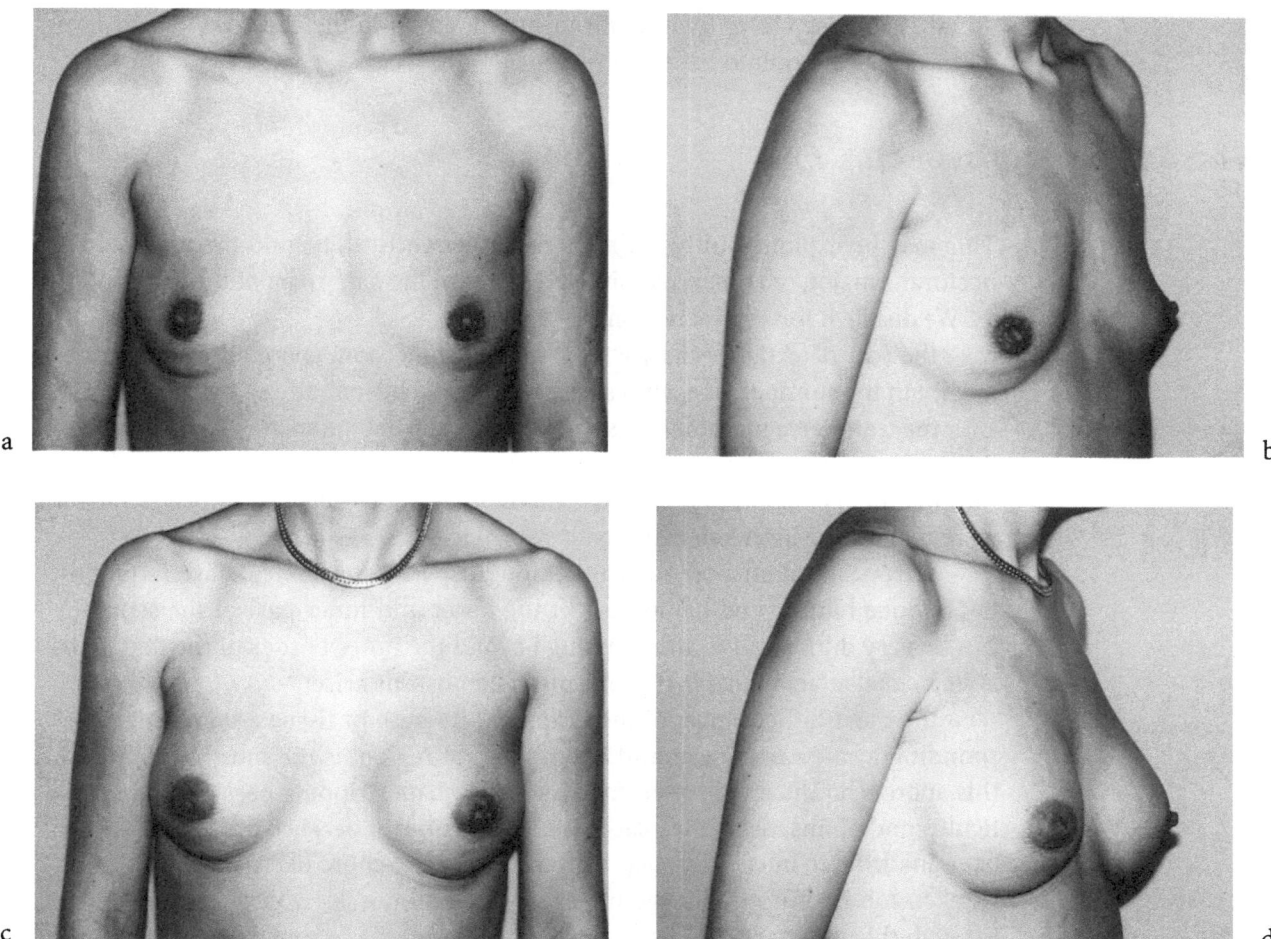

Fig. 170 a-d. Breast hypertrophy. Insertion of inflatable textured implants (Sebbin LS21) of 200 ml filled with 260 ml of normal saline in retropectoral position by inframammary route

to tether the deep layer (gland, infrapectoral fascia) to the chest-wall at the level of the crease in order to fix it.

The axillary approach

This may be exploited in two directions: either vertical, behind the fibers of the pectoralis major, or transverse, situated above in the hairy part of the axilla.

We dislike it for several reasons:

– the scar defect, especially with the vertical incision, is not altogether unobtrusive in the summertime, with sleeveless garnments or bathing costumes;

– the transverse incision necessarily crosses the hairy and sweat-gland zone of the axilla, where skin organisms are much more abundant than in the areolar or inframammary regions, and there is therefore less guarantee of asepsis, which is worrying for the insertion of a prosthesis;

– retropectoral stripping is easy (though special instruments are required), but is done blindly and hemostasis at the lower and inner part of the stripping can be very difficult. It is after passing beyond the inner border of the pectoralis at its medial attachments that problems of hemostasis arise;

– the most difficult part of the stripping, because of tissue adherence, corresponding to the same lower and outer pectoral region, is the most remote from this approach. The risk is of performing inadequate stripping because of this difficulty, and of unsatisfactory placement of the implant because the dissection has been inadequate inferiorly. Such malposition is also more likely if the dissection is taken too high up under the upper part of the muscle, which is so accessible through this approach. It is doubless for this reason that some surgeons have advised the use of considerable compression on the upper slope of the prostheses for a time to compel them to stay below the level of stripping and to prevent their ascent until the formation of the periprosthetic membrane has stabilised the position of the implant.

Pre- or retropectoral placement of the implant

Prepectoral placement

Prepectoral placement of the implant would seem at first to be the most logical, since it corresponds to a normal anatomic position of the implant, just behind the existing gland (figs. 171 and 172).

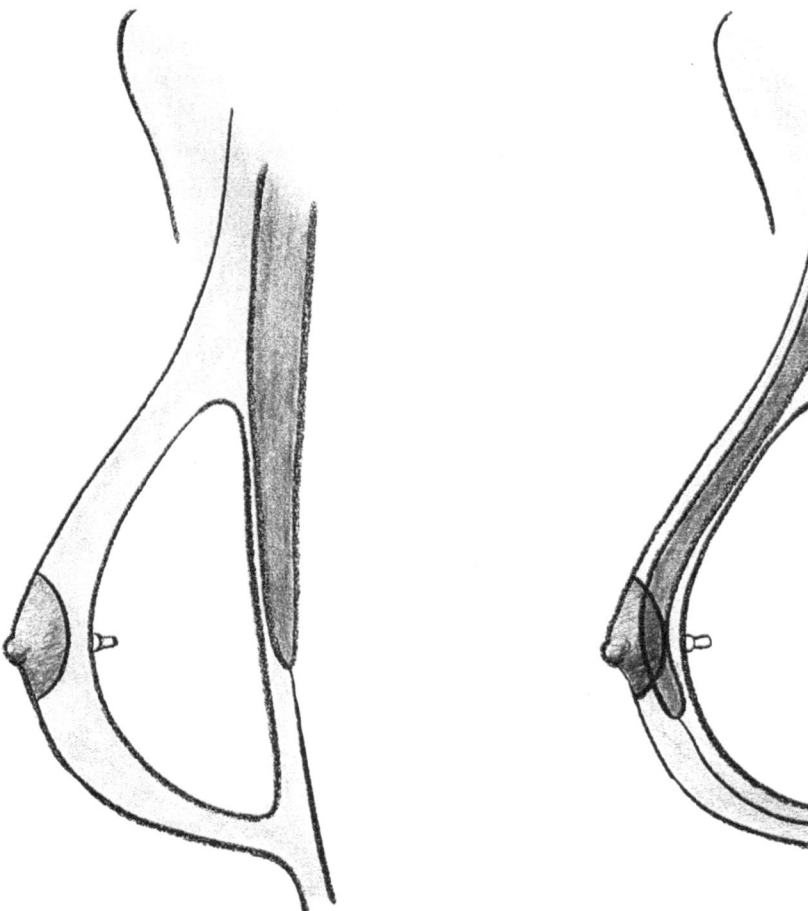

Fig. 171. Implant in prepectoral position   **Fig. 172.** Implant in retropectoral position

In practice, if the prepectoral tissues are sparse, which is the commonest case in hypoplasia, or if segment II is concave and empty of glandular tissue, as is usually found in atrophy, the contours of the implant risk being visible at the upper pole of the breast and the implant in its entirety is too easily identified on palpation (fig. 173).

A "wave effect" may also be observed if the implant is insufficiently filled and its compartment too big for it.

There is in our opinion only one preferential indication for prepectoral placement of the implant, ie when breast augmentation is for cosmetic reasons because the patient finds the volume inadequate to her liking, but when there is a certain amount of breast tissue uniformly distributed between the different parts of the breast, with skin of good quality, a normal or thick dermis, and a substantial subcutaneous fatty layer, particularly opposite what will correspond to the upper limit of the prosthesis.

Periprosthetic contracture, the risk of which can never be excluded, will be more visible and palpable if the implant is in prepectoral position.

Prepectoral stripping may also be done by the areolar route as well as by the inframammary approach. The choice thus depends on the size of the areola, the definition of the inframammary crease, the preference of the surgeon and the discussion with the patient. The axillary approach is not advised.

Retropectoral placement

The retropectoral position is the one best suited to conceal the implant from sight and touch, at least in its upper quadrants, since the breast base does not project beyond the muscle in the inferolateral quadrant and part of the inferomedial quadrant.

Therefore it is indicated when the breast is very hypertrophic, or when the fatty layer is thin under a fine skin. It is also the position of choice in the extreme situations posed by reconstruction after mastectomy and subcutaneous mastectomy.

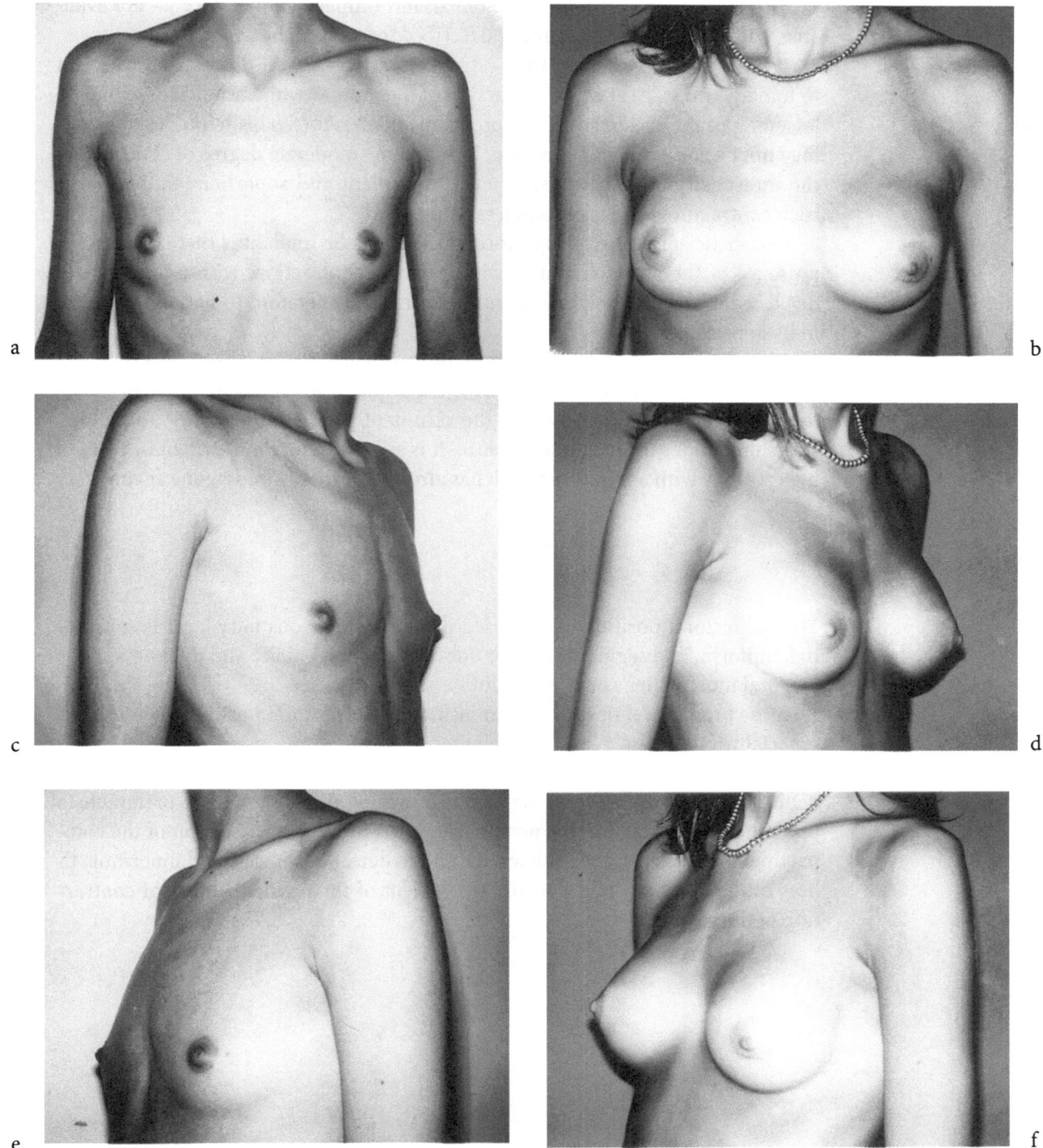

Fig. 173 a-f. Mammary hypoplasia: insertion by inferior hemiareolar approach, in retroglandular and prepectoral position, of smooth inflatable implants (Sebbin LS20) of 150 ml filled with 200 ml of normal saline.
Upper contours too visible because of prepectoral position

The three approach routes — areolar, inframmary and axillary — are available, with the implications already described for each of these.

It has been suggested that the retropectoral position of the implant causes it to undergo massage at each contraction of the muscle, which would contribute to lessening of the incidence of periprosthetic contracture. This hypothesis may or may not be correct, but in any case, for the same moderate degree of contracture, the interposition of the muscle between implant and superficial plane makes such contracture less visible and less palpable.

One criticism of the retropectoral position of the implant is that it makes the presence of the latter obvious during pectoral contraction, with a tendency to displace the implant downward and outward, and therefore to flatten the breast in its upper quadrants.

This phenomenon, which is not constant (fig. 174), is observed especially when the compartment is too large for the implant, when the stripping has been taken too far laterally, and when the skin is of poor elastic quality and allows stretching under the smallest pressure. It is seen therefore more often in cases of hypertrophy with a thin skin which has already inevitably undergone ageing.

Summary

The prepectoral position can be used if the subcutaneous fatty layer is substantial, uniform, and segment II is not unoccupied, the tonicity and thickness of the pectoral muscle then counting for little.

If the prepectoral tissues are thinnish, the retropectoral position is preferable, especially if the muscle does not seem too powerful.

The latter situation is a tricky one; the tissues are not very thick, the subcutaneous fatty layer is slight and the muscle powerful. All the same, it is preferable to place the implant behind the pectorals, but to ensure that dissection of the compartment is not taken too far laterally, and to detach the lowest and innermost fibers of the muscle, while warning the patient of the possible effects of contraction of the muscle.

Fig. 174 a-h. Mammary hypoplasia: trans-nipple approach, retropectoral placement of two textured inflatable Sebbin implants filled to 180 ml. Skin of good quality, compartment adapted to size of implant: elevation of the arms (g) and pectoral contraction (h) do not deform the breast

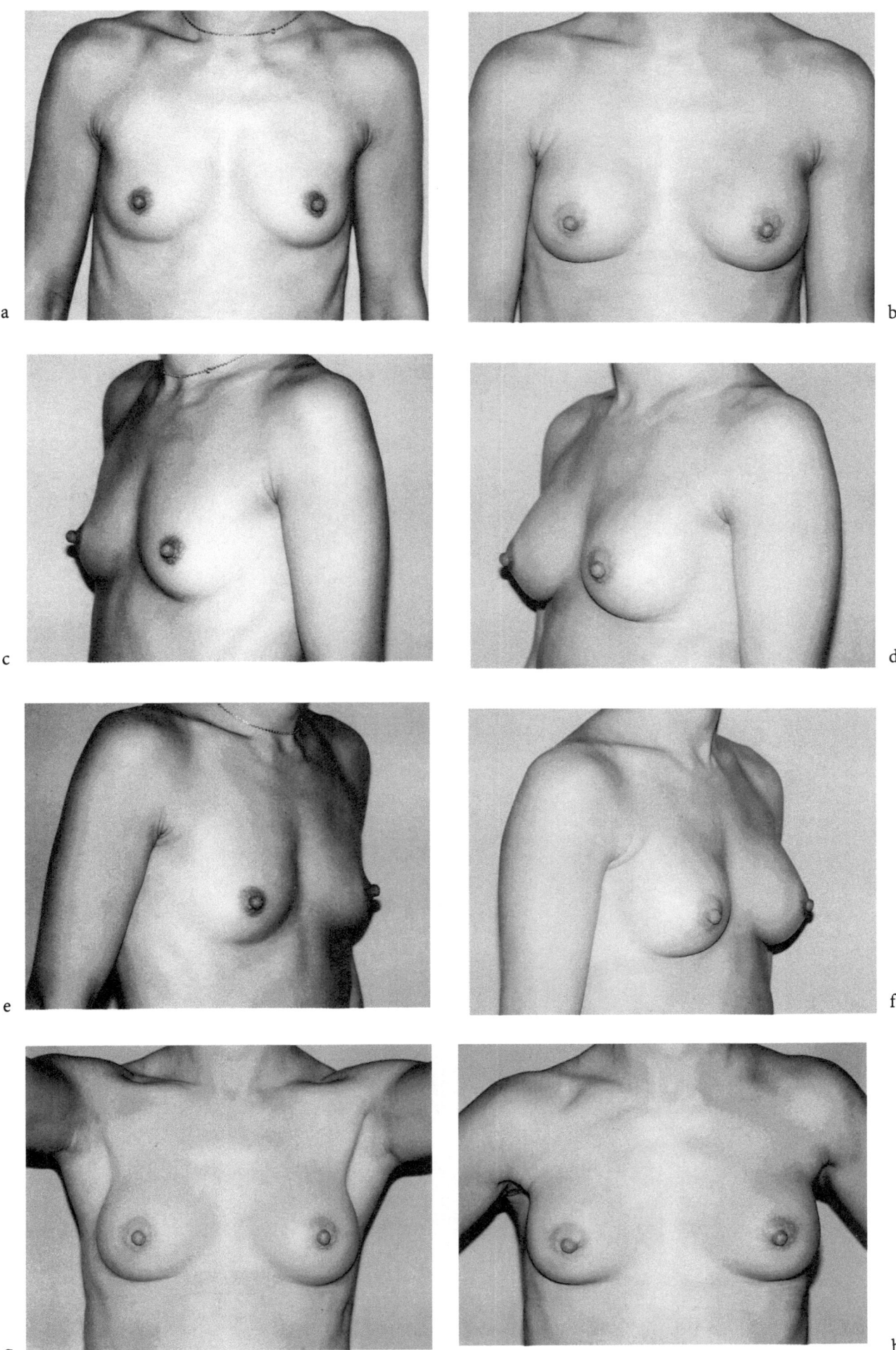

a

b

c

d

e

f

g

h

Operative technique

Strict asepsis is essential because of the introduction of a foreign body. The axillae are shaved, even if the approach is not an axillary one; the patient has a shower on the morning of the operation using antiseptic soap. We use disposable adhesive drapes which give maximum protection to the operative field. Though the no-touch technique is virtually inapplicable in breast implantation, the gloves are changed to manipulate the implant (rinsing them to get rid of any particles of talc which might excite inflammatory reaction) and we avoid any manipulations that might compromise the asepsis (removal and reinsertion of implant, undue exposure to the air in the operating room).

Finally, the anesthetist is asked to give an antibiotic injection by infusion from the start of the operation; this is the only injection unless there is a revision procedure, when antibiotic treatment is continued for three days.

Operative position

The operation is performed under general anesthesia. The patient is installed in a half-seated position, with the legs slightly raised to improve the stabilty of this position.

Landmarks

A design is made, related to the diameter of the implant chosen, centered on the nipple and exceeding the limits of the implant by about 1 to 2 cm. The compartment intended to receive the implant should not be lower than its base, for if the implant is not correctly spread out, the shape obtained will be unsatisfactory (the breast will from the outset resemble a retracted breast), and in particular the implant will form creases which predispose to fatigue of its envelope and a risk of perforation after a variable period.

Depending on the distance between the nipple and the inframammary crease, this design will descend below the latter to a varying degree. Unlike the situation in mammoplasty, where reduction of the content is essential and gives the breast its shape, here it is the content, ie the implant, which will impose its constraints on the skin by direct thrust from within outward. While it is imperative to respect the anatomic fold in cases of hypertrophy and ptosis, here this is not important since the thrust of the implant will obliterate the former crease if this is placed higher then the lower border of the implant (fig. 175). The important factor is not to pursue the inferior stripping lower than the chosen level, and for it to be symmetrical.

Dissection of the compartment and insertion of the implant

The dissection is made by the route chosen, combining stripping with the finger for the easily stripped planes and scissors for the more adherent regions and, in the case of a retropectoral compartment, possible detachment of the lowest and innermost muscle fibers.

Careful hemostasis is particularly important.

We routinely insert a suction drain, but not usually for longer than 48 hours.

The gloves are changed and rinsed to handle the implant, which is always filled with normal saline in our practice. At one time, it was suggested that antibiotics and/or corticosteroids should also be injected into the implant, the former to limit the risk of infection and the latter to limit the degree of periprosthetic contracture. In fact, if antibiotic cover is desired, systemic administration from the start of the operation is more effective, since it reaches the implant by way of the bloodstream and is better diffused. Introduction of corticosteroids into the implant is inadvisable since this may favor infection and, in the long term, atrophy of the skin with dermal thinning; in some cases, apart from deformation of the breast due to its tendency to migrate downwards, this has led to the ultimate complication of extrusion of the implant through skin ulceration.

A first filling will expel any air bubbles and test the implant; this initial filling is completely emptied so as not to infringe on the definitive filling. The implant is inserted, avoiding any instrumental contact, and then filled, always with overinflation relative to the manufacturer's norms; this varies but remains moderate for the reasons already given: consistency of the implant and the risk, if the pressure is too great, of seeing the volume reduced by equilibration of internal and external pressures until a balance is reached.

The position is checked: good spread of the base, absence of creases, anterior and medial situation of the valve; the filling catheter is removed and closure made.

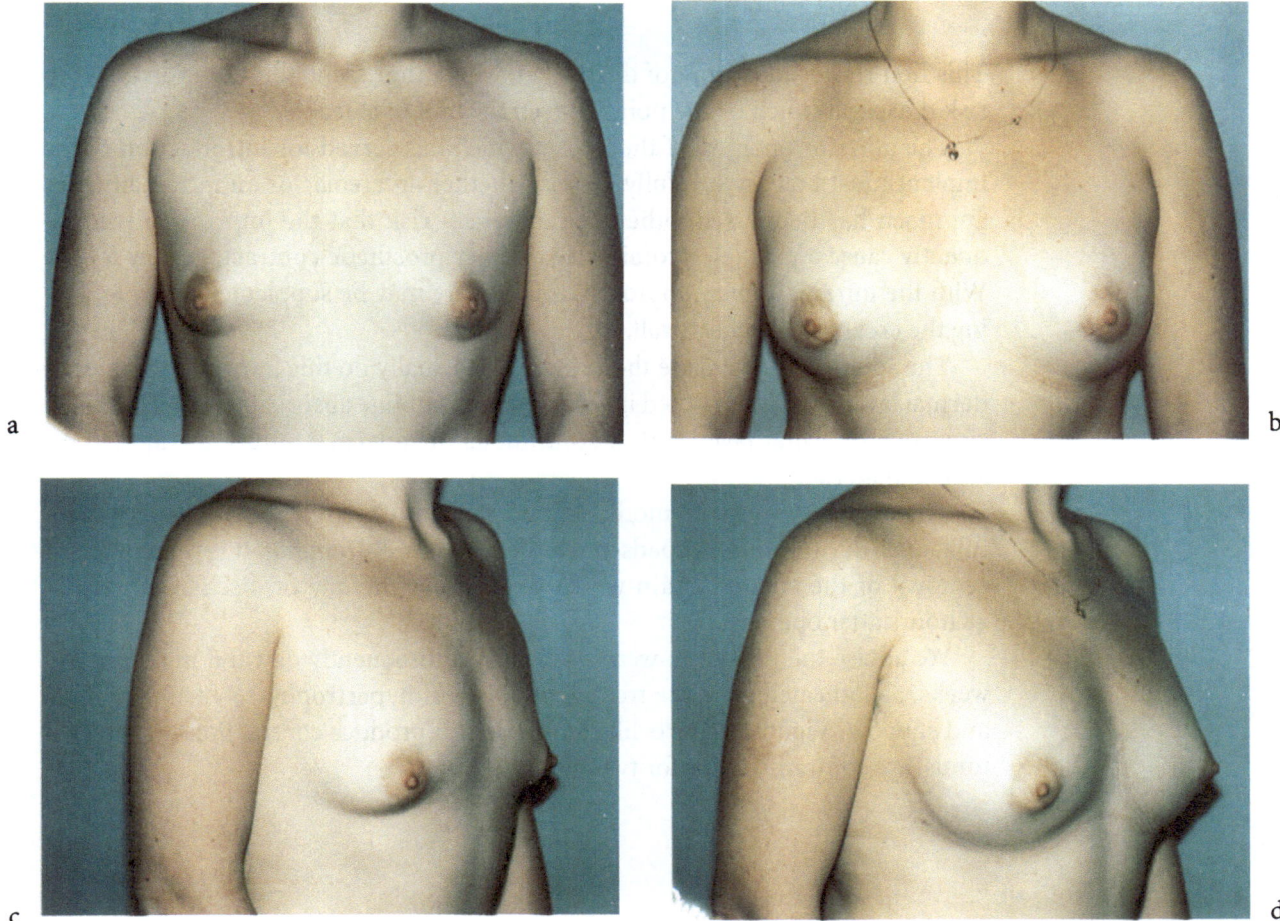

Fig. 175 a-d. Mammary hypoplasia with very short distance between areola and fold (3 cm). Insertion by inferior hemiareolar route in retropectoral position, with dissection of the compartment down to 4.5 cm below the lower border of the areola, of two textured inflatable implants (Sebbin LS21) of 200 ml filled to 275 ml

Closure

This first relates to closure of the pocket, where the essential precaution is not to risk the least scratch by the point or even the butt of a needle.

The anterior opening of the pocket which has served for introduction of the implant must be very carefully closed, whether an areolar or an inframammary approach has been used; otherwise there is a risk that the implant will subsequently cause a palpable prominence and periprosthetic contracture may follow. With the inframammary approach, this closure may be supplemented by attaching the crease to the chest-wall.

The superficial layers are then closed. We usually do this in two layers: a deep dermal layer with interrupted inverting sutures of fine absorbable material, and a superficial dermal layer with a continuous intradermal suture of rapidly absorbed material.

The dressing, which is modeling and moderately compressive, is done with tulle gras, dry (absorbent) pads and adhesive elastic strapping. It is retained until removal of the suction drain which determines the day of discharge (usually 48 hours after operation).

We advise the patient to wear a brassière subsequently day and night for two weeks, as indicated after the treatment of breast hypertrophy, to ensure comfort and support. Vigorous sports like tennis, which produce contractions of the pectorals, are contraindicated for two months.

Immediate complications

Postoperative pain

This is not strictly speaking a complication as it forms part of the usual consequences of any surgical procedure.

It may be a moderate nuisance, felt especially at the mobilisation of the pectorals, almost constant during the first few days when the implant is retropectoral, or it may be more severe, amounting to a feeling of cramp, either spontaneous or provoked by the least movement In this case the unpleasantness is effectively relieved by the administration of an antispasmodic.

Postoperative effusion

This is first sero-sanguineous and then serous and of variable extent, but is always present and seems to be rather more with textured than with smooth prostheses. This is why we prefer to insert a suction drain plus a moderately compressive dressing, for fear that persistence of the effusion may lead to a more serious inflammatory reaction.

If it is bloody and extensive, this is evidence of inadequate hemostasis, leading at worst to a hematoma; this is disquieting even if of moderate size and if the clinical features do not call for reoperation, since the formation of a hematoma is one of the known factors in periprosthetic contracture.

Infection

This is finally a very rare complication in breast augmentation for cosmetic reasons, doubtless because the tissues are healthy; it is so much more to be feared when a foreign body is implanted that the greatest attention must be given to asepsis; for it may be so dramatic as to require removal of the implant.

Doubtless, it is seen slightly more often when the implant is used for reconstruction after mastectomy, but we believe that this complication occurs especially in the latter situation when the indication has not been well-founded: the fragile tissues due to impaired laxity and the vascular sequelae of irradiation are intolerant of the additional tension imposed by the implant and are not resistant to bacterial multiplication, their portal of entry having possibly been created at the time of the mastectomy. We are far here from the operative conditions of a simple hypoplasia, an operation of first intention on healthy tissues.

Implant rupture

This is due to technical error: either a defect in manufacture, which is why its integrity should be checked before insertion, or injury at the time of implantation, due to difficulty caused by an exposure initially too small, or to perforation by an instrument or a needle.

The rupture is rapidly obvious with an inflatable implant, since the normal saline is immediately reabsorbed, less obvious with a prefilled implant but certainly with more serious complications in the middle and long term.

Other complications

These are usually secondary to another problem:

– exposure or expulsion of the implant is seen after a hematoma under tension, or an infection which may of course be secondary to this hematoma;

– exceptional skin or nipple damage may be the result of excessive tension exerted by the retractors when access is restricted, or if there is a hematoma or infection.

Malposition of the implant

This forms part of the immediate complications when it is due to a technical error.

To resemble a natural breast, the prosthetic volume must be centered on the nipples, even if these are divergent.

The least ugly malposition is found in situations where the areola is situated too high, displaced towards the upper slope of the breast, as this simulates a glandular ptosis. It is associated with excessive downward stripping, which may have been secondarily aggravated by skin distension under the weight of the implant. An implant cannot actually displace or migrate spontaneously, for the space allotted to it is rapidly fixed by the formation of the periprosthetic membrane.

If the implant is placed high up, segment II is longer and more convex than segment III, and the nipple faces downward. This situation may be seen when the initial distance between the nipple and the inframammary crease is short and less than the radius of the implant, and when the surgeon has not dared to take the stripping lower than the natural crease. Now, we have seen that, where hypoplasia is concerned, the position of the natural crease can be ignored, as it will be obliterated by the thrust exerted by the implant on the superficial layers.

Finally, implants which are eccentric outward give the breasts the unsightly appearance of a divergent squint. This complication is due to too large an initial outward stripping, often with an over-large compartment, the malposition being aggravated when the implants have been placed behind the pectorals and when the skin is atonic, each pectoral contraction displacing them outward into the zone of least resistance.

Secondary complications

Periprosthetic contracture

This is the dominant complication, which is responsible for what is called — improperly, but graphically — the "shell", or rather more correctly the "hard breast". We have already discussed the mechanism, which is no more than the outcome of the foreign body reaction to a supple implant, also the physiopathologic hypotheses.

Clinique

The classification of Baker allows us to assess the degree of periprosthetic contracture in four stages:

– stage I: this corresponds to a normal appearance, the implant not being detectable by inspection or palpation;

– stage II: the appearance of the breast is normal, but palpation reveals slight induration;

– stage III: the contracture is visible and palpable, but the deformation is minor;

– stage IV: the breast is deformed, its shape approaching the spherical; it is hard and may be constantly painful, and cold.

This classification has the merit of simplicity, though intermediate stages are possible, and the assessment is to some extent a subjective one on the part of the examiner. Naturally, the degree of contracture may vary to some extent from one examination to the next.

However, there does not currently exist any simple and widely used objective method for assessment of this phenomenon.

What is finally most important is to assess the effect on the shape obtained, the patient's tolerance, and when to suggest and discuss a revision procedure.

The crucial point is between stages II and III: a degree of firmness without marked deformation will be well tolerated, especially if bilateral. If unilateral, it produces an asymmetry which is much less tolerable.

The operative, radiologic and histologic findings show that the thickness of the periprosthetic membrane in cases of contracture is very variable, that it consists of fibrous tissue, and may calcify in some cases; also that it can pose difficult therapeutic problems in cases where the membrane cannot be left in place because it is palpable under the thinned superficial layer. Excision of this fibrous layer is often hemorrhagic, but there are cases where it has to be removed, notably when it is asociated with a ruptured prefilled implant, the risk being of leaving residues of gel.

The development of periprosthetic contracture is revealed in the great majority of cases before the end of the third postoperative month, but it may not become manifest or stabilised until the sixth month, or even a year or two after the operation. There have also been reported contractures of delayed development, several years after operation, where the breast had previously seemed quite normal. In these cases one looks for a cause, often without success: a local injury or an infection (local or remote) which may promote secondary contracture through a bacteremia. This is why many surgeons advise against breast-feeding after the insertion of an implant. But none of these hypotheses has been proved so far.

Physiopathology

It is difficult to list the causes of periprosthetic contracture since, even if some of the provocative factors are known, the essential one is yet to be found, if only to explain the development of unilateral contractures when the nature of the procedure and the immediate postoperative course seem to have been comparable on both sides.

We have already seen that the nature of the implant plays a not insignificant part. Implants filled with normal saline cause less periprosthetic contracture than "standard" implants prefilled with gel, and the development of textured walls seems to have brought a marked decrease of contractures. An average incidence of 15 to 20% was normal with smooth implants, and this incidence would seem to have fallen below 5% with textured implants.

However, the improvement in the tolerance of implants is difficult to evaluate in the long term, since changes have occurred very rapidly in recent years as regards the characteristics of their walls, their degree of permeability and their content. It is to be hoped that all these changes will work towards a constant improvement of the systems available to us.

Infection certainly plays a part, not so much an acute infection, which is obvious clinically though uncommon, as a subclinical infection which is determined by the presence of so-called saprophytic skin organisms, and perhaps at the expense of those commonly present in the lactiferous sinuses. For some workers this is a reason to avoid the transareolar route, but there is no certainty in this matter. On the other hand, subclinical infection may perhaps better explain unilateral contractures.

Some workers regard a hematoma as responsible for contracture, though others dispute this. In any case, it seems preferable to prevent it by scrupulous hemostasis combined with drainage, if only to prevent reintervention, an easier source of infection and hence of contracture.

It seems equally important to combat serous effusion, which is difficult to define as the cause or consequence of inflammatory reaction, but either factor may succeed the other in time. Two measures can prevent its formation and persistence: (a) drainage (obviously, a small-caliber suction drain whose track is obliterated by gentle massage after withdrawal is preferable to a simple rubber drain whose exit orifice, if too large, is itself a port of entry for infection) and (b) moderate compression postoperatively.

Others have incriminated the tension exerted by an implant that is too bulky or over-filled. Unfortunately, if one tries to deflate an implant secondarily, or to replace it with a smaller implant, the contracture is very often reproduced with the reduced size, probably because in this case the process of contracture is not yet stabilised.

Prevention and treatment

With our present uncertainty as to the causes of periprosthetic contracture (there is certainly no single mechanism, but possibly some terrains are more susceptible than others to different local factors), we are relatively incapable of preventing such contracture and of combating it.

Prevention may consist of:

– the most atraumatic dissection possible, preventing tissue damage responsible at least for an exacerbation of the inflammatory reaction, and possibly leading to cutaneous or glandular necrosis requiring exposure of the implant, or to an infection;

– rigorous hemostasis;

– drainage;

– irrigation of the compartment to eliminate clots, debris of textile fibers and particles of talc, if need be with an antiseptic diluted in normal saline;

– antibiotherapy, if used at all, seems more logical by the systemic route and from the start of the operation;

– and, as far as the implant is concerned, the future will reveal if the hopes based on textured walls confirm the currently promising results; in any case we prefer to use inflatable rather than prefilled implants, while realising that it is not possible altogether to eliminate transudation of the gel or rupture.

The treatment of periprosthetic contracture is uncertain for the same reasons. However, when contracture has developed around a prepectoral pocket, the implant can be replaced behind the pectorals in the hope that the quasi-permanent massage and mobilisation of the implant by the muscle will decrease the risk of contracture, or more simply that its retropectoral position will make it less perceptible. If the implant is already retropectoral, one can try to enlarge the prosthetic compartment by making it a very little bigger than necessary. The hypothesis is that the contracture has every chance of recurrence, but with lesser intensity because over a smaller surface, and that the operative damage is less severe. This may be effective.

Such open capsulotomy seems preferable to maneuvers of "capsuloclasis" (the "squeezing" of the English-language literature), often ineffective or even impossible to perform or followed by a recurrence of the contracture. Besides, this is a possibly dangerous maneuver on a prefilled implant, which risks being split or ruptured by a violent maneuver.

However, if capsuloclasis is nevertheless intended, it should be done without anesthesia and with moderate pressure.

If there is the least doubt, radiologic monitoring should be requested to check the integrity of the implant.

There is no obvious reason, when contracture has developed around a smooth implant, to expect that simple replacement by a textured implant will lead to disappearance of the contracture, doubtless because it is already formed.

Survival of the implant

It is difficult to be specific about the survival period of an implant; we have all seen cases where implants have been in place for ten years or even longer without problems, but we have also had to change implants at shorter intervals for various reasons.

An implant filled with normal saline does not need to be changed routinely. A change is made only when a problem arises, as in deflation.

This does not of course apply to prefilled implants, especially if their wall is not very thick, not so much because of the risk of transudation of the gel, which is always present, but because of simple wear of the wall at its margins, leading to perforation and then tearing of the implant. Clinical and ultrasonic monitoring of these patients must certainly be frequent. Some workers have even asked if it may not be necessary to change prefilled implants routinely, but no-one is capable of stating at what intervals.

Breast implants and cancer of the breast

The insertion of a breast implant involves no risk as regards the development of cancer of the breast, and it is of course a technique often used for reconstruction after mastectomy.

In fact, these patients will be even better monitored than others, since they often benefit from preoperative examinations at an age earlier than that of routine screening, and from subsequent regular surveillance.

In the hands of a trained radiologist, using mammography, ultrasound or even xerography, the presence of an implant will not prevent the detection of a breast lesion, a problem posed mainly by non-palpable lesions and one more difficult with a prefilled gel implant which is not radio-transparent than with an implant filled with saline. The latter is much less of a hindrance. A retropectoral position of the implant also favors radiologic study.

Finally, we should recall that diagnosis by needle aspiration is contraindicated in the presence of an implant.

Atrophy and ptosis

The treatment of atrophy associated with ptosis brings into the foreground, if it were necessary, the interdependence of mammary container and content, which cannot and should not be considered separately in the context of either analysis or treatment.

Clinical examination

This will first assess the degree of glandular insufficiency in order to evaluate the size of implant required, not overlooking the presence of any asymmetry.

Particular importance attaches to examination of the skin envelope:

– the extent of the envelope;

– the position on it of the areola, chiefly the distance from the areola to the suprasternal notch and the inframmary crease, and the relative sizes of these two measurements;

– the dimensions of the areola;

– definition of the inframammary crease, which is usually well-marked when there is glandular shrinkage;

– the elasticity of the skin, presence of striae, quality of the dermis (whether thinned or not).

Clinical examination is followed by radiography in order to exclude any lesion that might call for another preliminary or concomitant procedure to the cosmetic operation.

Operative procedure

The first stage is that of restoration of volume, to which the skin envelope is subsequently readjusted. This is a logical way to proceed from several viewpoints:

– the priority accorded to manipulation of the implant is preferable in terms of asepsis;

– it is only when the implant is in place that it is possible to assess the extent of redundant skin, since if the elasticity of the skin is poor the skin stretching will be seen to be aggravated by insertion of this additional weight;

– finally, the areola must be properly situated, at the apex of the reconstructed volume, and this can only be determined when the implant is in place.

Positioning

The patient is positioned as usual in the half-seated position, with the shoulders horizontal and the arms beside the body (we do not use the axillary route).

The axis of the breast is drawn from a point situated on a horizontal line at 5 cm lateral to the suprasternal notch; the inframammary crease is defined by a fine line (fig. 176).

Insertion of the implant

For this purpose we prefer to use the inframammary approach (fig. 177) because:

– apart from the initial ease of passage by this route to the retroglandular and retropectoral planes, the exposure for hemostasis is excellent;

– the scar defect is minor, since the fold is well-marked in ptosis;

– in any case, in the great majority of cases the secondary procedure of skin reduction will end with the lower margin of this incision coinciding with the horizontal resection;

– however, one should be content with an incision not exceeeding 4 cm in length, so as not to risk transgressing what will correspond to the subsequent resection.

Correction of ptosis: basic technique

Once the implant compartment has been closed, correct placement of the areola is designed by centering it on the axis of the breast.

Two points are important to define initially: the upper point, and the most medial limit of the de-epithelialisation, marked out symmetrically on both sides. The circle of de-epithelialisation is then traced; we again use a Dufourmentel ring, but one much less open than in the treatment of hypertrophy as the subjacent skin resection is extensive. The opening of the ring virtually corresponds to the diameter of the areola (fig. 178).

The dimensions of the areola are verified, and if need be reduced, the nipple-bearing flap is de-epithelialised (without a mammostat) and the subareolar vertical is incised. Then the two vertical skin flaps are lightly stripped to allow placement of the clamp. Here, the posterior aspect of the gland is not stripped from the deep muscle plane.

The areola is constructed, and the clamp is placed without excess tension, simply reapplying the skin envelope to the prosthetic volume with uniform tension along the whole length of the clamp (fig. 179).

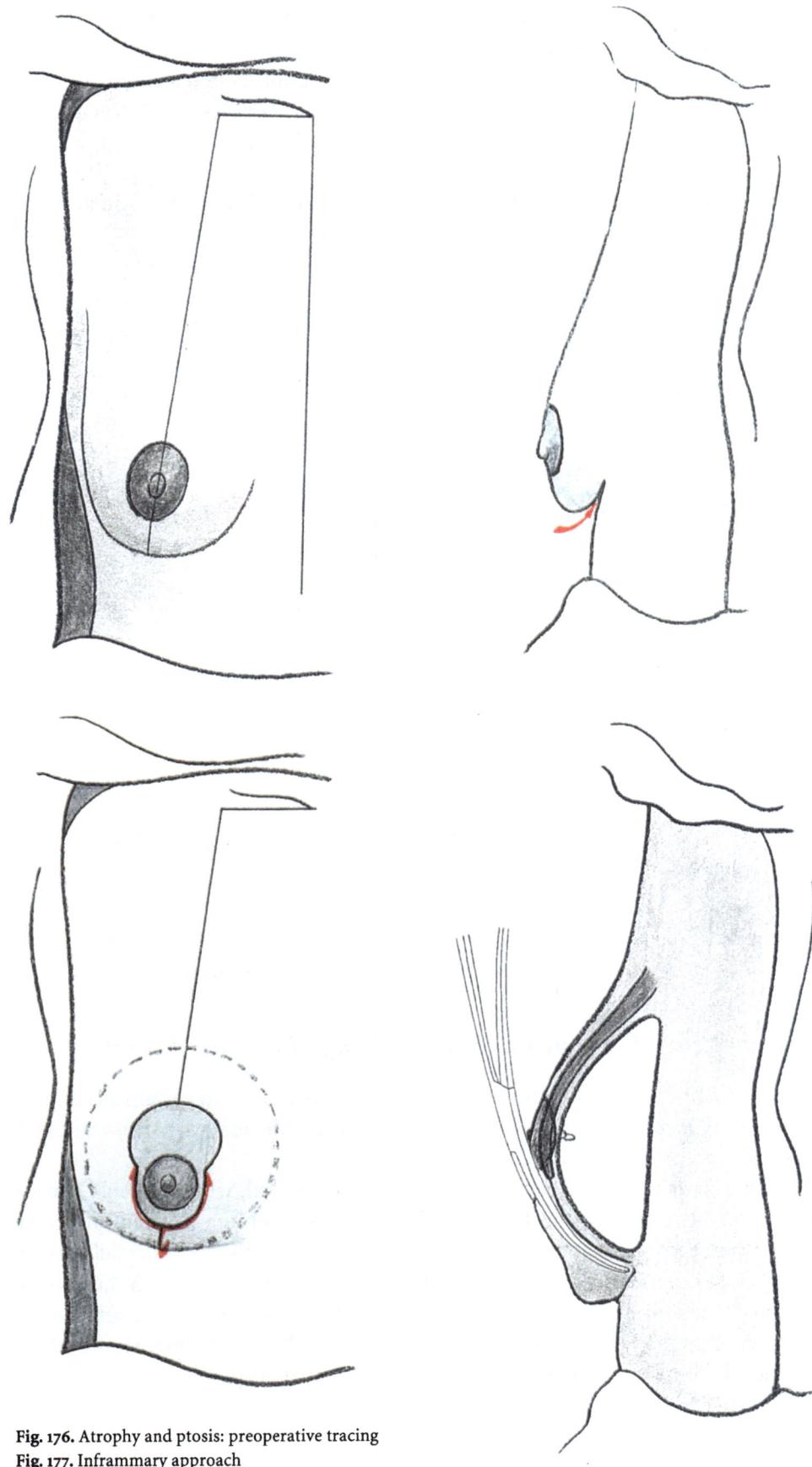

Fig. 176. Atrophy and ptosis: preoperative tracing
Fig. 177. Inframmary approach
Fig. 178. Siting of zone of periareolar de-epithelialisation
Fig. 179. Application of clamp and readaptation of skin envelope

The excess skin is resected and the subareolar vertical is sutured. At this stage, supplementary de-epithelialisation is sometimes needed to round off the inferior alveolar circumference. Then the horizontal resection is determined, so as to place the inframammary scar, also without tension, opposite the lower pole of the implant (fig. 180). If excessive vertical traction is exerted at this stage of the procedure, there is a risk of seeing the horizontal scar reascend on the lower slope of the breast immediately after the resection or during the following weeks.

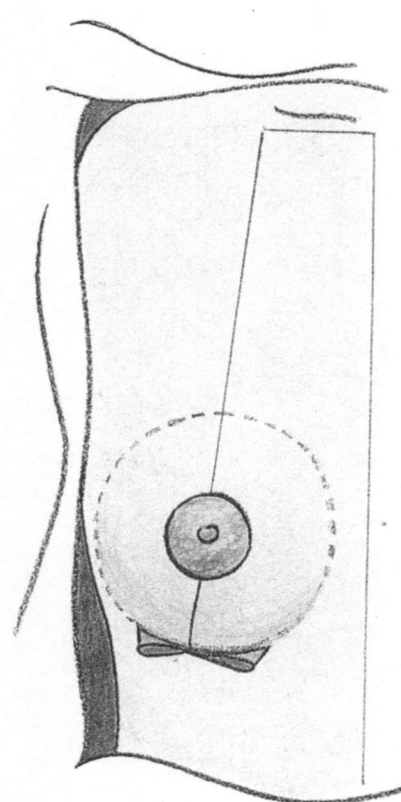

Fig. 180. Horizontal resection in the inframammary crease

Correction of the ptosis: minimising the scar defect

This manner of proceeding is the one we use in most cases. In certain situations, much more rarely encountered, the scar defect is a little less extensive, without a vertical scar.

This occurs in cases where the excess skin is minimal, with an areola simply situated a little too low on the breast (this is almost more a problem of breast shape than a true ptosis with skin stretching), and an initially short subareolar distance of around 4 cm. Here only a periareolar de-epithelialisation may be attempted, the aim being to slightly ascend the areola and to round it off, the ascension of the upper point not exceeding 2 or 3 cm (hence the importance of inserting the implant through a short incision). It is then preferable to place the implant via an inferior hemiareolar incision to avoid the inframammary scar.

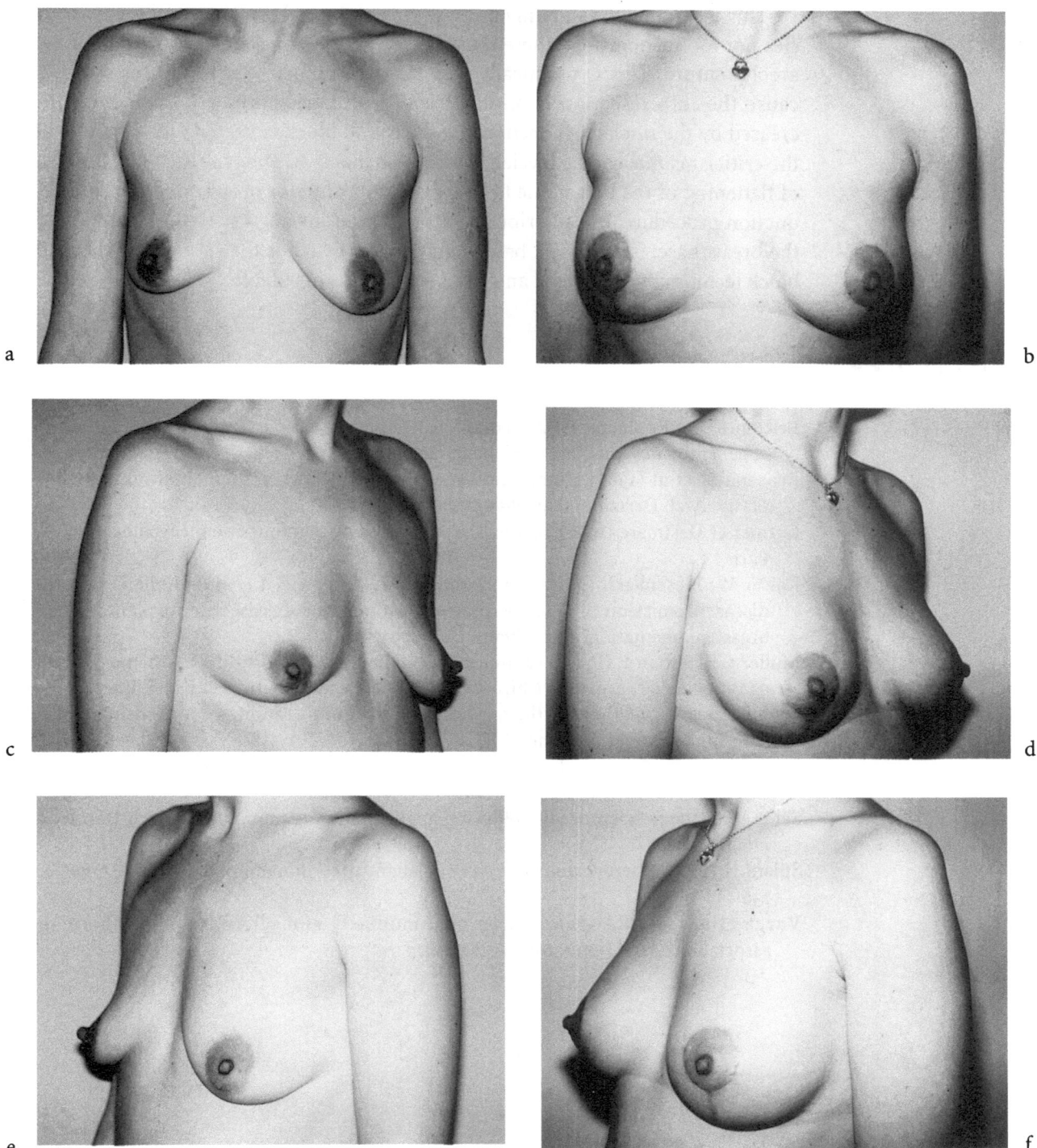

Fig. 181 a-f. Atrophy and ptosis after two pregnancies (32-year-old). Insertion of two smooth inflatable Sebbin implants of 150 ml, filled with 180 ml right and 170ml left. Preoperatively, right areola 18.5 cm from suprasternal notch, left 19.5 cm; both distances reduced to 17 cm

This technique is valid only if the skin is of the right quality, and the two circles not too incongruent; there must be virtually no puckering at the end of the areolar suture. This is practically a "mini-round block", useful in this case because the skin resection is minimal and the anterior projection has been increased by the implant. Indeed, when the round block is used on its own, one of the criticisms that can be leveled against it is that it ascends the areola at the cost of flattening of the breast due to decrease of its anterior projection. In a skin reduction procedure, the anterior projection varies inversely with the reduction of the breast base; if the breast base is untouched, which is the case with the round block technique, decrease of anterior projection is inevitable.

References

Bricout N, De Roquancourt A, Saouma S, Servant JM, Banzet P (1988) Risques locaux et généraux des implants de silicone. Chirurgie 114: 538-544

Brozena SJ et al (1988) Human adjuvant disease following augmentation mammoplasty. Arch Dermatol 124: 1383-1386

Garnier et Delamare (1966) Dictionnaire des termes techniques de médecine. Maloine, Paris,

Kaiser W, Biesenbach G, Stuby U, Grafinger P, Zazgornik J (1990) Human adjuvant disease: remission of silicone induced autoimmune disease after explantation of breast augmentation. Ann Rheum Dis 49: 937-938

Muller GH, Sitbon E (1991) Les implants mammaires. Rapport du XXXVIème congrès de la Société Française de Chirurgie Plastique, Reconstructrice et Esthétique

Nightingale SL (1989) From the food and drug administration: safety considerations with silicone breast prostheses. JAMA 261 (3): 350

Roux H et al (1987) Pathologie auto-immune et chirurgie esthétique ; à propos d'un cas. Rev Med Int 8: 475-480

Sahn et al (1990) Scleroderma following augmentation mammoplasty. Arch Dermatol 126: 1198-1202

Spiera H (1988) Scleroderma after silicone augmentation mammoplasty. JAMA 260/2: 236-238

Varga et al (1990) Augmentation mammoplasty and scleroderma. Is there an association? Arch Dermatol 126: 1220-1222

Reconstruction of the breast

General considerations

Although the conservative management of malignant tumors of the breast has been very widely used in recent years, mastectomy remain indicated when it constitutes the only reasonable local treatment because of the size or histologic type of the tumor, or when there is a risk of multifocal lesions.

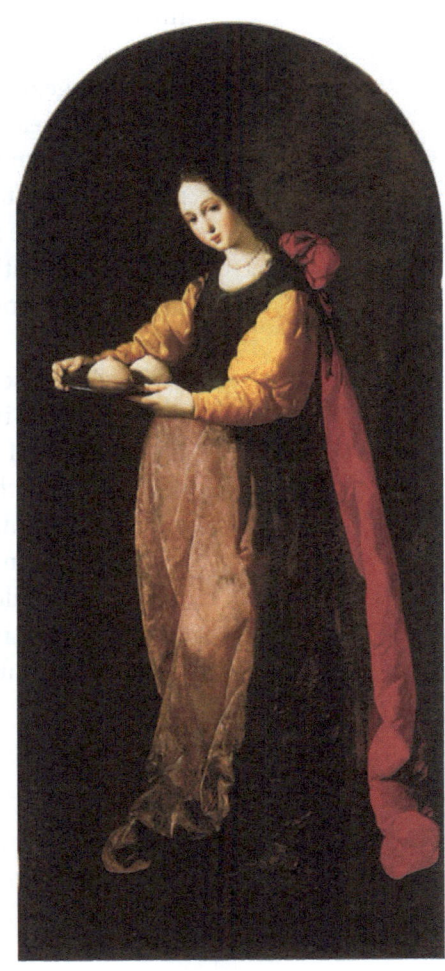

Fig. 182. Saint Agatha, Sicilian martyr, patron saint of wet-nurses (Francisco Zurbaran [1578-1664], Musée Fabre, Montpellier)

Since the heroic epoch when the sole procedure regarded as satisfactory for eradication of carcinoma was developed by Halsted, consisting of en bloc sacrifice of skin, breast and pectoral muscles together with an axillary nodal clearance which took little account of the need for lymphatic drainage of the arm, or for preserving the nerves and hence the function of the latissimus dorsi and serratus anterior, mastectomy perfomed by the Madden-Patey procedure has become a procedure more respectful of the skin envelope, lymphatic drainage and upper limb function.

Although the sequelae of an operation of this type are functionally and cosmetically much less disastrous than the frightful mutilation left by the Halsted operation, the loss of a breast is always a major psychological trauma for the woman who suffers it, as this mutilation is very obvious evidence of the damage to her physical integrity and feminine identity.

The very idea of the possibility of reconstruction, whether immediate or delayed, suggested at the initial stage of treatment, often secures better acceptance of the need for mastectomy and for possibly associated treatments.

In this context, the surgery of breast reconstruction is an integral part of the treatment of breast carcinoma. It is to be discussed with the oncologist to decide on the opportune time (the reparative procedure must not hinder or delay the treatment program) and to ensure joint surveillance of the postoperative course and subsequent developments.

Plastic surgery continues to advance and to bring forward increasingly refined techniques.

This is, indeed, a field where the surgeon must master, not just one, but a whole range of techniques which will allow him to choose the most suitable combination for each case.

It is without doubt one of the most exciting fields of reparative plastic surgery, since it is constantly being added to under esthetic demands. It is not enough to reconstruct the size; the shape must also be satisfactory and it must be in harmony with the patient's build and with the opposite breast, which itself also often has to be remodeled and adapted to the model imposed by the reconstructed breast.

In this sense it demands a long apprenticeship and a considerable degree of experience, as it requires the surgeon to have a perfect understanding of breast morphology, of the plastic surgical techniques appropriate to it, and of the future of an operated breast, which once more involves the ineluctable concepts of the qualities of container and content. However, the plastic surgeon must not be content with confining his knowledge and the operative indications to the reparative procedure, while neglecting the oncologic aspects of the problem, which he must always bear in mind. Although everything is changing very rapidly in this field, he must continue to keep himself fully informed.

The factors involved

The morphologic sequelae of a mastectomy combine three factors:
- the absence of breast contour,
- the reduction of the skin envelope,
- the presence of a scar across the side of the chest.

The relative importance of these three factors varies with the extent of the skin sacrifice necessary during the mastectomy, and with possible sequelae associated with the radiotherapy, but also with the quality of the tissues and the patient's build.

Skin sacrifice: this will have been more extensive when the lesion was bulky and remote from the areola; of course, without being at all critical, some surgeons are more economical than others as regards the skin substance, even though the indications are comparable. The amount of skin available is sometimes surprising, as in the performance of a subcutaneous mastectomy where skin sacrifice is limited essentially to a spindle circumscribing the areola, compared to other cases where the tissues are extremely stretched and obviously require the provision of supplementary skin.

The sequelae left by associated radiotherapy are also variable, not only because of the program used but also because of the quality of the tissues, whose tolerance of the irradiation varies, especially as concerns the possibility of sclerosis. The chief factors here are the thickness of the subcutaneous fatty layer and the tension existing at the time of closure, before carrying out the radiotherapy.

Finally, if the mastectomy is done after some other procedure, such as a tumorectomy combined with radiotherapy, even if there has been no notable skin sacrifice and if this combined treatment does not seem to have left obvious sequelae, there will as a rule be marked loss of elasticity and laxity after the operation.

The choice of the most suitable reconstruction technique is based on scrupulous analysis of these various factors. Plastic surgery is fortunately rich in resources and never ceases to suppy new solutions as regards both the quality of the material and the art of using the tissue stock available.

The objectives of breast reconstruction

These are three in number and of varying difficulty:
- to restore the missing volume,
- to ensure symmetry with the opposite breast,
- to recreate an areola and a nipple.

Restoration of volume

Different methods can be used and depend on the amount and quality of the overlying skin:
- when this is of good quality, well-vascularised and sufficiently lax, it is possible to reconstruct the volume in a single stage by provision of an implant, filled at the outset to its definitive volume;

– when the skin cover is of good quality, and substantial in thickness but a little insufficient in amount to tolerate the stretching due to insertion of an implant filled immediatetly to its definitive volume, the device of an expansion prosthesis may be used. This is an implant possessing a system resembling the arrangement used for chemotherapy, which makes it possible to obtain the desired volume gradually by percutaneous injections in parallel with the tissue distension;

– when the laxity is quite inadequate, and/or when the quality of the tissues leaves something to be desired, it becomes necessary to apply a flap; the flaps most commonly used, because the most reliable, are the myocutaneous flaps (so called because the vascularisation of the cutaneous layer is ensured by perforating branches from the muscle acting as pedicle) from the latissimus dorsi and rectus abdominis. We shall see that the first method nearly always necessitates the use of an implant, whereas the main advantage of the second is that it allows reconstruction of sufficient volume in the great majority of cases even without an implant, since it employs the excess of subumbilical skin and fatty tissue. Each method has its own indications.

The opposite breast

The plasty of the opposite breast may be the reduction of a hypertrophy, usually associated with that of a ptosis, but also the treatment of pure ptosis, or even — more rarely — the correction of an atrophic condition.

The procedure will depend mainly on the state of the residual skin, but also on the technique employed for the reconstruction:

– very commonly, a procedure is necessary at the opposite breast when the missing breast has been reconstructed with an implant, which must create a breast of satisfactory volume in relation to thoracic and general morphology (if it remains too small because of local conditions, it means that the indication for reconstruction by a simple implant was injudicious, and that it would have been better to use another technique). But this reconstructed breast will be without ptosis;

– on the other hand, it is less often necessary to deal with the opposite breast when the reconstruction has been made with a rectus abdominis flap, as the possibilities of modeling of this flap allow the construction of a breast of very natural shape.

Areola and nipple

The creation of an areola and nipple constitute the final procedure in a reconstruction, without which the restored volume, even if very satisfactory in shape and symmetry, cannot claim to represent a breast. Though acting as a center of attention, it cannot however be considered as a minor procedure and it would be wrong to ignore its importance. One of the important factors concerns its place on the reconstructed breast, which depends not only on its shape and size but also the size and position of the nipple-areolar plaque of the opposite breast. This is why we usually reconstruct it last, once the reconstructed breast is stabilised and the opposite breast perhaps improved.

Two operative stages are usually needed to perform this reconstruction, done after a few months' interval. The first consists of reconstruction of the missing shape and volume. The interval between the two procedures, usually around 4 months, is necessary for stabilisation of the shape of the reconstructed breast. The second operation combines the procedure on the opposite breast with reconstruction of the nipple-areolar plaque, and with possible adjustments to the reconstructed breast. Some prefer to do everything in one stage. We prefer two-stage reconstructions, even if this may seem more troublesome for the patient, as it seems difficult to predict the precise development of all the factors involved in this combination of procedures, the coordination of which goes to ensure the quality of the reconstruction, while still insisting on the importance of proper placement of the areola.

Both stages usually require general anesthesia, except when the second stage is reduced to no more than reconstruction of the nipple-areolar plaque, which may then be done under neuroleptoanalgesia.

Preoperative examination

Clinical examination

This is primarily the assessment of the sequelae of the mastectomy.

History

This must be complete and cover the history of the disease of the breast and the different treatments carried out, the medical, surgical and gynecologic antecedents of the patient, and the medical treatment presently applied. Even if the patient's documentation is very complete, we conduct this interrogation very carefully since it is this first contact with the patient that allows one to establish a relationship and to assess her motivations. This is a branch of surgery where the human quality of the relationship and the confidence established between the reconstructive surgeon and the patient will play a great part in the outcome.

Local examination

The scar
This is judged not so much on its length as its quality: breadth, transverse marks of sutures, suppleness, and adherence to the deep plane.

Fine supple scars not adherent in depth do not necessarily require to be excised throughout their extent. But if the scar is broad and adherent, excision must be performed if only for the cosmetic appearance of the result; otherwise, if this procedure is neglected, a contracture may develop locally under the effect of the thrust exerted by the implant. This excision will in many cases prevent having to compensate the effect of a contracture by a Z plasty at the outer end of the scar, which may certainly give a good resul but will aggravate the visible scar defect.

Skin cover

An assessment is made of the quality of skin cover: its trophicity and suppleness, its degree of laxity and the amount available, not forgetting to look for the sequelae of badly tolerated irradiation, ie tissues that are sclerosed and poorly mobile on the deep plane or more obvious sequelae such as telangiectases.

The subcutaneous fatty layer

Its thickness is evaluated, and especially its uniformity throughout the area of the mastectomy, in particular on either side of the scar. If the layer is thinned at the scar edges, this must be allowed for in choosing a reconstruction technique as it may indicate two phenomena: either major tension has been exerted on the margins to allow closure, or the dissection was more superficial at that site, which is troublesome since this will correspond to the zone of greatest anterior projection and therefore of greatest tension during the insertion of an implant.

This may therefore be a — relative — contraindication to the simple insertion of an implant or an expansion prosthesis. If this thinning is accompanied by a lack of laxity, it is better to prefer the provision of a flap. If, on the other hand, skin laxity is good, it will be necessary to excise the thinned zone so as to suture margins of uniform thickness.

The muscles

The integrity and functional quality of the pectoralis major muscle must be checked: is it of good bulk throughout its extent or, on the contrary, is it atrophic? It is important to examine it not only at rest, but also when making it contract, a procedure which may reveal disappearance or atrophy of the inferior head secondary to nerve damage during nodal eradication.

Also to be checked are the state of the latissimus dorsi and its contractility, assessed by palpating it at the mid-portion of its anterior border to avoid confusing its contraction with that of the teres major. Here, too, if contraction is absent or minor, there should be caution in considering the use of a latissimus flap, since the absence of contraction indicates a nerve lesion, usually associated with injury of the pedicle. This is not a formal contraindication to use of this flap, as will be seen, but calls for primary checking of the pedicle and it is essential to preserve the thoracic branch.

The opposite breast

This is carefully examined: its degree of hypertrophy or ptosis, quality of content and container, suppleness and elasticity of the skin, presence or not of striae, shape and position of the inframammary crease, palpation of the gland (not forgetting the axillary fossa) to assess its suppleness and to avoid missing a palpable anomaly. One should note the dates of the most recent supplementary investigations — mammography, ultrasonography — which must be repeated if more than a year back.

General examination

Note:

– the presence of other scars, particularly abdominal;

– the shape of the chest (whether long or short, which affects in part the orientation of the lower border of the pectoralis major and therefore the cover its surface may be expected to give to a possible implant);

– the general build (tall or short), weight, height, whether the distribution of any overweight is uniform or not.

Supplementary investigations

These are those of the preoperative assessment required before any surgical procedure, together with those required for oncologic surveillance.

Reconstruction by implant

The implant

Type of implant

Just as in the surgery of augmentation, so in breast reconstruction, we remain faithful to inflatable implants and for the same reasons:

– suppleness of use associated with adaptable and variable volume,
– least foreign body reaction,
– innocuous content: normal saline has the further advantage of being radio-transparent, unlike silicone gel which makes radiologic surveillance more difficult.

It seems to us even more important in this field to be prepared to vary the anterior projection and volume for a given size of breast base as may be required. This breast base is chosen more in relation to the area of implantation of the breast to be reconstructed than to the opposite breast, which will often be the subject of a plastic procedure at a second stage. This procedure, which is most often a decrease in volume or correction of ptosis, will be accompanied by a varying degree of reduction of the breast base.

On the other hand, the theoretic choice of volume may bring some surprises. In some cases one will be — relatively — limited by the suppleness of the tissues; in other cases, however, it may be possible to fill the implant more than was expected. Despite considerable experience with reconstruction, we remain unable to predict the definitive volume of an implant within 50 ml, and this margin, though relatively small, may greatly influence the appearance obtained.

We use the same types of implants as those chosen for breast augmentation, with a relatively spread base and an anterior valve, but obviously of greater volume, The implant is always over-inflated compared with the theoretic norm laid down by the manufacturer. In the model we now use, the suppleness of the elastomere of the wall allows quite large variations in relation to the basic volume, and the more so when the implant is bigger. However, it is important not to abuse this possibility, to avoid creating an excessive internal pressure which may result in secondary decrease in volume until the pressures on either side of the membrane reach a new equilibrium.

Choice of implant

This is based on various factors, local and general:

Local factors

The chief factor is the determination of the necessary breast base, which will decide the volume of the implant and which is arrived at by first defining the horizontal diameter. This corresponds approximately to the distance between the inner ends of the intercostal spaces and the anterior axillary line (fig. 183). This distance is then carried vertically from the presumed inframammary crease, drawn symmetrically with the opposite breast except in cases of very marked hypertrophy. The diameter of the implant is ultimately a compromise between the breadth of implantation of the breast to be reconstructed and the extent in height conditioned by this measurement, which constitutes the limiting factor. It is important that an over-large implant should not place the upper limit of the reconstructed breast at too high a level.

Other local and regional factors are involved here, such as the shape of the thorax; a longilinear thorax, with a rather low area of breast implantation, may accept an implant of larger diameter than will a short thorax.

General factors

These are represented essentially by the degree of overweight; the greater this is, especially with abdominal obesity, the more the opposite inframammary crease will be displaced upward and horizontalised by the supra-umbilical fat. The diameter of the usable implant, and therefore its volume, will be correspondingly reduced (fig. 184). This is of less importance if the subcutaneous fatty layer has also remained substantial, since its thickness will participate in the volume of the reconstruction; here, the implant will supply mainly a central anterior projection, rather than a globally spread-out volume.

It is much more of a hindrance if the fatty layer has been very thinned by the mastectomy and the possible effects of supplementary treatments, and when it has become much smaller than the general build of the patient would require. In such a situation, the use of an implant alone risks giving a mediocre result, even if the suppleness of the tissues would allow the simple provision of a prosthesis. For the global volume, it then becomes necessary to provide a flap to supplement the subcutaneous fatty layer over a large part of the breast area (eg the skin and muscle supplied by a latissimus dorsi flap). The other solution is to resort to a flap that itself ensures the whole of the volume without reliance on a prosthesis, as with a rectus abdominis flap, its volume being more easily adjustable.

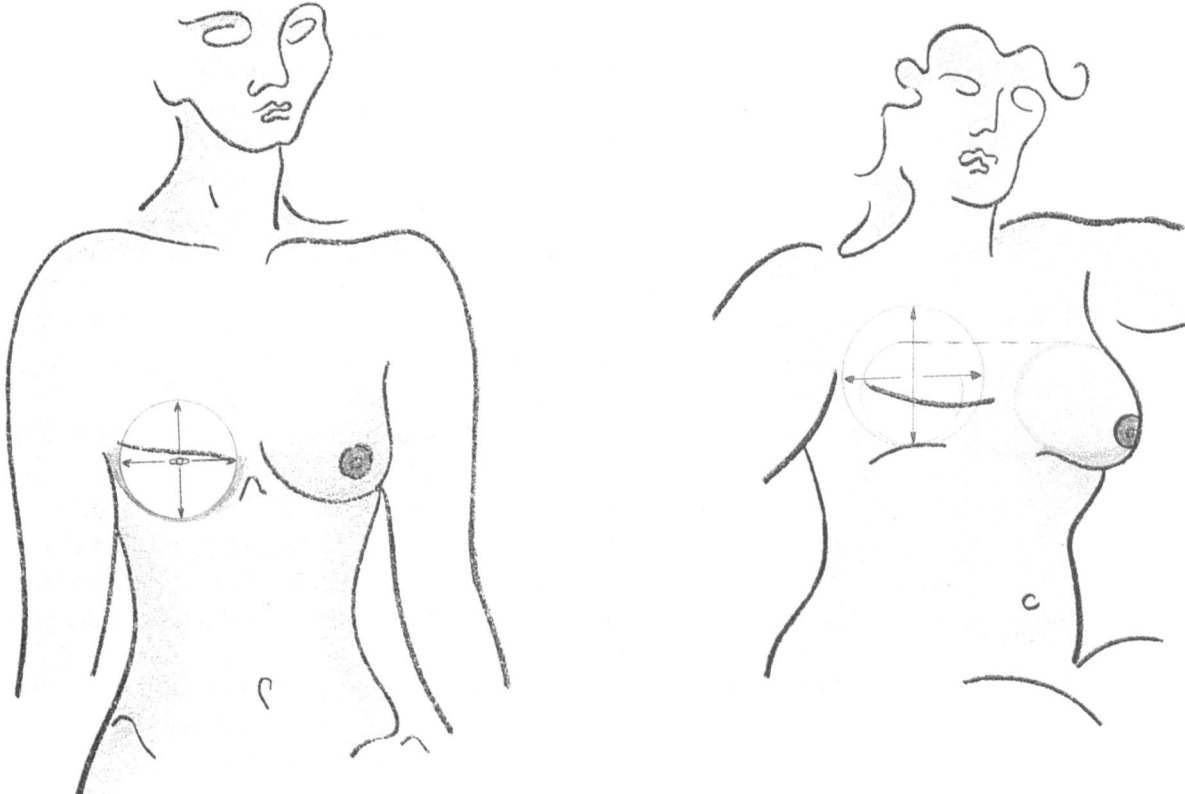

Fig. 183. Determination of diameter of implant, a compromise between the necessary size and what is acceptable in the vertical direction in relation to the thoracic level of the opposite inframammary crease

Fig. 184. The problem posed in obesity:
– the necessary diameter in the horizontal direction has too great a vertical distance, with the upper limit of the implant situated too high, because of ascent and horizontalisation of the inframammary crease produced by the abdominal fat
– if the subcutaneous fatty panniculus has been over-thinned, the diameter acceptable in the vertical direction risks providing a globally insufficient volume, and the transverse spread is too reduced

Position of the implant in relation to the pectoralis major

The insertion of the implant in a retropectoral position (fig. 185) is preferable in breast reconstruction for different reasons:

– the presence of the muscle in front of the implant better isolates the latter from the superficial layers, often not very thick, especially in what will correspond to the upper quadrants of the reconstructed breast;

– for the same reasons the thickness of the muscle renders the implant less obviously visible and palpable, particularly at its upper limit;

– the implant will also be better isolated from the scar, which is usually projected over the muscle almost throughout its extent, and which constitutes a rather more vulnerable zone;

– the presence of the muscle in front of the implant slightly flattens its upper, retromuscular, part, while allowing rounding-off of its lower inframuscular and subcutaneous part; this contributes to giving the reconstructed breast a more natural shape, whereas the spontaneous shape of the implant is regularly rounded.

In practice, the implant is never entirely retropectoral for anatomic reasons:

– the lower border of the pectoral, oblique downward and inward, crosses the area of breast projection at an angle which varies with the shape of the thorax (the lower border of the muscle is more oblique when the woman is lanky and more horizontal when she is stocky), and with the natural level of breast implantation which determines the position of the inframmary crease (as assessed in relation to the other side);

– but, in any case, the inferolateral quadrant and a variable portion of the inferomedial quadrant are situated below the pectoralis major muscle;

– some workers consider that the risk of periprosthetic contracture is less when the implant is situated behind the muscle, because of the effect of the constant massage produced by muscular contraction on the implant during ordinary movements. What is more certain is that a moderate degree of periprosthetic contracture is bound to be less obvious and palpable when the implant is behind the muscle. Finally, the retropectoral position of the implant facilitates clinical and radiological surveillance of the breast.

The sole indication for prepectoral implantation may be in cases where the subcutaneous fatty layer is very thick, in a fat woman, where the essential requirement is that the implant should ensure central projection and not be flattened by the muscle. This is a rather exceptional situation. Further, considerable laxity must exist, without any sequelae of radiotherapy which might involve a threat to the scar, the more dramatic since the implant becomes immediately exposed.

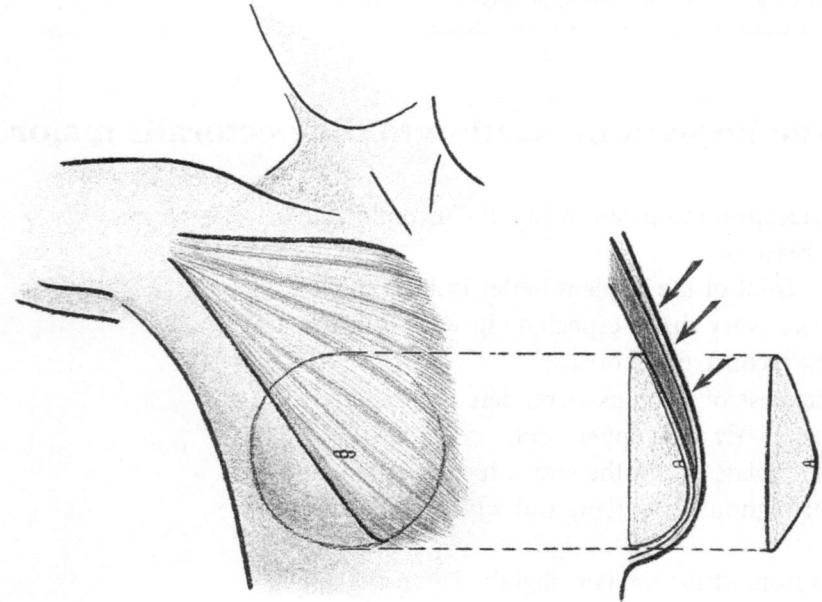

Fig. 185. Insertion of the implant in retro- (and infra-) pectoral position is the situation best suited to breast reconstruction

Operative technique

Positioning

The operation is performed under general anesthesia with intubation and in the semi-seated position, shoulders horizontal and arms beside the body, while ensuring that the pelvis is square. The drapes expose the clavicles above, the midaxillary line laterally and just exclude the umbilical zone below.

Design

A line drawn in ink frames the scar if this is to be excised, as is usually the case, since, unless it is linear and very supple, there is a risk that it may tauten to give the affect of a very unsightly transverse bridge once the implant is in place.

The inframammary crease is then drawn symmetrically with the opposite side, thanks to a first horizontal landmark tangential to the central dependent part of the existing crease (fig. 186). It is only when the opposite breast is very bulky and therefore very heavy, and when some slight ascent is expected after resection of the excess, that the new crease is drawn for reconstruction at a very slightly higher level.

Then a second trace is made below the first, defining a crescent. This line is about 3 cm away from the first at its center and joins it at both ends. It serves to obtain the "suspension" of the inframammary crease, a device we employ whenever possible, which supplies a little more tissue stock in the lower part of the reconstructed breast. This contributes to giving it a more natural appearance from

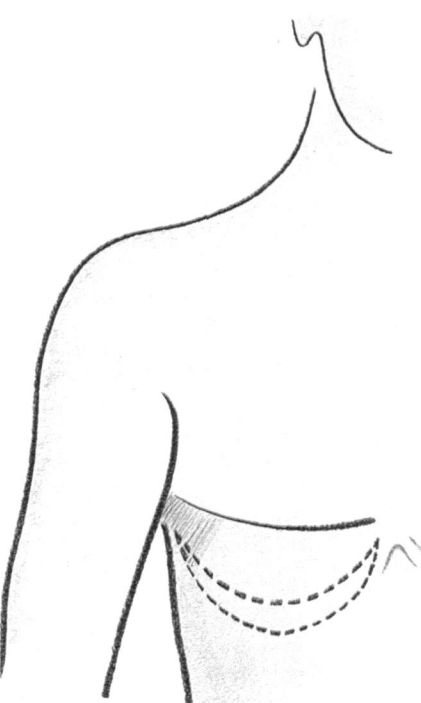

Fig. 186. Preoperative design:
- location of the inframammary crease, symmetric with the opposite side.
- crescent-shaped lower line about 3 cm below, for suspension of the crease
- below and lateral to the lower border of the pectoralis major (hatched area) there is a fibrous zone which often needs to be slashed with deep incisions to relax it

the outset, one more convex in its lower part than in its upper part, and also helps in the proper marking of the inframammary crease.

Whether or not it is decided to perform a suspension of the breast, it is very important to the end-result that the crease of the reconstructed breast be situated no lower than that of the opposite breast. This defect, difficult to make good, is much more obvious and more unsightly when the crease is sited a little too high up; it hinders the wearing of a brassière more than the converse fault (since the crease marked out by an implant is relatively fixed on the chest wall, whereas the natural crease retains a certain degree of mobility which allows it to ascend, thanks to the support of a brassière, but not to descend more than is due to the effects of gravity.

Approach

This follows the mastectomy scar, which is usually excised almost completely. The skin is excised with the underlying scar fibrosis down to the muscle plane; the muscle is then incised boldly and directly at the same level and parallel to the skin incision, without respect for the direction of its fibers, since this would require stripping of the skin and subcutaneous tissue from the anterior aspect of the muscle. This incision is made through the entire thickness of the muscle down to the precostal plane (fig. 187).

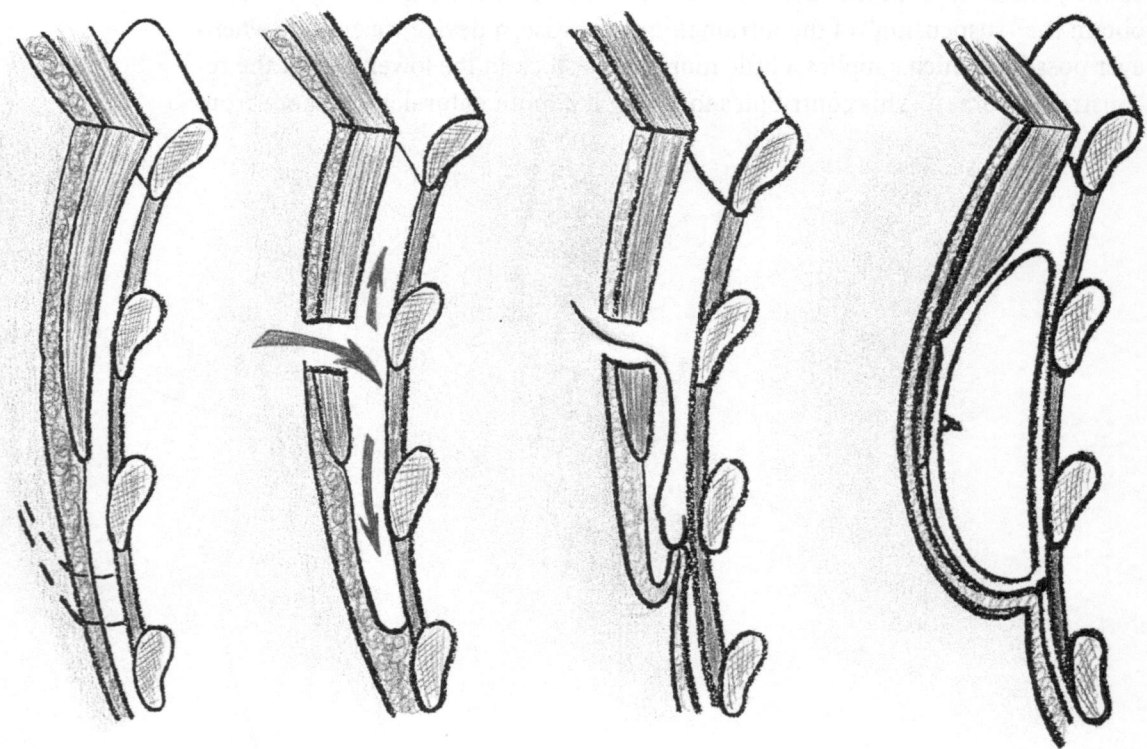

Fig. 187. Excision of the scar: direct transmuscular approach, retromuscular stripping, suspension of the crease

Creation of the compartment

The freeing of the deep aspect of the muscle is made differently at both margins of the incision:

– under the upper margin, the muscle is not adherent to the chest wall and stripping can be done almost entirely with the finger, taking care not to take it any higher than is required by the dimensions of the implant selected;

– under the lower margin, the dissection is carried out with scissors as one very soon encounters the lowest and innermost attachments of the pectoralis major, which must be partially detached on their deep aspect, and, especially below the lower border of the muscle, adhesions of the subcutaneous layer to the chest wall.

This detachment of the lowest and innermost muscle fibers is made from the depths to the surface and is complete for the muscle fibers but respects the continuity of the superficial aponeurosis.

Under the outermost part of the stripping are found the digitations of the serratus anterior, but between these digitations and the pectoral fibers there is a plane without superficial muscle fibers where it is important not to enter behind the aponeurotic plane of the intercostal muscles, nor, more medially, under the aponeurosis of the very uppermost part of the rectus abdominis muscle. These two aponeurotic planes are thick and rigid and do not submit to rounding off by the lower pole of the implant, which tends to be displaced upward.

Laterally, the stripping will not transgress beyond the anterior axillary line, so as to prevent subsequent outward displacement of the implant by the pressure of pectoral contraction to assume a too lateral position, which would be evidenced by medial flattening. In the outermost and uppermost zone of this plane, just below the site where the pectoral fibers start to come together to form the tendon, there often exists a fibrous zone which is inextensible and rigid and often marked by adhesion to the muscle plane. This is associated with postoperative adhesion of the subcutaneous plane at the parietal plane, and corresponds to the junction beween the end of the mastectomy and the lower end of the axillary nodal clearance. To restore a degree of freedom at this region, one can slash the fibrosis on the deep aspect throughout its thickness until the yellowish layer of the subcutaneous fatty layer is encountered. We prefer to perform this procedure, which is often adequate and effective, rather than to perform a Z plasty at the outer end of the scar, where the scar defect is more obvious.

Beyond the lower border of the pectoralis major, the skin and subcutaneous tissue are stripped flush with the parietal aponeurotic plane, this stripping being pursued as far as the lower tracing of the inframammary crease.

Hemostasis must be scrupulous, checking in particular the region of the perforating intercostal branches which may have been damaged when detaching the lowest muscle heads. To prevent retraction of these vessels, thus complicating hemostasis, it is better not to detach these heads at periosteal level but to divide the muscle fibers a little beyond their origin.

Suspension of the inframammary crease

We have now reached the stage of suspension of the new crease (fig. 187).

A number of sutures are passed on the deep aspect of the stripping using undyed slowly-absorbed 2/0 material and held with forceps. These U stitches grasp the entire thickness of the dissected margin from the depth outward so as to catch the deep aspect of the dermis, corresponding to the lower tracing of the crescent. This procedure is begun medially and then continued by lateral sutures at intervals of about 3 cm. Three to five sutures usually suffice, as the crease does not need to be marked out as far as its extremities (the application of the tissues to the implant by the suction drain and the postoperative scarring will deal with this).

When the sutures have been passed, they are taken up again one by one to be tethered higher up, this time to the parietal plane, seizing solid support on the aponeurosis or the periosteum.

By using packs in the lower part of the compartment, it is verified that the new crease thus created is of harmonious shape, and especially that it is placed at the same level as the opposite crease. The packs are removed, hemostasis checked again, and a Jost suction drain placed in the depth of the dissection.

This procedure gives a more natural shape to the reconstructed breast from the outset, while providing a tissue excess in the lower part of the compartment, which, together with the retropectoral position of the implant, helps to give the lower slope of the reconstructed breast a more marked convexity than its upper slope, which is slightly flattened by the muscle. It is only in obese patients that we do not do this, and for two reasons:

– the wall is too thick to be easily mobilised upward and for passage of the sutures to be possible;

– this procedure creates a new fold concave upward, whereas the inframammary crease in an obese patient is horizontal or exhibits an inverted curvature, concave downward.

Closure of the compartment

This is done simply leaving a central opening for insertion of the implant. To close the compartment almost completely before inserting the implant limits the risks of injuring the latter by any awkward movement of the needle, and in particular it allows a better assessment of the volume necessary for filling. Suture of the muscle plane, if the muscle is of normal substance, is not done through its entire thickness; the X sutures made with undyed slowly-absorbed material, like those used for suspension of the fold, seize only the superficial aponeurosis and part of the thickness of the fibers. This "tenting" suture allows the muscle to spread out and helps to somewhat increase the space available to the implant on its anterior aspect.

Insertion of the implant

The implant is removed from its packing after a change of gloves, which are rinsed to get rid of particles of talc; irrigation may also have been done in the pocket itself, using a mixture of normal saline and polyvinylpyrrolidone (unless the patient is sensitive to iodine).

The filling catheter is applied, the air completely expressed, and a first filling made with 50 ml of saline to expel any air-bubbles and allow the detection of any malfunction. The catheter is clamped and the unit is inserted into the compartment, and the implant inflated with normal saline up to the desired volume, which will always be more than the theoretic volume indicated by the manufacturer. This prevents the formation of creases and ensures that the valve is watertight, but without causing excessive pressure. Before withdrawing the catheter, a check is made that the implant is properly spread out in its compartment and that the valve is correctly placed, at the middle of the anterior surface. After withdrawal of the catheter, one must check that the little lid situated under the flap covering the valve is properly applied over the opening of the latter.

Closure of the muscle plane is completed with great care not to graze the implant, even with the butt of the needle, so as not to risk damaging or fragilising it, which could produce a perforation after a varying period. Suture of the superficial plane is made in two layers, the deep dermal layer with interrupted inverting sutures of slowly absorbed material, and the superficial dermal layer with a continuous intradermal suture that is rapidly absorbed.

If it is desired to perform a reduction plasty for hypertrophy or ptosis at this same operative stage, which is not our habit, the implant is inserted first, if only for reasons of asepsis, but at the stage of closure a small opening is contrived for passage of the filling device. Clamped and left in place until the procedure on the opposite breast is completed, this allows modification of the necessary volume as required.

Dressings and postoperative course

A well-modeled and slightly compressive dressing is constructed with tulle gras, dry packs, and hypoallergenic elastic adhesive strapping. The first adhesive bandage marks the inframammary crease and the other bandages are then applied, taking care to flatten the upper slope of the implant and to hold it towards the midline. This dressing is retained until removal of the suction drain, on average at 4 to 5 days. After removal of the drain and dressing, it is sufficient to protect the scar with Steristrips for some ten days; showers are allowed daily using antiseptic soap, and a well-supporting elastic brassière is worn day and night for two weeks.

We prescribe no other treatment except analgesics as needed and anti-staphylococcal) antibiotic cover begun at the start of operation and continued for 72 hours.

With smooth-walled implants, it was our practice to have the patient massage the implant as soon as possible in an attempt to combat the risk of periprosthetic contracture, by applying the palm of the hand flat against the reconstructed breast and mobilising the implant upward, downward, inward and outward, but this no longer seems indicated with textured implants.

In sum, the important points are:
- *the retro- and infrapectoral position of the implant;*
- *detachment of the inferior heads of the pectoralis major;*
- *suspension of the inframammary crease;*
- *a "tented" muscle suture;*
- *moderate overinflation of the implant.*

The fate of the reconstructed breast

The result in a breast reconstructed with an implant is not stabilised for several months, as the shape and consistence depend on several factors of differing importance, some with opposing effects.

These are:
- the shape of the thorax, which influences the position and orientation of the pectoralis major;
- the trophic state of the pectoralis;
- the level of implantation of the opposite breast;
- the site of the scar;
- the amount of subcutaneous fatty tissue;
- the quantity and quality of skin left after the mastectomy;
- the capacity for skin stretching;
- the fate of the periprosthetic membrane.

Shape of thorax and position of pectoralis major

Although the attachments of the pectoralis major are constant at the sternum and first five or six costal cartilages, the shape and spread of the muscle and the direction of its lower border vary from one woman to another. The lankier the patient, with wide shoulders and a thorax narrowed at its base (fig. 188), the more the lower border of the muscle will run obliquely downward and inward, exposing a more extensive part of the implant, which at that site will be directly subcutaneous.

The stockier the woman, with narrow shoulders and a short wide thorax, the more the lower border of the muscle will be horizontal and the more it will cover the implant in uniform fashion.

Trophic state of the pectoralis major

The upper contours of the prosthesis will be better concealed, and the upper slope of the reconstructed breast will have a more natural appearance, ie less convex than its lower slope, when the muscle has retained good pliability and good trophicity.

It is important, after mastectomy, to regain good function and flexibility of the shoulder, if need be by appropriate rehabilitation, and above all great care is required at the time of nodal clearance to respect the innervation of the pectorals. It is not uncommon to find, not a complete atrophy, but a wasting of the lower heads of the muscle, which is reduced to a mere superior functional relic

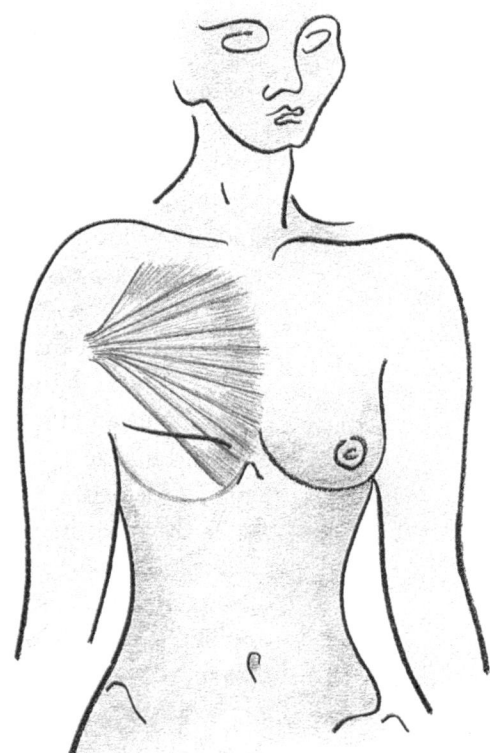

Fig. 188. The covering of the implant by the pectoral muscle depends on the build of the patient: the longer the thorax, the more the implant will be exposed in the inferolateral quadrant

whose lower border, horizontal and too highly situated, is clearly visible on contraction.

This situation, if accompanied by a subcutaneous adipose layer of poor quality, risks producing a reconstruction of very poor quality if one is content to insert an implant. This is an indication for the provision of a myocutaneous flap of the latissimus dorsi with good muscular overlap to line the defective subcutaneous layer, the small skin flap serving mainly to give more breadth to the inferolateral quadrant. It may even be enough to manage with a simple muscular lining without any supplementary provision.

Implantation of the opposite breast

The breast base is implanted at a variable level on the thorax, which will determine the level of the inframammary crease and thus its position in relation to the lower border of the pectoralis major. This factor will therefore also have an effect on the surface of cover of the implant by the muscle in its lower quadrants.

Position and direction of the scar

Although mastectomy is a controlled procedure, the placement of the scar will vary depending on the site of the initial lesion, its size, and the extent of skin sacrifice in relation to the envelope of the entire breast.

Depending on the site of the lesion, the surgeon will have to extend the skin incision more widely in one or other direction and, particularly in lesions of the upper quadrants, to displace the excision upward, which places the upper margin in a zone with finer and less lax skin, making it necessary to close with a wider stripping of the lower margin on the abdominal slope. It is in this type of excision that residual laxity is most reduced and the two margins are of unequal thickness as regards both the dermis and the fatty panniculus, which is often marked by a kind of fibrous rim just under the scar. The higher the scar, the less the laxity required for suspension of the inframammary crease and the more difficult it is technically.

Scars sited at the middle of the breast base are bordered by skin of uniform quality at both margins. The lower the scar, the thicker and more elastic are the integuments and the subcutaneous fatty layer is also thicker; this depends on the general build of the patient, but also on the way in which the mastectomy has been performed.

On the other hand, the appearance of the reconstruction may be ill served by the position of the scar, for which there is no remedy since it depends on the conditions in which the mastectomy was performed. Ideally, in reconstruction by implant, there will be a horizontal scar (fig. 189) projected at the level of the future nipple-areolar plaque; thus it will be interrupted visually by the reconstructed areola and less obvious, the eye being attracted by the areola, which will play its role of optical "deception" better if it is well-placed on the reconstructed breast and symmetric with the opposite side. It is one of the reasons why we attach such importance to this and do not perform reconstruction at the first operative stage (fig. 190).

Capacity for skin stretching

This depends on the amount of skin left after the mastectomy, but also on its elasticity and its tolerance of radiotherapy.

The position of a well-suspended crease will not be altered, but above this the superficial layer will undergo a variable reaction under the thrust of the implant. Some skins can stretch so much — though this is rare — that it is necessary to excise a little skin on either side of the scar at the second stage, or to fill the implant a little more, which may be considered as an expansion in two stages.

In other cases, it is the skin coverings which will not stretch sufficiently, even if they have not undergone radiotherapy, the reconstructed breast retaining too spherical an appearance and with insufficient convexity below and laterally. Perhaps it is commoner to find this situation when the scar is low (lesion of the lower quadrants) or especially very oblique downward and inward, which has been produced at the time of the mastectomy by stripping the tissues extensively below and laterally to ensure closure.

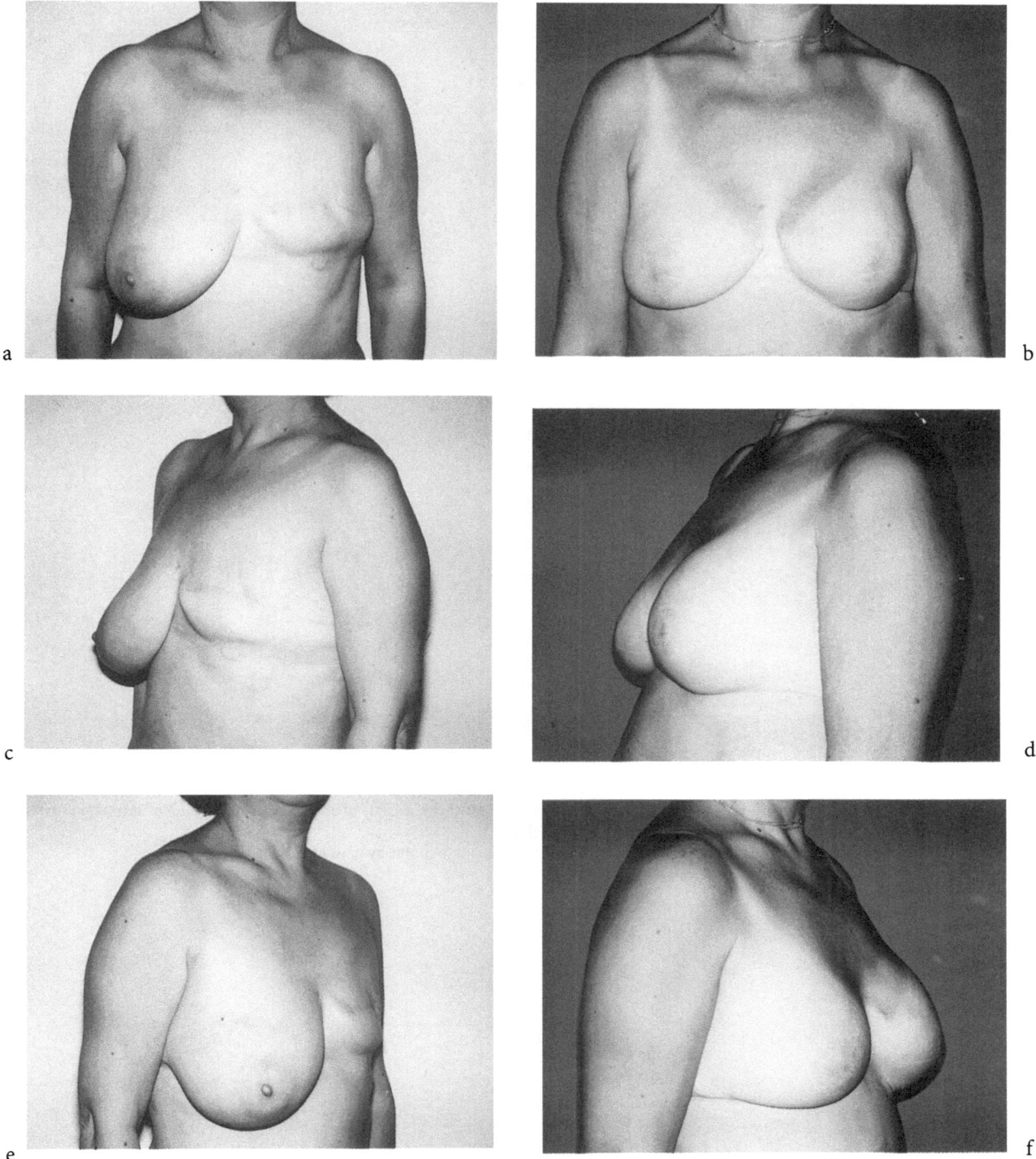

Fig. 188 a-f. Reconstruction by implant.
Stage 1: insertion of a smooth inflatable implant (Sebbin LS20) of 300 ml with suspension of the inframammary crease, filled with 350 ml of normal saline.
Stage 2: reduction plasty of opposite breast and reconstruction of areola by grafts from the inguinal region and the opposite nipple

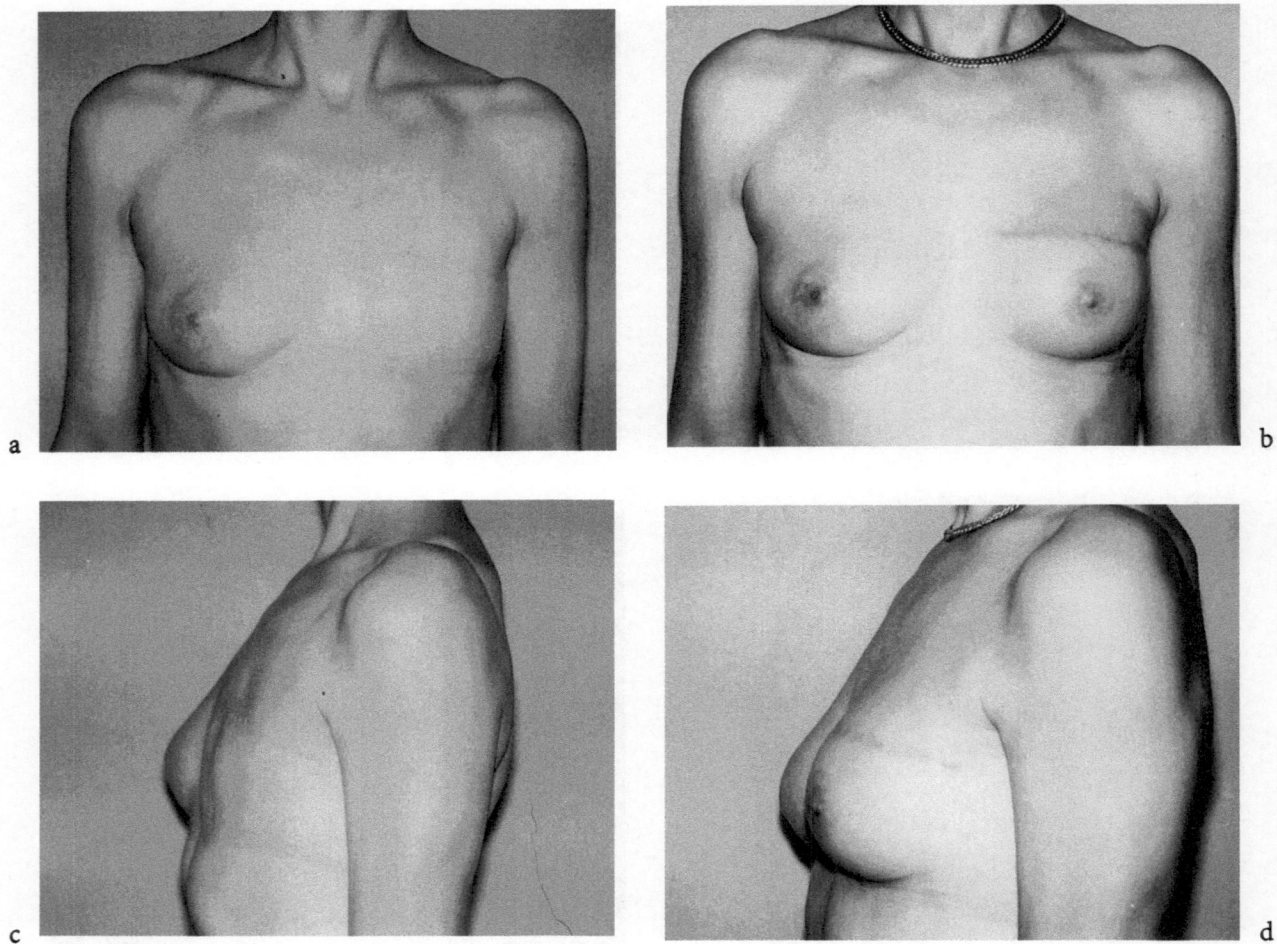

Fig.190 a-d. Reconstruction by implant.
Stage 1: insertion of textured inflatable implant (Sebbin LS21) of 200 ml with suspension of inframammary crease, filling with 250 ml of normal saline.
Stage 2: reconstruction of areola by tattooing and of nipple by graft of earlobe

These very oblique scars, with the skin cover more stretched at the inferolateral margin than the superomedial margin, should arouse caution since they often give a poor result with an implant alone, which remains too high and too medial. On the other hand, they lend themselves very favorably to the placement of a flap, with or without an implant, as its skin component will fit naturally into the opening of the scar, whose lower margin often reaches the level of the inframammary crease without the need for supplementary excision.

The fact that radiotherapy has been given subsequent to the mastectomy is not in it a contraindication to the placement of an implant if the skin shows no obvious sequelae and exhibits a good trophic state and sufficient laxity (fig. 191). It is particularly important for the skin to have uniform elasticity and flexibility over the whole extent which will project in front of the implant, and for the subcutaneous fatty layer to be of uniform thickness.

However, there are cases where the ability to stretch is not uniform everywhere, particularly towards the middle of the scar, which is then associated with less substantial and more rigid integuments. This is evidence of a zone of excessive tension during closure, which for vascular reasons has been less tolerant of the radiotherapy, leaving as a sequel a secondary localised sclerosis (fig. 192). This rigidity will be revealed still more with the implant, the reconstructed breast exhibiting a more rigid and flat appearance and lacking in anterior projection.

One should be much more cautious when the radiotherapy has preceded the mastectomy, as when it has been used to supplement a previous tumorectomy. Even if the lack of substance is not obvious, the lack of elasticity and even a degree of tissue damage will be revealed after the procedure, the relaxation in front of the implant being insufficient.

In our experience, the combination of tumorectomy and radiotherapy, followed at a varying interval by a supplementary mastectomy, is nearly always an indication for a flap.

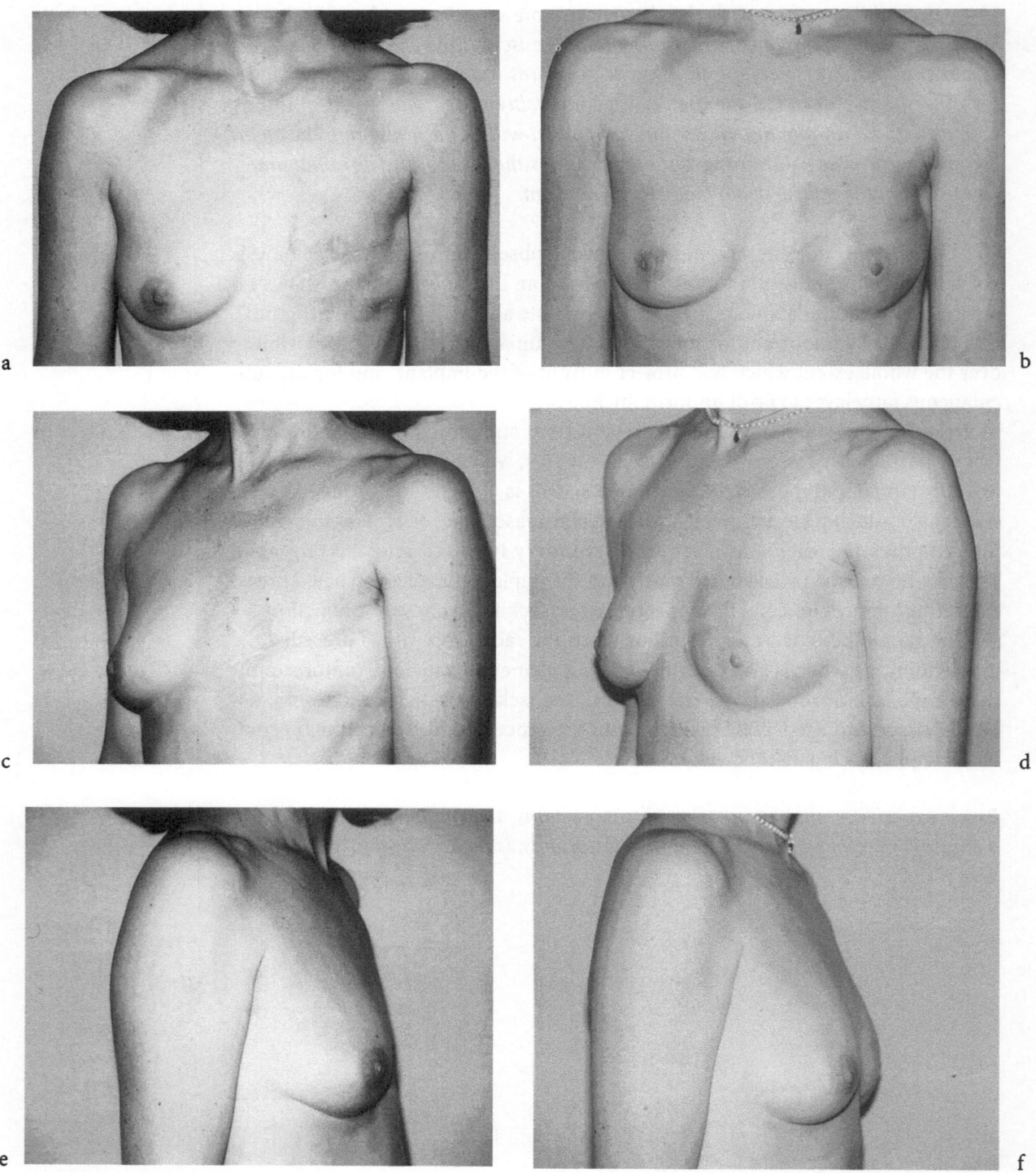

Fig. 191 a-f. Reconstruction by implant after mastectomy followed by radiotherapy (to breast and medial thoracic areas). Sebbin LS21 textured inflatable implant of 175 ml, filled with 200 ml of normal saline. Secondary reconstruction of areola by tattooing and nipple graft, treatment of inner thoracic telangiectases by diathermy during procedure

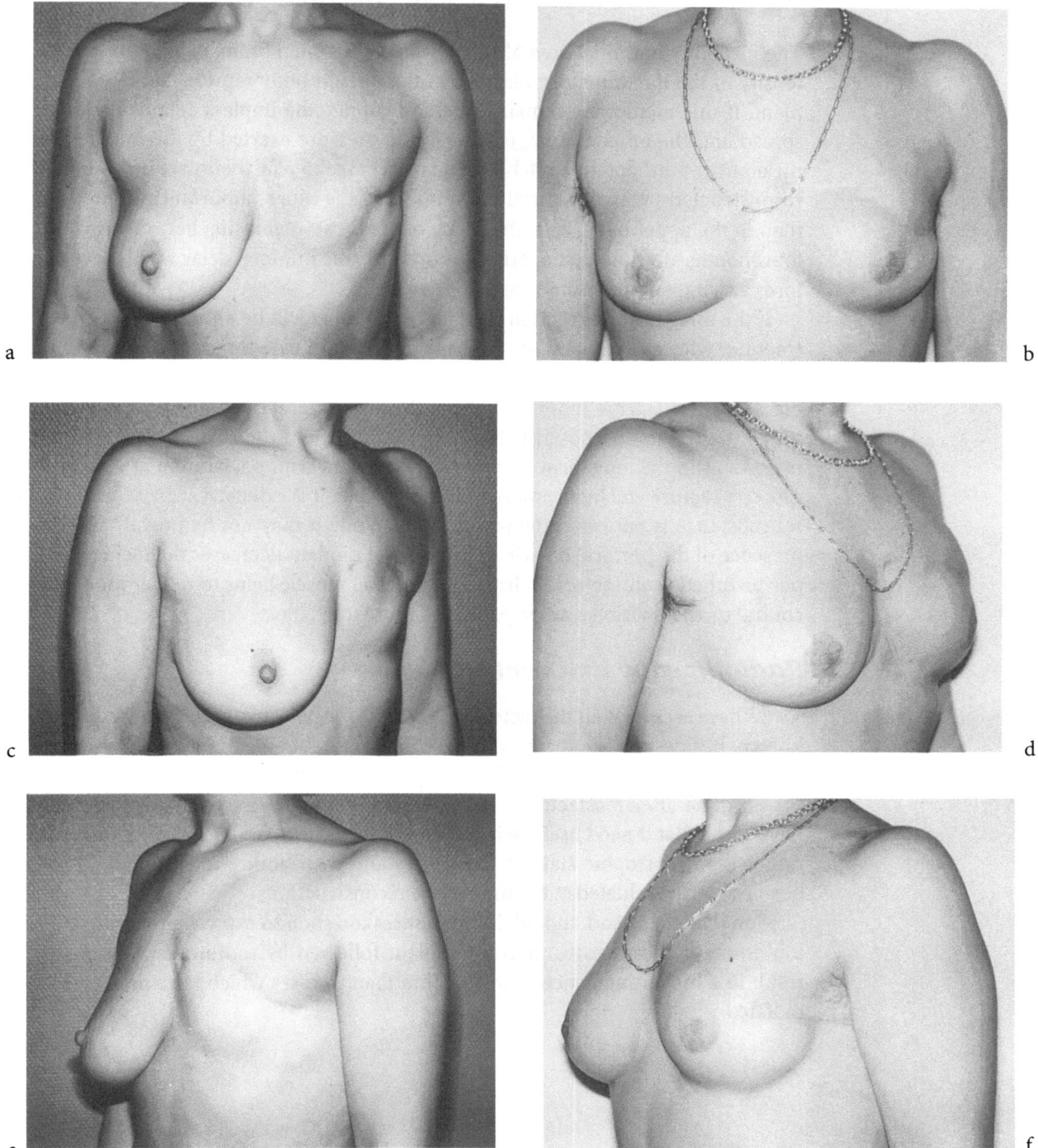

Fig. 192 a-f. Mastectomy followed by radiotherapy. Reconstruction by smooth inflatable AHS implant of 225 ml, filled with 275 ml of normal saline, reduction mammoplasty (100 g) of opposite breast, reconstruction of areola by inguinal graft and lower half of opposite nipple. The radiotherapy is probaby responsible for the lack of flexibility of the tissues on either side of the scar, the zone where the greatest tension is exerted post-operatively

Periprosthetic membrane and contracture

The flexibility and thickness of the periprosthetic membrane depend on the intensity of the inflammatory reaction to the foreign body represented by the implant. If this membrane remains fine and supple, the implant retains its initial spread and the other factors, especially the pressure exerted by the muscle and the ability of the skin to stretch, will be better able to play their part in giving the reconstructed breast a natural curvature. This is more important in the lower than in the upper quadrants, the shape of the breast stabilising between two and four months after the first operative procedure, the minimal delay we observe before carrying out the second stage (fig. 193).

If the foreign body reaction is exaggerated there will be a periprosthetic contracture, whose disadvantages we have already discussed: reduction of the implantation base, an over-spherical shape, exaggerated firmness, the formation of creases. These last are more palpable in the inferolateral quadrant, where there is very little tissue interposed between the implant and the surface; such creases may result in the long term in wear of the implant with perforation at this level. The contracture will be the more unesthetic when it is extensive, when the pectoral substance is poor and the patient thin. While it may not be proven that the presence of the pectoral muscle in front of the implant decreases the incidence of periprosthetic contracture, at least a substantial muscle helps to render moderate contracture less visible and palpable and more tolerable.

Radiotherapy and contracture

As we have seen, not all the factors responsible for periprosthetic contracture are known. Besides those already considered in discussing the indications for breast augmentation, it seems that radiotherapy plays a part:

– if done after mastectomy, in the case of secondary reconstructions,we do not believe that it need itself be incriminated in the formation of contracture, but rather that the trophic state of the tissues and their ability to stretch have not been properly evaluated at the time of the reconstruction;

– on the other hand, though it is doubtless too soon to express a definite opinion, immediate reconstruction by implant followed by radiotherapy seems to result in a higher incidence of contracture than in cases which have not been irradiated.

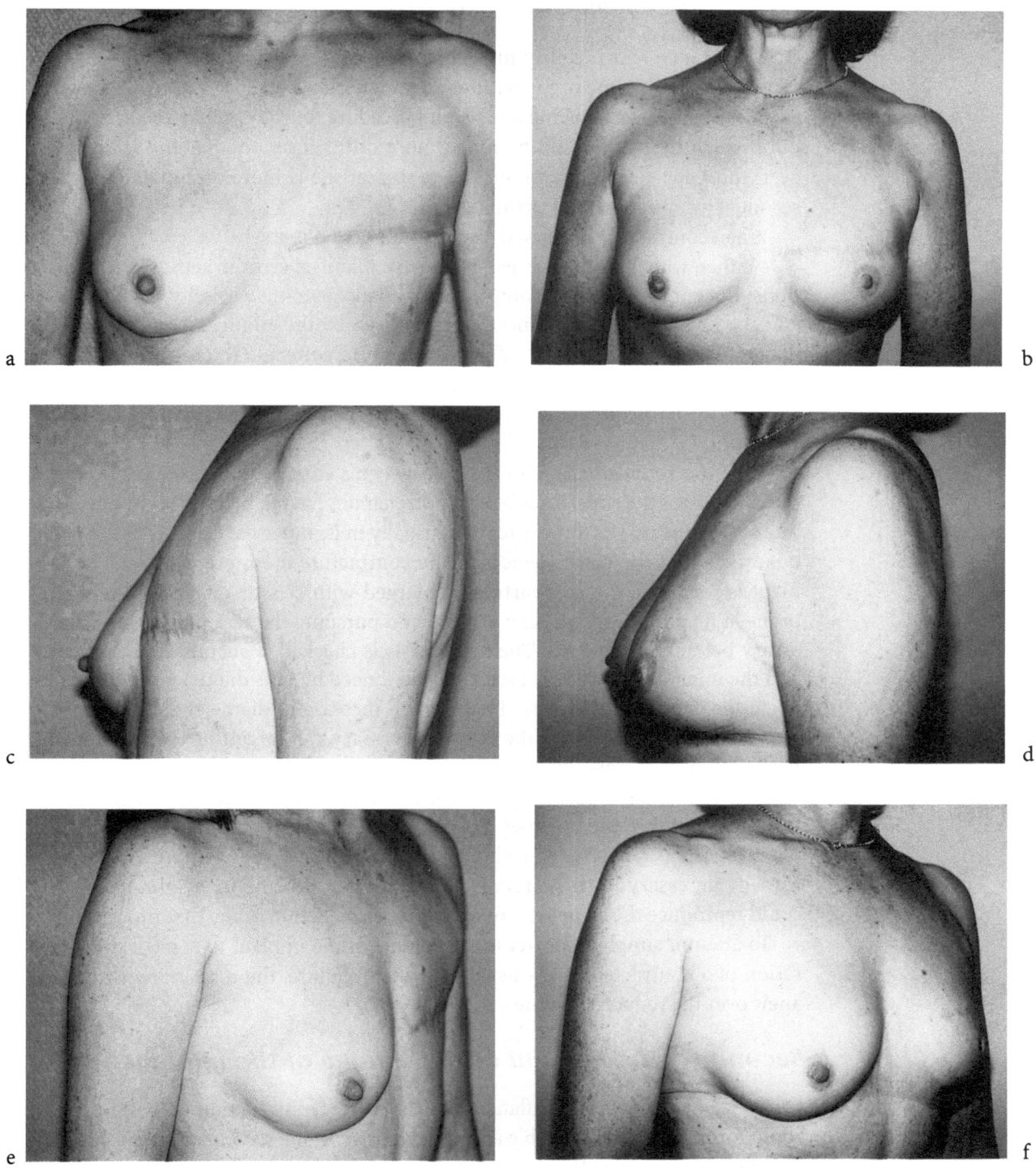

Fig. 193 a-f. Reconstruction by implant.
Stage 1: reconstruction, with suspension of inframammary fold, by smooth inflatable Sebbin LS20 implant of
225 ml, filled with 275 ml of normal saline.
Stage 2: 4 months later, reconstruction of areola by tattooing and graft from opposite nipple

The management of contracture

Our ignorance and inability to predict the risk and severity of periprosthetic contracture is also one of the reasons why we perform the procedure in two stages, the second stage allowing a revision procedure for the compartment, a procedure which by itself would be much more difficult for the patient to accept if everything has been done in one stage, so that she is more disappointed by the secondary development of asymmetry.

When contracture is marked, two attitudes are possible:

– either, which is rare, it is partly due to a manifest error in settling the indications: the contracture is accompanied by inadequate distensiblity of the tissues and the reconstruction will need to be revised by the addition of a flap. In this uncommon situation all our efforts will tend to complete the reconstruction in one stage — flap, plasty of the opposite breast and reconstruction of the areola — so as to rid the patient's mind of the failure of reshaping at the first operative stage; or:

– the too rounded shape of the breast seems entirely due to the contracture, the capacity of the superficial layers to stretch not having been brought into play. The scar of the mastectomy is revised, usually in its outer part, as it is in the outer quadrants that the consequences of the contracture are more evident. The implant is removed, the compartment enlarged with scissors, splitting the membrane at its periphery in whole or part, and pursuing the stripping as far as necessary below and outward. The hemostasis is checked, a suction drain inserted and the implant replaced, or even changed if need be if its diameter seems inadequate for the new breast base. However, an increase in diameter should be considered in conjunction with the volume necessary, not forgetting that the implant must always be at least slightly overinflated.

This enlargement of the compartment, made on a part only of its surface, often has a positive effect; either the contracture does not recur, or it recurs but with lesser effect, and the morphologic outcome proves much improved. It is not actually necessary to try to remove the entire periprosthetic membrane, as this could reproduce the same type of inflammatory reaction as the first procedure.

To attempt simply to decrease the volume of the implant to combat the induration of a contracted breast usually results in failure, the membrane shrinking anew over the reduced volume.

Secondary adjustment of the volume of the implant

One of the advantages of inflatable implants in reconstruction is that a certain room for maneuver is available as to the volume. At the second operative stage, if the volume seems insufficient, and if the implantation base is of correct size, it is possible, while remaining within reasonable limits, to increase the filling by means of a short reopening of the scar at the level of the valve. On the contrary, if the breast is too round and firm because the implant has been overfillled, and not because contracture has developed, one can perform the converse maneuver, since the capacity for cutaneous distension remains present, but with caution. This is because a compartment that is supple but too large, over an implant that may have been correctly filled but with insufficient volume, risks producing a wave effect clearly visible in the upper quadrants, the remedy for which can only be skin excision, and this is an overplus as far as the reconstruction is concerned.

Special features of immediate reconstruction by implant

When the amount of tissue material available permits the technical performance of an immediate reconstruction, there are some precautions to be respected:

– the stripping of the deep aspect of the gland must respect the aponeurosis of the pectoralis major muscle, and especially the fascia that prolongs it at the lower border of the muscle, and which alone can ensure continuity in front of the implant in a zone of varying extent devoid of muscle fibers situated between the lower border of the pectoralis major medially and the digitations of the serratus anterior laterally;

– the implant compartment can also be created by a transmuscular approach, but the incision will be made on this occasion in the direction of the fibers since the subcutaneous plane is already widely stripped. The upper stripping at the deep aspect of the muscle is also easily made with the finger, and similar care must be taken not to carry it too high, to avoid secondary malposition of the implant.

The difficulty concerns the inferior and outward stripping, again respecting both this fascia and the digitations of the serratus anterior, much more delicate than those of the pectoralis.

The lower limit of the stripping must correspond to the level of the inframammary crease. The aim is to ensure a continuous covering for the implant, both muscular and fascial, as in a subcutaneous mastectomy, isolating it completely from the superficial plane.

– When the flexibility of the superficial plane allows (and the fatty panniculus is not too thick), the stripping is pursued subcutaneously to allow suspension of the crease (fig. 194). The deep dermal support sutures are tethered to the chest wall at the level of the lower border of the compartment. These sutures are fixed before placement of the implant to eliminate any risk of perforation (fig. 195).

– Drainage is double: a suction drain in the compartment, placed at its lower border and brought out at the outer end of the crease, and another suction drain in the zone of superficial stripping, also placed low down between the compartment and the superficial layer, which ascends to the axillary fossa to ensure simultaneous drainage of the nodal clearance and of the mastectomy, and is brought out at the inner end of the inframammary crease.

– Closure of the different planes presents no particular feature.

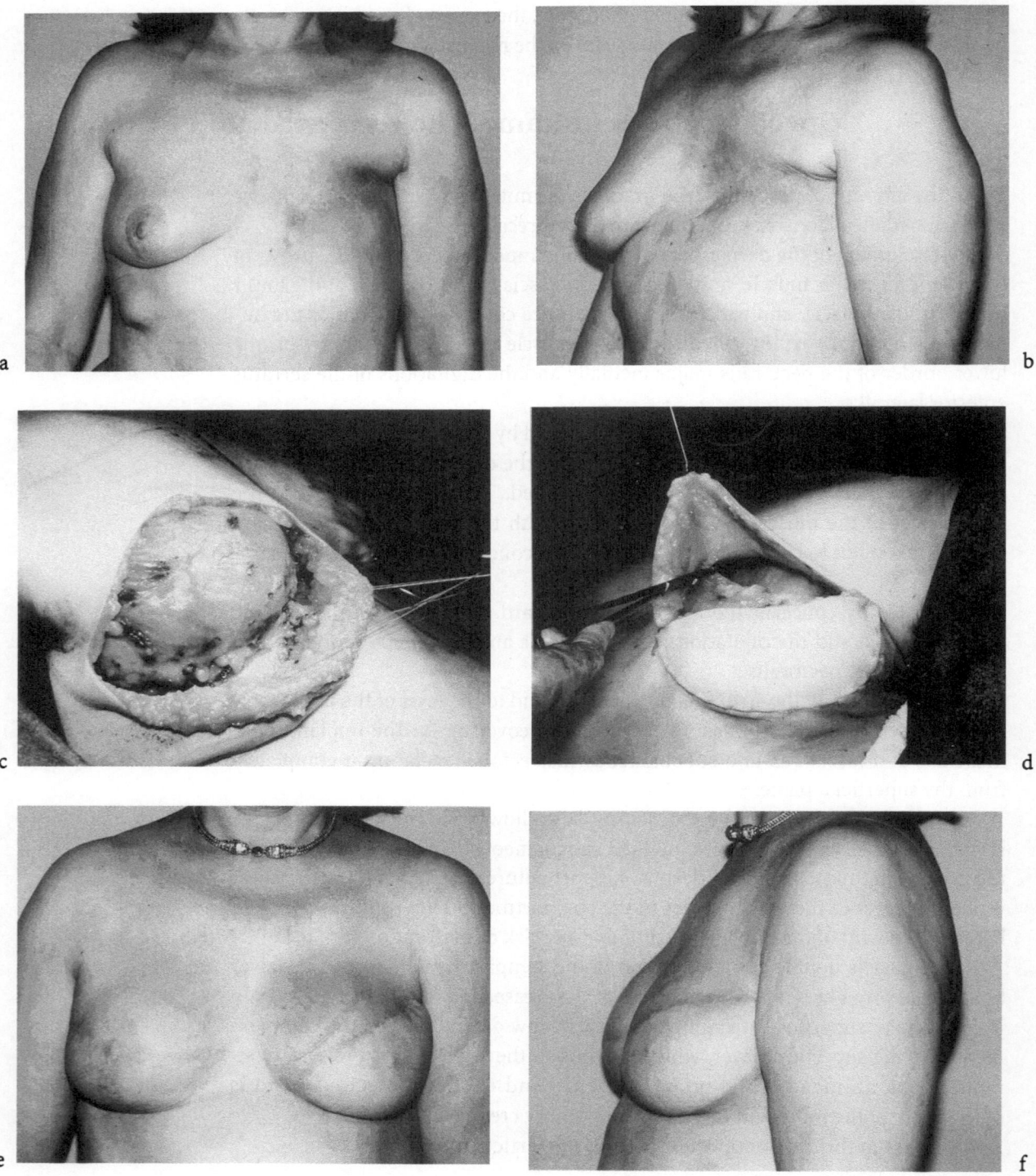

Fig. 194 a-f. Mastectomy of right breast with immediate reconstruction and simultaneous reconstruction of left breast by latissimus flap. **a** The swelling visible under the left breast is that of an implantable device for chemotherapy; **b** 3/4 left view: the indication for the latissimus flap was loss of laxity of the skin cover, the sequelae of irradiation and atrophy of the lower heads of the pectoralis major; **c** continuous retro- and infra-muscular compartment, LS20 implant of 200 ml filled to 300 ml. The lower margin has been stripped on the abdominal slope and advanced so as to perform suspension and fixation of the crease; **d** fixation of the muscle overlap of the latissimus dorsi to the pectoralis major. Implant LS20 of 200 ml filled to 270 ml; **e** reconstruction of areola by tattooing (too pale) and earlobe grafts

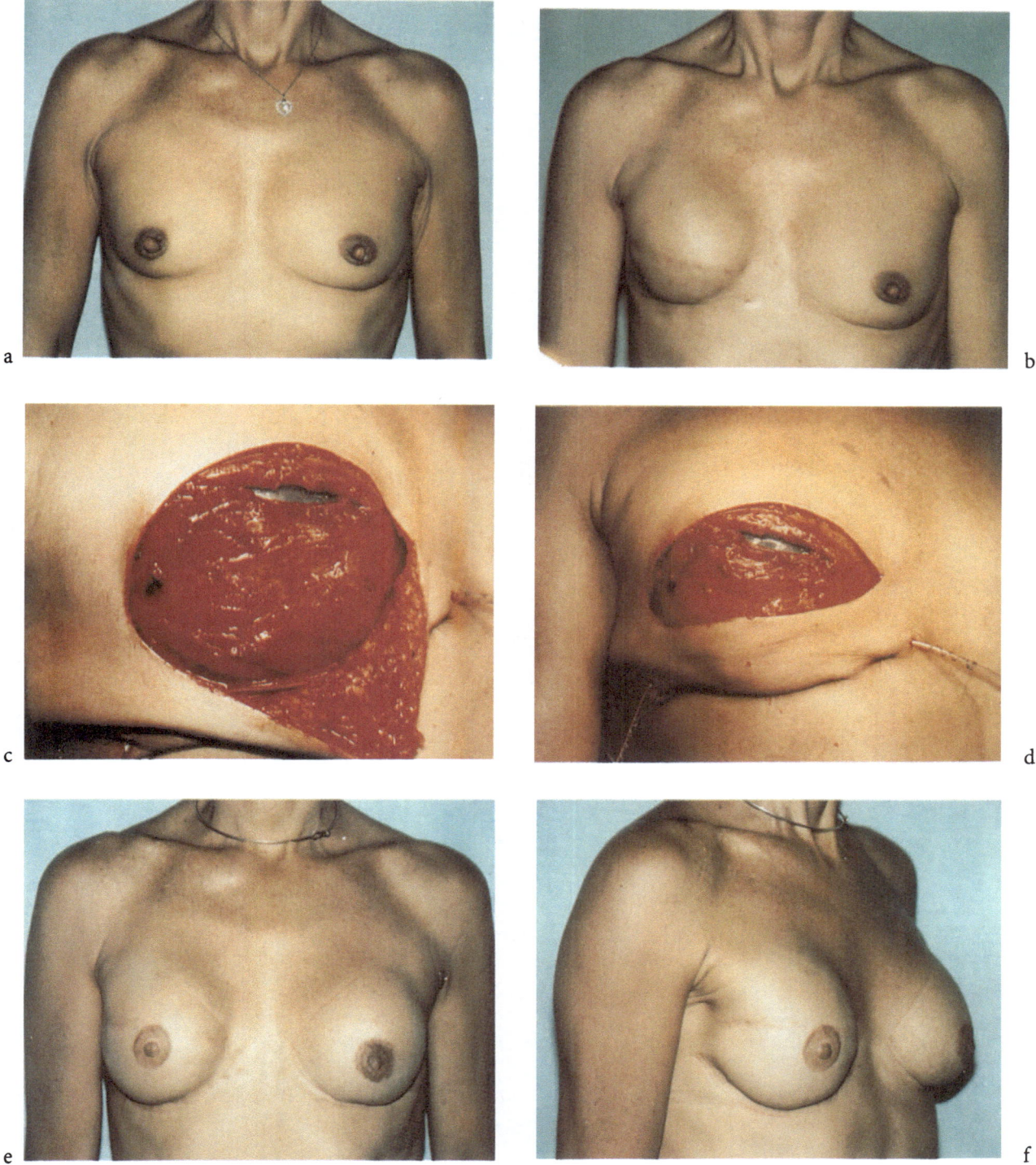

Fig. 195 a-f. Mastectomy of right breast with immediate reconstruction (no postoperative radiotherapy), with suspension of inframmary crease, Sebbin smooth inflatable implant of 150 ml filled with 175 ml of normal saline. Second operative stage: enlargement of compartment below and medially, change of implant for one of 175 ml filled with 230 ml, insertion on left side of LS20 implant of 100 ml filled with 120 ml, reconstruction of areola by tattooing and of nipple by graft of lower half of opposite nipple

Expansion procedures

The principle of cutaneous expansion consists of increasing the available tissue stock in a given region by placing under the tissue selected an implant of a particular type furnished with a valve. This expansion prosthesis is filled gradually by percutaneous injections adjusted to the tissue tolerance until the desired surface increase has been obtained.

The initial idea came from G. Neumann, by analogy with the natural abdominal expansion seen during pregnancy and with the customs of certain tribes: in Chad, the women develop the circumference of their lower lips in an impressive manner by inserting plates of increasing size. In a Burmese tribe, the women likewise obtain a major stretching of the soft structures of the neck by the progressive superimposition of metal rings; this cosmetic practice is also double-edged, since the punishment of an adulterous woman consists of taking away her rings!

The essential observation of Neumann (1957), which concerned an ear reconstruction, remained a singularity for a long time because of the poor quality of the material employed.

The idea was revived and widely developed by Radovan in 1976 in several parts of the body, particularly in breast reconstruction following mastectomy.

There are two ways of envisaging tissue expansion in breast reconstruction:
– in situ, directly beneath the tissues left by the mastectomy,
– or remotely, beneath the donor zone of a flap which is then transferred to the reconstruction site.

General principles

Whether in the reconstruction of a breast or in some other application, skin expansion must is subject to a certain number of general principles:
– the expansion can only be done under tissue of good quality, supple, well-vascularised and sufficiently thick such as the scalp, or possessing a substantial and above all a uniform subcutaneous fatty layer.

If the skin is too thin, insubstantial, or sclerosed, or if its blood-supply is inadequate to adapt to such a stress, the gain in distension obtained will be mediocre, or at worst unachievable because of tissue damage which may result in skin necrosis or disruption of the surgical approach route, exposing the prosthesis and preventing further continuance of the expansion;
– the expansion prosthesis is a foreign body which, no matter what the implant, requires working under strict aseptic conditions, the conduct of rigorous hemostasis, drainage of the compartment in order to prevent the formation of a

hematoma or an effusion, a source of additional tension and a possible focus of infection which would necessitate premature removal of the implant;

– in principle, the access route should be situated lateral to the zone of expansion and at right angles to the lines of greatest tension, so as not to be too stressed by the tension exerted during filling before complete healing has occurred.

Features specific to breast reconstruction

Expansion in breast reconstruction has some special features which sometimes run counter to the principles cited above, and which risk limitation of its application:

– when the expansion is performed at the actual site of mastectomy, the prosthesis is properly placed beneath the tissue previously dissected, which is not therefore healthy tissue as it exhibits the fibrosis of the healing process to which may be added the effects of radiotherapy.

Obvious sequelae evidently contraindicate the use of this technique, but the problems may only make their appearance during the expansion, ie when it may seem to have been reasonably attempted on apparently supple tissues, but when the trophic effects of combined surgery and radiotherapy do not emerge until the distension;

– this zone is moreover the site of the mastectomy scar, which is rather less supple than the adjacent tissue and which risks creating a contracture unless excision is performed;

– the approach route is therefore by definition that of the mastectomy scar, which is removed in whole or part. Its direction is obligatory and it may not be situated lateral to the expansion zone.

Equipment

There are several types of expansion prosthesis, depending on their shape, texture and filling device.

Shape

In reconstruction, round or "tear-drop" expansion prostheses are employed for expansion in situ, ovoid ones for expansion beneath a flap (fig. 196). It has been suggested that other, ovoid, shapes of prosthesis be used for in situ expansion, analogous to certain implants proposed a few years ago in the surgery of breast augmentation but which were not of proven superiority. Their use seems rather illogical since their shape, and therefore that of the periprosthetic pocket, does not correspond to that of the definitive implant.

Some manufacturers have proposed prostheses with differential expansion, which undergo less deformity in their lower and central parts. We cannot believe in their efficacy, since the shape assumed by the stretched tissues depends, in our

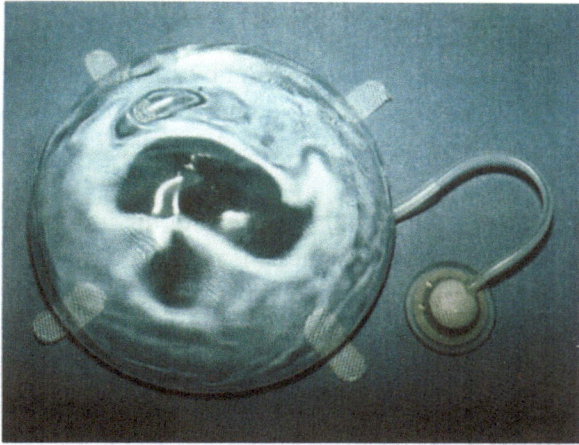 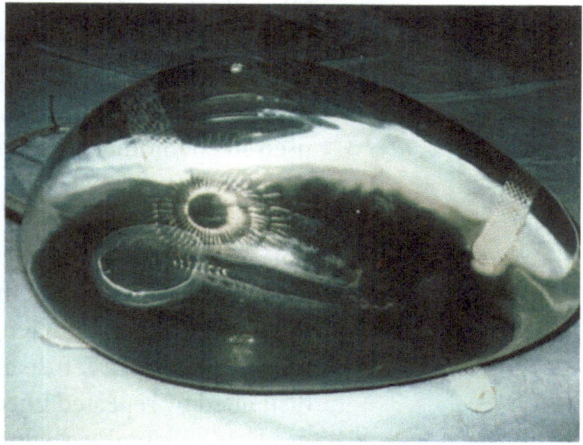

Fig. 196. a Round expansion prosthesis, remote valve, used for expansion in situ; **b** "teardrop" expansion prosthesis, remote valve, used for expansion under latissimus dorsi flap (Sigma Dow Corning)

opinion, more on their elasticity and their capacity for distension, and on features specific to the periprosthetic membrane and the effects of gravity, rather than on the characteristics of the prosthesis itself, which, if it is hemispherical in shape, will always favor the development of anterior projection if the tissues allow.

In simple expansion prostheses with one compartment the membrane consists of an elastomere of silicone, finer than that used in standard implants, to allow its proper distension. The first models had a smooth structure, but now the same prostheses are proposed in a roughened version, also with the intent of combating the formation of a periprosthetic membane. This is because, unfortunately, and contrary to initial hopes, progressive distension does not exclude the development of contracture, whether this be rapid and inimical to continuation of the expansion, or secondary and not excluding the risk of induration.

When this type of expansion prosthesis is used, it must be replaced at the second operative stage by the definitive implant.

Other expansion prostheses (such as Becker's) have a thicker wall made of two thicknesses, separating a central compartment which is the expansion compartment inflatable with normal saline from a peripheral layer containing a layer of silicone gel. The filling device can be withdrawn, leaving the implant in place, which has the advantage of using only one implant, but the disadvantages are represented by the presence of a peripheral compartment containing silicone gel, whose impermeability may prove imperfect in the long term once the filling device has been withdrawn.

The filling device

The valve may be situated remotely, connected to the implant by an intermediate catheter, this arrangement being quite comparable to the implantable chambers used in chemotherapy, or it may be directly incorporated at the implant surface. We prefer the former.

In practice, finding the right point of puncture on the dome of the implant is not always easy, especially when the expansion prosthesis is placed beneath the thickness of the pectoral muscle, and the risk of accidental perforation cannot be excluded. Some manufacturers have suggested a system of magnetic location to guide the puncture. It seems to us equally illogical to traumatise the tissue to be distended by repeated injections, especially as there is a risk of causing a hematoma by accidental vascular puncture. Lastly, these expansion prostheses with a central chamber remain flat and rigid opposite the chamber, a region where the expansion will therefore be less, and yet which corresponds in the reconstruction to the very zone where the greatest anterior projection is desired

Expansion prostheses with a remote valve call for some precautions during their placement. The valve compartment must be separate from that of the prosthesis and placed sufficiently remotely not to risk coming into contact with the prosthesis during the expansion and causing a perforation. The connecting tube should have a smooth curve, or should be shortened, so as avoid kinking which would make filling impossible, nor should it pass above the valve. Certain devices can be shortened by an intermediate metal connection. We prefer one-piece systems, even if this requires a somewhat longer connecting tube, so as to eliminate any risk of disconnection.

Expansion in situ

Choice of expansion prosthesis

Expansion prostheses are not subject to the same filling constraints as definitive implants. Therefore their volume is not of the first importance for two reasons: if the theoretic volume is not achieved, this underinflation is unimportant since the implant will be changed in the near future; and on the other hand, because of the more elastic structure of its elastomere wall, this type of prosthesis can tolerate considerable overinflation.

The expansion prosthesis will therefore be selected in terms of its useful theoretic diameter and not of its volume. The diameter, determined as for a definitive implant in terms of the thoracic base and the position of the inframammary crease and of the opposite breast, must be virtually that of the definitive implant intended to replace it. Too small a diameter will make it necessary at the second stage procedure to split the periprosthetic membrane over its entire periphery to spread the base of the implant, and this would sacrifice one of the advantages of expansion,which is to form a continuous periprosthetic membrane from the outset. Too great a diameter carries the risk of an over-large compartment in which the definitive implant risks floating and creating a wave effect, even if correctly filled, due to maladjustment between container and content, especially if the periprosthetic membrane does not contract down on the new compartment. Unfortunately, the future dimensions of the compartment after expansion depend on a barely predictable factor, as will be seen.

Operative technique

Approach

This is the same as for the mastectomy, the scar of which is revised and partly or wholly excised depending on its quality; if this is fine and supple it can be partially excised laterally or at its middle; if broad and fibrous it is better to excise it completely.

The pectoral muscle is also incised to create a retro and inframuscular compartment, the stripping being made as for simple insertion of an implant but without suspension of the inframammary crease. But the access to the muscle need not be as wide as the skin approach if the whole scar has had to be excised. The muscle approach can be direct, by incision of the fibers parallel to the skin incision. Some workers recommend stripping the skin, if the scar is horizontal, to allow incision of the muscle in the direction of its fibers, and the least superimposition of the two incisons. We have tried both procedures, without problems, provided that the tissues are of good quality (always an essential to the success of this technique) and that the repair stage is carefully carried out (fig. 197).

Compartment and sulcus

The lower limit of the stripping forms part of the controversies relating to expansion. Some advise that the stripping be taken lower than the desired definitive inframammary crease, having noted that the crease may ascend after insertion of the definitive implant. Others do the same, but are often led to excise an inferior crescent of the capsule at the second stage procedure to reascend the crease, which remains too low, and to tether it in place..

We have also noted that the proper level of the crease forms one of the hazards of expansion-reconstruction, and when it ascends it is doubtless associated with an excessive difference in size between the expansion prosthesis and the definitive implant, secondary readaptation of the compartment on the implant accompanying this phenomenon of ascent.

Two attitudes one may be adopted towards the inframammary crease:
– either the initial stripping is extended deliberately lower than the crease intended, in the knowledge that a secondary suspension is obligatory to fix it in good position, and that this will not be easy if the tissues are thick, so that this procedure is best reserved for tissues that are very supple and not too thick; or:
– the stripping is not taken any lower than the intended crease, which is logical when the tissues are thick, but it must be expected that the crease is not very well defined, and it is important to precent secondary ascent that the filling should not greatly exceed the definitive volume intended.

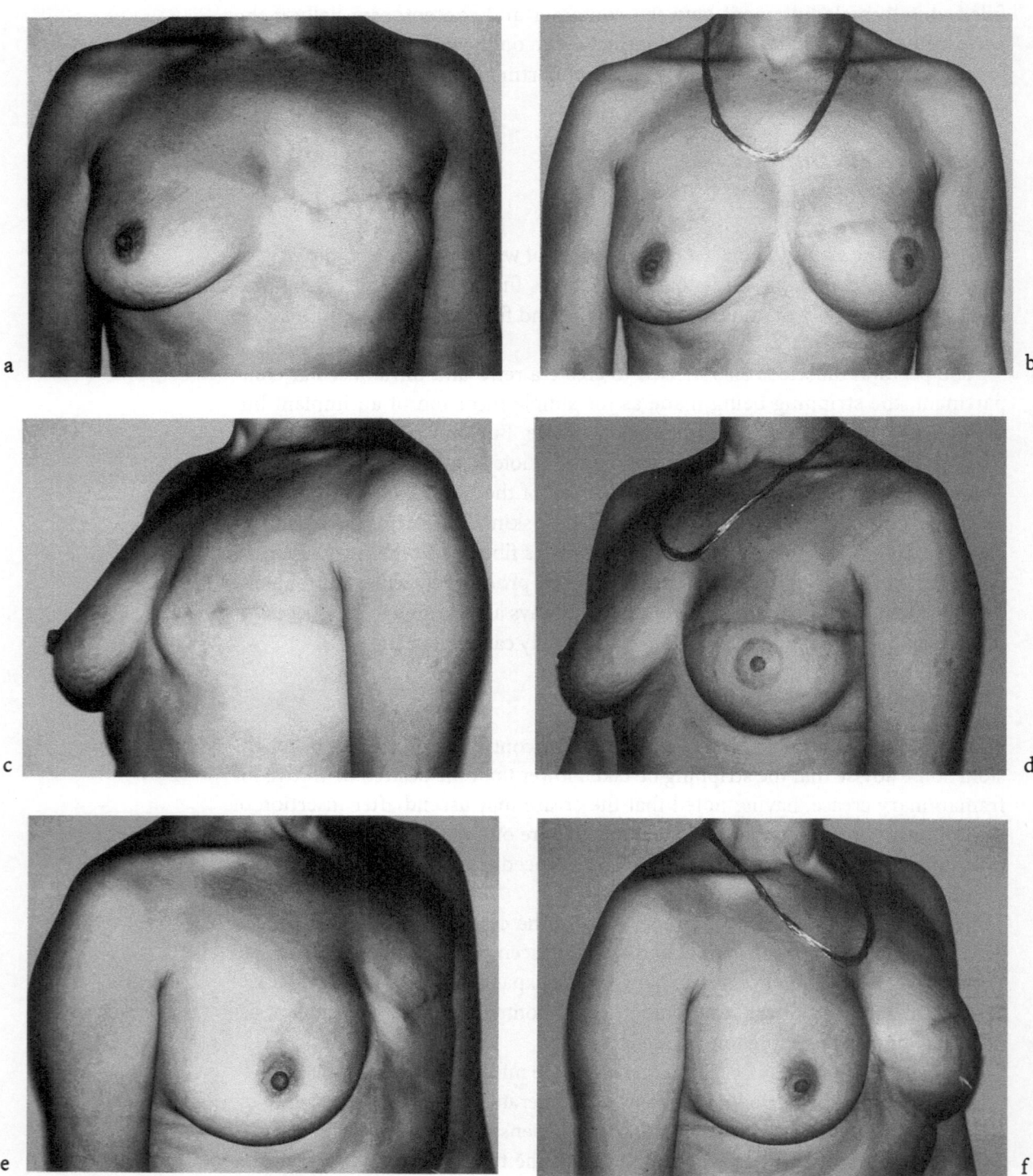

Fig. 197 a-f. Reconstruction by round expansion prosthesis (Sigma Dow Corning), remote valve, theoretic volume 600 ml. Initial filling 300 ml, expansion taken to 500 ml. Replaced at 2nd stage by an inflatable smooth Sebbin LS implant of 350 ml, filled with 470 ml of normal saline, with reconstruction of the areola by tattooing and grafting from the lower half of the opposite nipple

To receive the valve, a small pocket is dissected with scissors, usually in the lateral thoracic subcutaneous plane, but avoiding placing it at the same height as the strap of the brassiere, which is uncomfortable.

The prosthesis is removed from its packing after taking the usual aseptic precautions and changing gloves.

It is emptied of its air, and inserted already slightly filled to ensure that its base is well spread. It is not at this stage filled as much as the tissues allow, so as not to hinder closure, and the valve is checked to ensure that it is readily accessible and that the connecting tube is not kinked. The valve can be fixed with a subcutaneous stitch passed round the origin of the intermediate tube, but without compressing it. This stitch is useful to prevent displacement of the valve in the first fortnight. Subsequently, of course, the valve is immobilised by development of the periprosthetic membrane which is formed around every foreign body.

Closure

As always, this must be particularly careful, after having checked the hemostasis and inserted a suction drain; apposition of the muscular and dermal margins must be as meticulous as possible if one hopes to obtain good quality healing allowing the rapid conduct of expansion.

When closure is completed, and before applying the dressing and waking the patient, filling is completed by percutaneous injection as far as the state of the tissues permits, ie without undue tension. This maneuver, which takes pace in conditions identical with the subsequent injections, provides a last opportunity for checking the proper functioning of the system.

Filling

The frequency of the injections is quite variable, and depends solely on the capacity for tissue stretching; not uncommonly, we perform the first injection on removal of the dressing just before taking out the drain if the tissues appear sufficiently relaxed.

The rate of injection is about once a week. Frequency and amount injected are guided by clinical tolerance; the filling is stopped as soon as the patient feels the tension as painful, or if the appearance of the tissues greatly changes, appearing taut or changing color by becoming pale or reddened. Persistence of one of these features means that the injections must be more spaced out.

How far should the expansion be taken?

It has been suggested that the definitive volume desired should be greatly exceeded, even to twice its amount, in the hope of creating a ptosis giving a more natural appearance to the breast reconstructed by such a procedure.

This seems unreasonable in view of the uncertainty about the fate of the tissues thus distended; in some cases they will completely contract again on the definitive implant, and this is then accompanied by a very irritating modification of the position of the crease.

In other cases, the tissues have lost their elasticity, and the degree of ptosis exceeds expectations. In addition to a wave effect in the upper quadrants, and an implant obviously situated too low down, too mobile and therefore too prominent whenever the patient changes position, the result is as unpleasing as when an attempt is made to correct a ptosis merely by using an implant (fig. 198). Once again, the content must be perfectly adapted to the container.

In practice, we do not exceed the volume which seems indicated for the definitive implant or only slightly. If we do push the expansion, it is without exceeding the predicted definitive volume by more than a third.

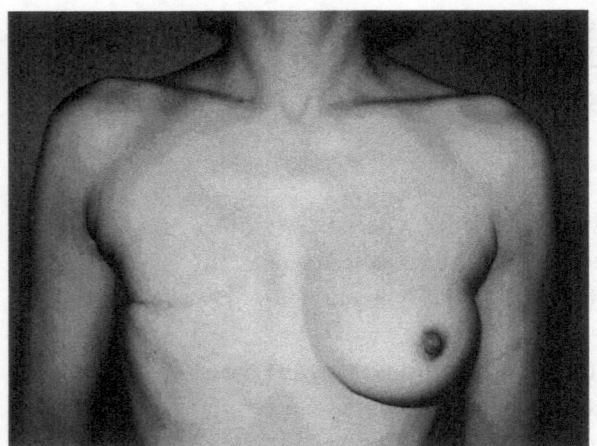
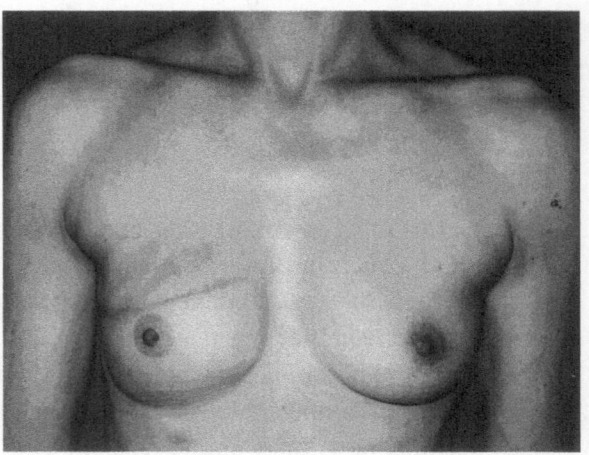

a   b

Fig. 198 a,b. Reconstruction by round expansion prosthesis, remote valve (Sigma Dow Corning) of theoretic volume 400 ml, initial filling 105 ml, expansion taken to 350 ml. Replacement by smooth inflatable Sebbin LS20 implant of 200 ml, filled with 220 ml of normal saline. The implant has retained a satisfactory consistence and has not decreased in volume; the presence of skin creases in the superior quadrants is due to excessive tissue stretching by the definitive implant.

When to change the prosthesis

Once filling has been completed, a delay of three months seems correct for stabilisation of the skin stretching.

As we do not use systems where the filling device can be removed, because of the presence of gel and because they do not seem impermeable in the long term, the temporary prosthesis is replaced by the definitive implant during the second operative procedure, which is also that of reconstruction of the areola and of any procedure on the opposite breast.

On this occasion the approach, still at the level of the mastectomy scar, is as limited as is compatible with removal of the prothesis and its valve (which is sometimes the most difficult step) and with insertion of the definitive implant (fig. 199). The access is necessarily wider if the procedure has to be done at the inframammary crease.

We do not interfere with the periprosthetic membrane unless the compartment has to be enlarged or the crease adjusted, so as not to lose the advantage of an existing membrane and one that is, hopefully, stabilised.

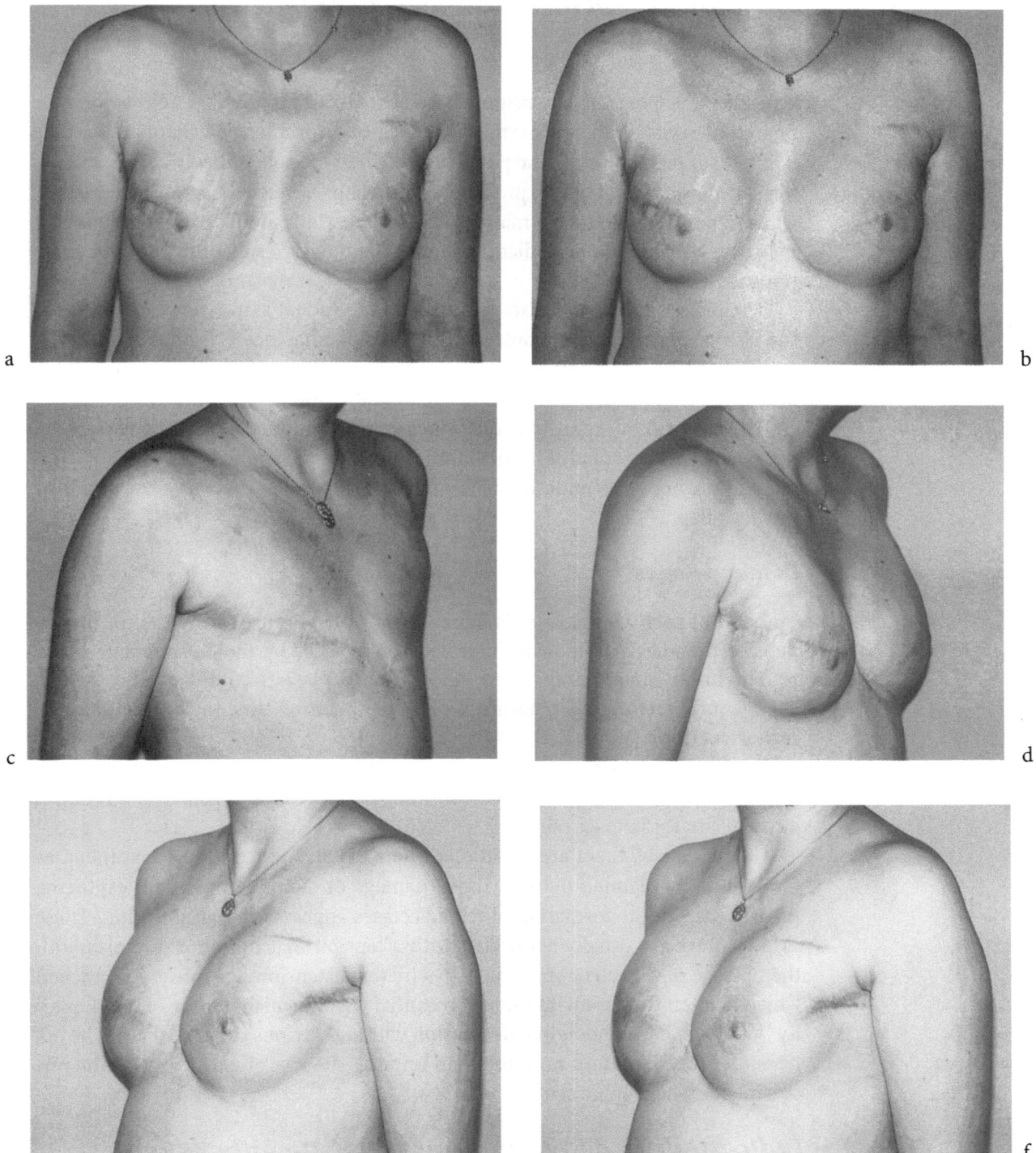

Fig. 199 a-f. Mastectomy with radiotherapy and chemotherapy. Bilateral reconstruction by round expansion prostheses, remote valve (Sigma Dow Corning) of 600 ml. Excision of scar, expansion taken to 300 ml. At 2nd stage, revision of scar only in its outer part, enlargement of compartments laterally, and insertion of inflatable Sebbin LS21 implants of 300 ml filled to 400 ml. Areolae reconstructed by tattooing and earlobe grafts

Advantages and disadvantages of expansion in situ

Advantages

The chief advantage of expansion in situ is not to add to the scar defect when the degree of laxity does not permit insertion of an implant of adequate volume without supplementary tissue provision, ie when the sole possible alternative before the development of this procedure was a flap. Nevertheless, we shall see that, while expansion allows the management of a certain number of situations that may be qualified as intermediate, it cannot claim to be a substitute for the indications for a flap.

The original hope was also, because of the gradual skin stretching, to lessen the risk of periprosthetic contracture. This hope has been disappointed in the first generation of smooth-walled expansion prostheses. Only the future will tell if textured expansion prostheses change this situation.

The use of skin expansion constitutes a gain in immediate reconstruction, in cases where the residual skin substance is not sufficient to accept a definitive implant and where it is undesirable to add to the operation and the scar defect by raising a flap.

Disadvantages

The cost of such a procedure is increased, if only because of the cost of the expansion prosthesis itself, which must later be replaced by another implant.

The breast must be operated twice, first to place the implant and then to change it. Therefore this does not lessen the operation time in cases of deferred reconstruction.

The timing of the injections requires repeated visits.

The valve may be difficult to locate in obese patients and sometimes requires a counter-incision to extract it.

Unfortunately, there are situations where expansion cannot be continued as far as initially planned because tissue damage or simply a persistent erythema associated with the formation of telangiectases appears after an injection. These skin changes are usually associated with a tension that does not diminish with the passage of time. The maximal capacity for distension has thus been reached which is often the case with quite substantial tissues which appear of good quality but which have undergone irradiation without obvious consequences. The expansion procedure does no more than unmask the loss of elasticity and the impairment of the trophic state.

Indications and limitations with in situ expansion

Skin expansion is primarily addressed to tissues of good quality and substance, but where the degree of laxity is not enough to permit the definitve volume desired at the outset. This situation obviously occurs more often in immediate reconstruction, in breasts of small size where the skin sacrifice is relatively major in relation to the global breast substance.

A good indication is also represented by situations where the skin envelope is not large enough to accept immediately an implant of definitive volume, but

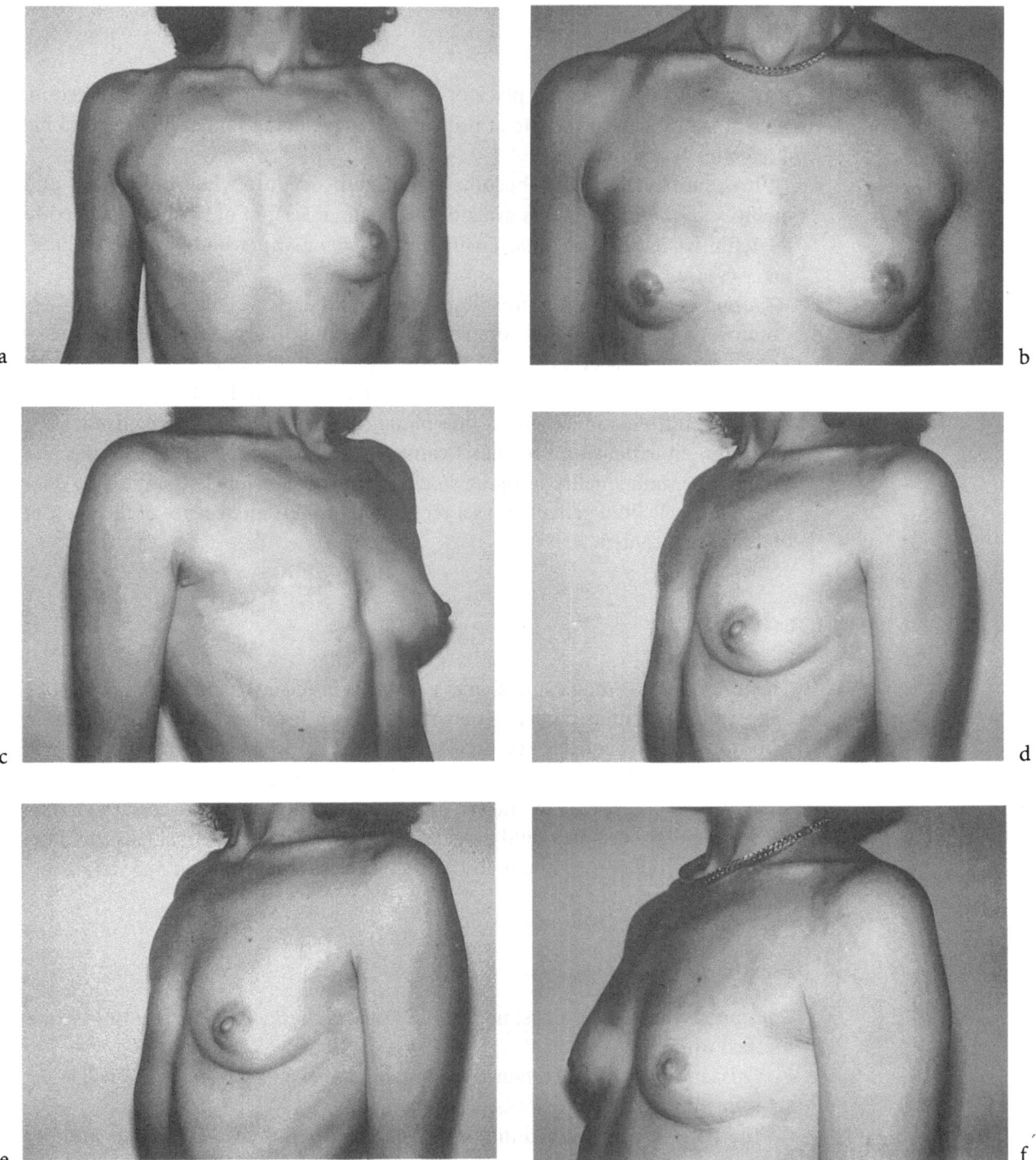

Fig. 200 a-f. Ist stage: excision of scar, insertion of Sigma Dow Corning expansion prosthesis, remote valve, of 300 ml filled initially with 80 ml. Expansion taken to 155 ml. 2nd stage: replacement by smooth inflatable Sebbin implant of 125 ml, filled to 140 ml, skin reduction plasty of opposite breast, reconstruction of areola with graft from the outer half of the opposite areola and the lower half of the nipple where the presence of a large scar with "birdcage ladder" suture markings impair the cosmetic aspect of the reconstruction (fig. 200). In no case should an expansion prosthesis be used when a flap is indicated because of insubstantial tissues without evident laxity or showing trophic changes.

Conclusion

It is not easy to define the place of in situ expansion in breast reconstruction, since it is precisely at the site of previously damaged tissue that multidirectional elongation is sought.

It should certainly not become a routine procedure when the quality and quantity of the integuments available allow the insertion of an implant filled to its definitive level at the outset, using the device of suspension of the inframammary crease.

A number of expansion prostheses prove of little use when it is found that they can already be filled almost completely at the time of insertion, and that one or two subsequent injections suffice to attain the volume initially planned. On the other hand, we have seen that there is less certainty about the stability and definition of the inframammary crease thus obtained unless it is secondarily fixed.

Again, an expansion prosthesis cannot stretch damaged or taut tissues and provide the same quality of tissue stock as a myocutaneous latissimus flap does with its muscle lining effect, or as a rectus abdominis flap because of the amount of its skin/fat content.

Expansion at a distance

The idea of performing expansion at a distance in reconstruction of the breast by the use of a latissimus dorsi flap occurred to us for the first time with a patient in whom irradiation sequelae required resort to a flap whose skin component was necessarily very large. Of course, this lanky and very thin woman possessed no subumbilical excess of skin and fat, and the dimensions of the necessary skin island of a latissimus flap would have been incompatible with direct closure of the donor site, which is essential in the cosmetic employment of this flap.

Operative technique

First stage

The contractility of the latissimus dorsi muscle is checked and its anterior border marked with a felt pen.

This landmark can be retained throughout the expansion stage, and will assist subsequently in designing its skin component.

The patient is positioned in dorsal decubitus, with a rolled draw-sheet under the scapula to expose the lateral thoracic region.

In order not to add to the subsequent scar, and particularly not to risk subsequent inclusion in the expansion zone, the approach route follows the outermost part of the mastectomy scar, first verifying if necessary the presence of the pedicle. A wide stripping is taken as far as possible downward, straddling the anterior border of the muscle. This stripping is easy under the upper and middle parts of the muscle but more difficult in front of its anterior border, where care must be taken not to become involved under the serratus anterior, also below in the vicinity of the iliac attachments. The dissection is facilitated by the use of long strong scissors, such as those of Dubost.

Hemostasis is effected, a suction drain inserted, and the prothesis introduced. For this indication we use a "tear-drop" prosthesis with a remote valve, of 1000 ml theoretic capacity, the tapering pole of the prosthesis being placed below. The valve is placed in the anterior thoracic region and the incision is closed, isolating the compartment of the prosthesis above from the route of access by several anterior support sutures attaching the dermis to the chest wall.

The prosthesis is initially filled as much as possible, around 300 ml on average. This initial filling allows testing of the valve and decreases the risk of bleeding into the compartment.

The injections are continued at the rate one a week. It is not uncommon to be able to introduce 100 ml at a single occasion. Six to eight weeks are required to reach or even exceed the theoretic volume of the prosthesis.

Second stage

This is done one month after the end of the expansion. We do not exceed this delay because of the discomfort, especially from the clothing, that results from the presence of such a device on the outer side of the chest.

Moreover, as it is a matter of transferring a flap the expansion of which will be maintained by an implant of a different shape, it seems less important than in an in situ expansion to await the stabilisation of a shape which is not going to be the definitive one.

The design of the flap is centered on the anterior border of the muscle, and made before operation (fig. 201).

The patient is positioned in dorsal decubitus with a rolled draw-sheet under the scapula, the classical position for all latissimus flaps removed astride the anterior border of the muscle.

The position of this anterior border can be verified from above if there is any doubt when first making the approach. The easiest way is in fact to incise the anterior border of the skin layer immediately, situated 5 to 7 cm in front of the muscle border, while the expansion prosthesis is still in place. Still leaving the expansion prosthesis, the stripping is pursued a little forward so as to stagger the opening of the capsule. The prosthesis is then withdrawn and the incision of the skin of the flap completed below and behind, removing the largest possible skin layer to permit direct closure of the loss of substance.

The pedicle and its branches are clearly visible through the periprosthetic membrane, as well as the muscle bundles, layered and spread out by the expansion. The flap is isolated for greater security on a muscular and a vascular pedicle. The capsule is preserved, which is an advantage here as it will remain in contact with the implant.

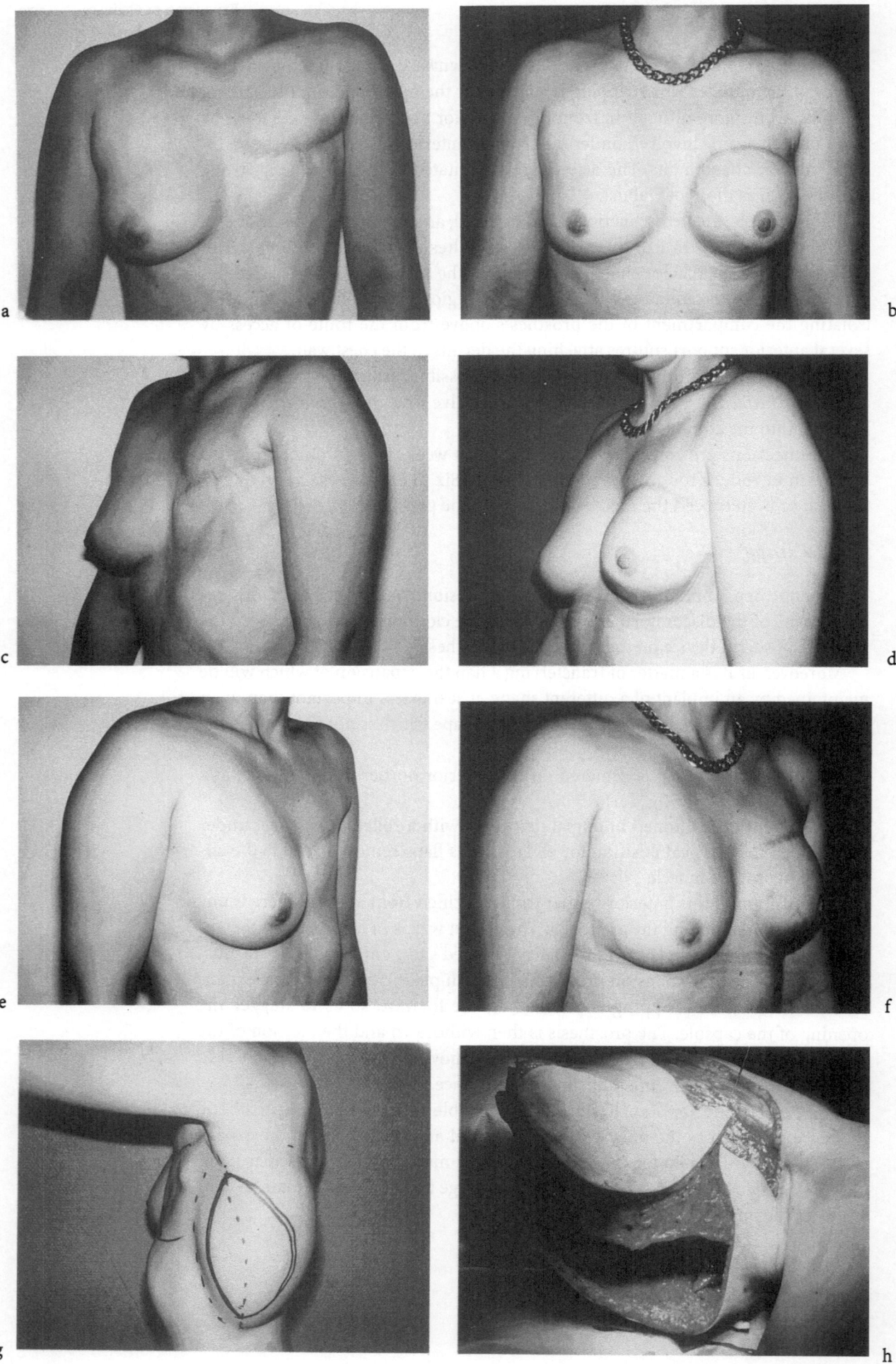

a b c d e f g h

The mastectomy scar is excised and the stripping of the lower margin begun; the flap is temporarily held in reserve on the anterior thoracic region while hemostasis is checked, a suction drain is placed in the stripping zone and the zone where the flap was raised is closed.

The sheet under the shoulder is removed and the patient is positioned half-seated for placement of the flap and introduction of the definitive implant.

The dressing is applied on the lateral thoracic region, but without compression of the flap, opposite which an opening is contrived to monitor its color. The arm is held very slightly away from the body to avoid compression in the axillary fossa.

Reconstruction of the areola is done at a third stage, together with any procedure indicated on the opposite breast.

Advantages and disadvantages of expansion under a latissimus flap

The use of expansion under a latissimus dorsi flap may as much as double the available tissue stock while remaining compatible with direct closure of the loss of substance, all being done under perfectly healthy tissue.

The gain in expansion so obtained is preserved by the immediate placement of the implant during transfer of the flap.

The raising of the flap astride the anterior border of the muscle, which is perfectly safe as regards vitality of that part of the flap situated in front of the muscle, allows concealment of the scar — which is a long one — in the lateral thoracic region level with the arm.

On the other hand, three operative stages are needed, with an interval of some 3 months between stages, and at the end of the expansion the bulk of the implant hinders adduction of the arm and complicates getting dressed. In some patients, elevation of the shoulder is also restricted at this period, no doubt because of the tension exerted on the latissimus tendon by the implant, since this difficulty disappears after transfer of the flap.

Dissection of the muscular and vascular pedicle is a little trickier at the upper part of the flap because of the hypervascularisation induced by formation of the periprosthetic membrane, which must not be excised for fear of damaging the pedicle.

◀ **Fig. 201 a-h.** Latissimus dorsi flap with previous expansion prosthesis (young woman, no children, no excess of subumbilical skin and fatty tissue)
1st stage: insertion of Sigma Dow Corning "tear-drop" expansion prosthesis, remote valve, theoretic volume 900 ml, 18 cm x 11 cm, filled initially with 350 ml of normal saline, expansion taken to 900 ml.
2nd stage: placement of flap with an inflatable Sebbin implant of 250 ml
3rd stage: reconstruction of nipple-areolar plaque by tattooing and graft of lower half of opposite nipple

Conclusion

This technique is useful when provision of a flap is necessary, when the tissue stock provided by a simple flap of the latissimus dorsi would be insufficient, and when a rectus abdominis flap is not practicable (fig. 202). However, because of the constraints imposed on the patient, we use it only exceptionally, when the flaps previously cited are contraindicated.

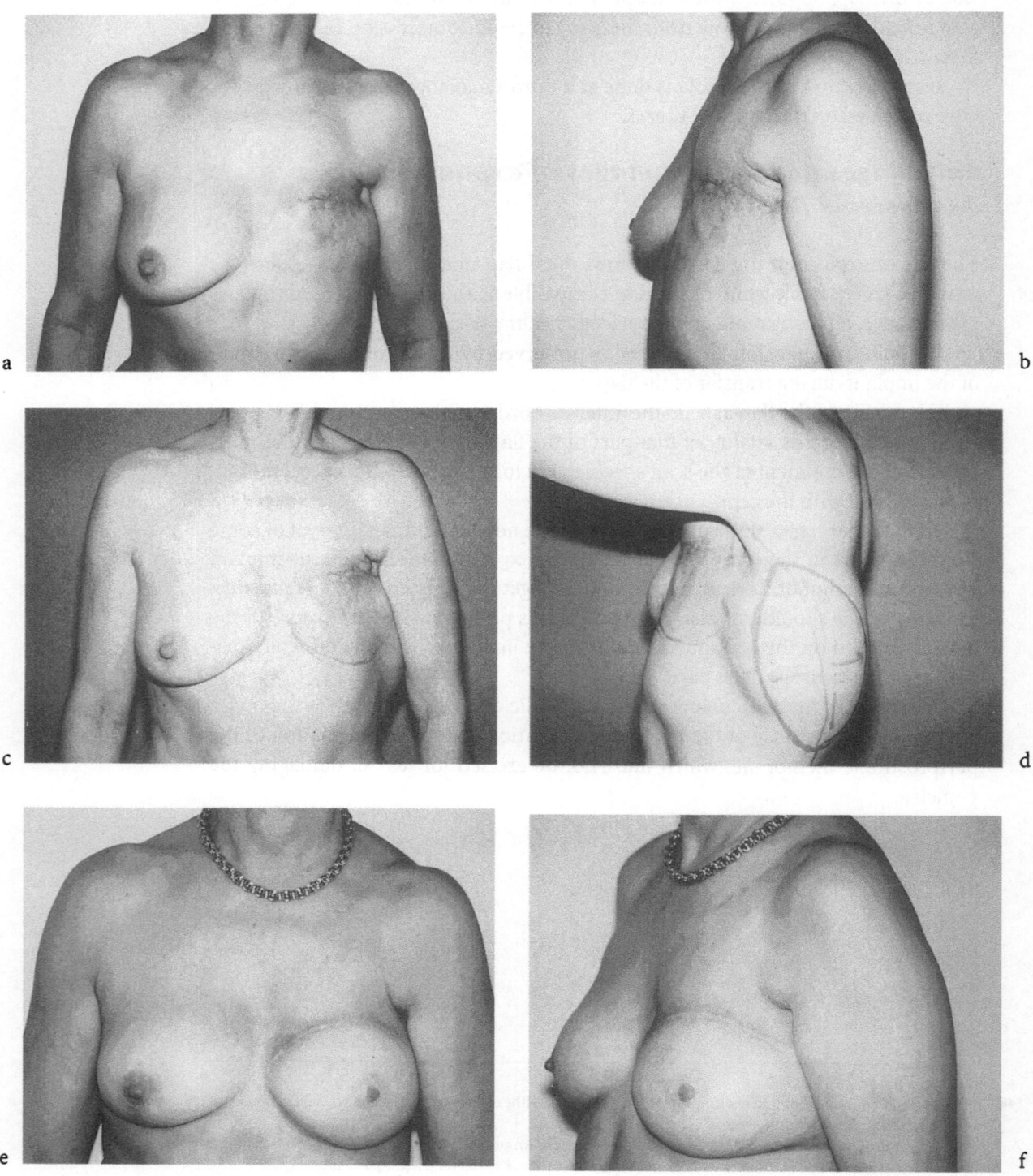

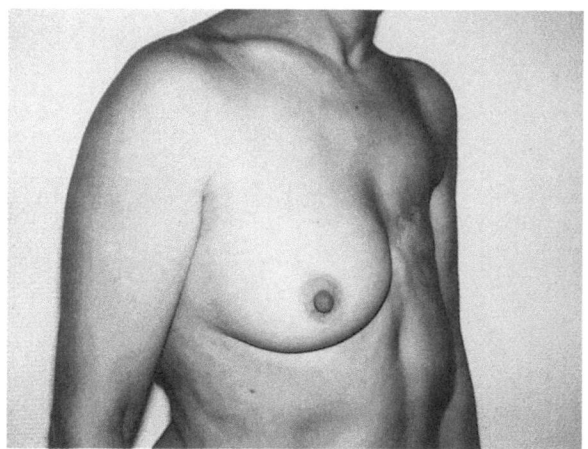

g

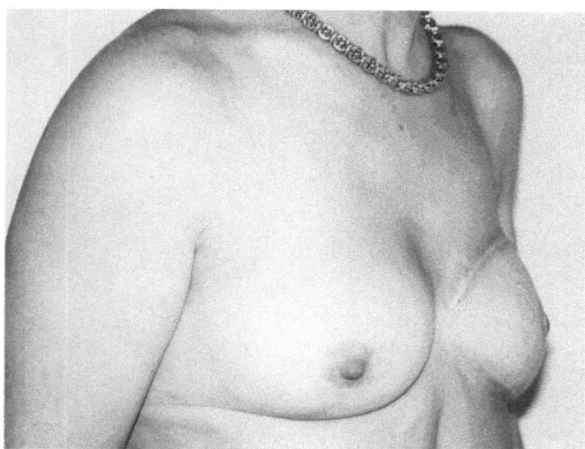

h

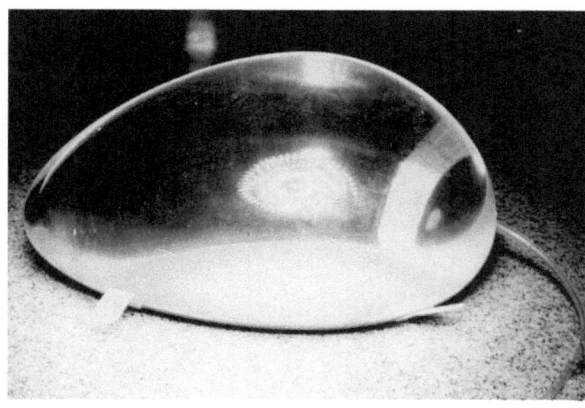

i

Fig. 202 a-i. Latissimus dorsi flap with previous expansion (major irradiation sequelae requiring excision of tissues between scar and sulcus; abdominal scars contraindicating rectus abdominis flap). "Tear-drop" Sigma Dow Corning expansion prosthesis, remote valve, theoretic volume 1000 ml, 19 x 14 cm, filled initially with 300 ml, expansion taken to 930 ml. Definitive smooth inflatable Sebbin implant of 175 ml, filled with 210 ml of normal saline

References

Becker H (1982) Breast reconstruction using an inflatable breast implant with detachable reservoir. Plast Rec Surg 73: 678-683

Maxwell GP (1989) Immediate breast reconstruction utilizing a textured silicone tissue expander. Plast Surg Forum 12: 146

Neumann CG (1957) The expansion of an area of skin by progressive distension of a subcutaneous balloon, Plast Rec Surg 19: 124-130

Bricout N, Servant JM, Banzet P (1987) Lambeau de grand dorsal "expansé" et reconstruction du sein: étude préliminaire. Ann Chir Plast Esth, tome 32, n°2: 174-176

Richard L (1987) L'expansion cutanée: application en chirurgie réparatrice. Thèse, Lyon

Radovan C (1982) Breast reconstruction after mastectomy using the temporary expander. Plast Rec Surg 69: 195-208

Vasconez LO, Lejour M, Gamboa-Bobadilla (1991) Atlas of breast reconstruction, J.B.Lippincott Company, Philadelphia

Flaps

The provision of supplementary tissue becomes necessary when the local integuments are of defective laxity (wide mastectomy with major skin sacrifice), or are insubstantial, or exhibit obvious trophic changes following a poorly tolerated combination of surgery and radiotherapy which has left sclerosed or fragile tissues, incapable of stretching or exposed to the risk of necrosis and disruption when they are placed under tension by the insertion of an implant, which may then be extruded.

Fascial and fasciocutanous flaps

The first step was that of the use of skin flaps, the most commonly used being the thoraco-epigastric flap described by Cronin and more recently repopularised in a fasciocutaneous version by Holmström (fig. 203).

The skin component of this type of flap, wider and longer in its fasciocutaneous version because more reliable in terms of vascularity, is raised transversely astride the inframammary crease and rotated to occupy a vertical position, usually interrupting the mastectomy scar.

The raising of this flap has the advantage of simplicity, but there is the disavantage that the implant is placed in direct contact with the subcutaneous plane

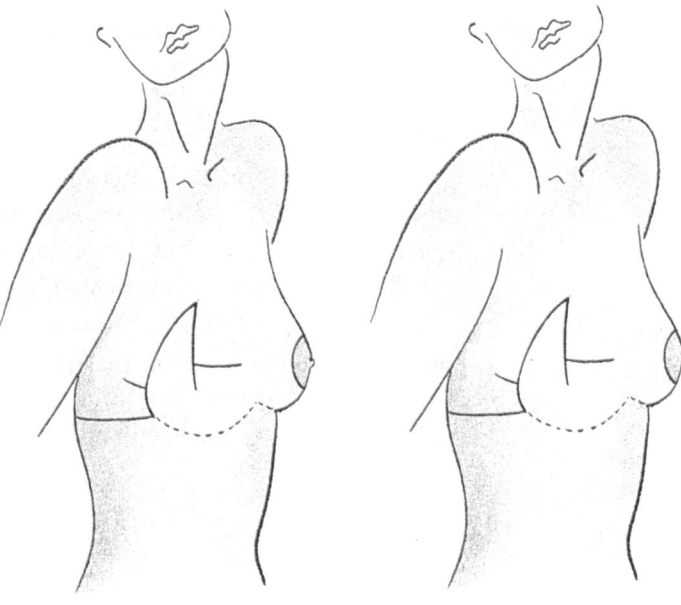

Fig. 203. Fasciocutaneous flap of Holmström

of the flap without any muscle interposition, which adds to the risk of peripheral contracture or at least makes it more obvious.

Although the examples of the thoracodorsal fasciocutaneous flap demonstrated by its author are very encouraging, we have been disappointed with this technique, having found in particular that proper position and good definition of the inframammary crease were not easy to obtain and that the flap lacked thickness in front of the implant.

In our view, these flaps cannot replace the unique advantages provided by the myocutaneous flaps.

Myocutaneous flaps

These are so called because the blood-supply of the skin component is ensured by perforating vascular branches derived from the subjacent muscle chosen as the vascular source; the use of these flaps in covering losses of substance in general and in the field of breast reconstruction in particular is considerable, since the vascular security and the possibilities offered are far superior to those of the classic skin flaps.

The oldest of the flaps used is that of the latissimus dorsi. Provided its pedicle has been preserved at the time of axillary nodal clearance, the technique of its construction is relatively simple; the difficulty consists mainly in knowing how to define the dimensions of the necessary skin layer, its position on the muscle and its proper positioning on the zone of the breast to be reconstructed.

Its disadvantage is the dorsal scar defect, though all flaps impose a supplementary scar associated with closure of the donor area, and especially the need to add a prosthesis, the quality of the result and its hazards being linked in great part to the reaction of the organism to this quasi-inevitable implant.

The other myocutaneous flap which shares the stage in breast reconstruction with the latissimus dorsi flap is that of the rectus abdominis, an inferior abdominal flap which exploits the excess of subumbilical skin and fatty tissue in a uni- or bipedicled version. Its technical performance is more demanding and rather more time-consuming than with the latissimus flap, and the morbidity greater, but its great advantage is that it allows reconstruction of a naturally shaped breast without the need for a prosthesis.

At various times and following fashion, one of these techniques has tried to prevail over the other. But in fact each of them has its elective indications and does not benefit solely from the contraindications to the other.

We cannot conclude this introduction to the myocutaneous flaps without mentioning the flap of the upper rectus abdominis, pedicled on the superior epigastric vessels. Raised in the opposite inframammary region, it was very useful for the quality of skin it provided, very similar to the breast skin, and because of the discreet scar defect concealed in the inframammary crease. But it is not usually large enough to dispense with an implant and, in particular, it has been virtually discarded because of the risk of total necrosis associated with the inevitable torsion of its pedicle during its placement.

References

Cronin TD, Upton J, Mc Donough JM (1977) Reconstruction of the breast after mastectomy, Plast Rec Surg, 59: 1

Holmstrëm H, Lossing C (1986) The lateral thoracodorsal flap in breast reconstruction, Plast Rec Surg 77, n°6: 933-941

Lejour M (1982) Reconstruction of the breast with a contralateral epigastric rectus abdominis myo-cutaneous flap. Chir Plast 7: 131-134

The latissimus dorsi flap

Of all the myocutaneous flaps, that of the latissimus dorsi is without doubt the oldest described and the most widely used, whether as a pedicled or as a free flap.

As a pedicled flap, its arc of rotation easily allows it to cover losses of thoracic substance. Isolated on its single pedicle, the cutaneous layer of the flap, judiciously placed, easily reaches the neck and lower third of the face and even the upper part of the middle third if the build of the patient allows.

As a free flap, the caliber and length of its vascular pedicle and its plastic qualities (wide flat muscular base, wide range of skin designs) make it the flap of choice.

But we must return to reconstruction of the breast. This is of course undertaken to cover large losses of thoracic substance after extended mastectomy with removal of the pectorals and sacrifice of skin ascending as far as the axilla. It was for this purpose that Iginio Tansini reported on its use in 1906. He had tried in 1896 (fig. 204) to cover this racket excision by a posterior skin flap with its apex at the axilla, but had observed partial necrosis of the distal flap in some of his cases. Anatomic studies led him to believe that preservation of the inferior scapular pedicle *(subscapular a.)* but also of the circumflex scapular pedicle *(circumflex scapular a.)*, was necessary to survival of this vast flap. His racket design for raising a posterior flap modeled on the dimensions of the anterior loss of substance, with its long axis oblique downward and backward and an axillary apex, is in fact that of a latissimus flap whose security is increased by preservation of the pedicle and part of a parascapular flap.

Tansini had also noted at that time the importance, not only of the vascular requirements, but of taking the muscle substance of the latissimus to fill in for the loss of substance left by sacrifice of the pectorals.

Subsequently long forgotten, despite the article of Este in 1912, this idea was reintroduced by Olivari in 1976, and then by Muhlbauer and Olbrich in 1977, who published the first applications to breast reconstruction; and it was further developed, notably by using skin islands of varying shape and situation without the need for preserving a skin bridge, by Bostwick in 1979 and Lejour in 1984.

However, the position of the skin island in the particular case of breast reconstruction is dictated by the cosmetic imperatives. The donor zone must be capable of direct closure, and the scar concealed as well as possible.

LAVORI ORIGINALI

CLINICA CHIRURGICA OPERATIVA DELLA R. UNIVERSITÀ
DI PALERMO

Nuovo processo per l'amputazione
della mammella per cancro
pel prof. I. Tansini

Comunicazioni Originali

CLINICA OPERATIVA DELLA R. UNIV. DI PAVIA (Prof. TANSINI)

SOPRA IL MIO NUOVO PROCESSO
DI AMPUTAZIONE DELLA MAMMELLA
del Prof. IGINIO TANSINI
Comunicazione al R. Istituto Lombardo di Scienze e Lettere
(seduta del 22 febbraio 1906)

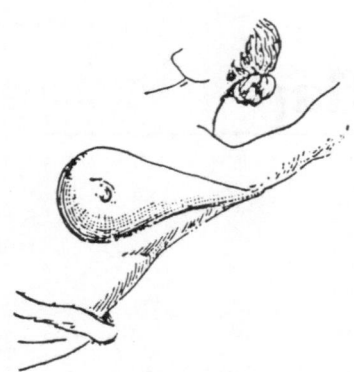
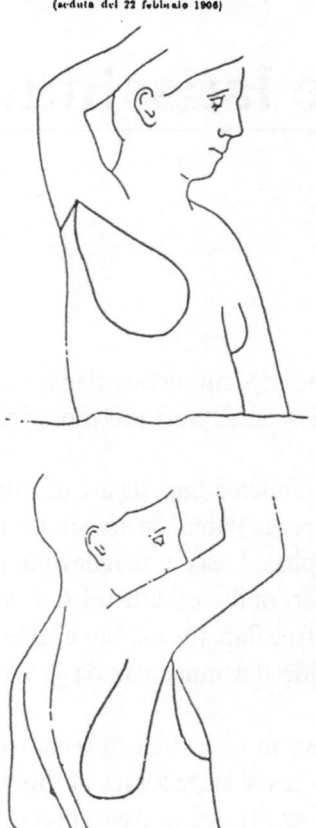
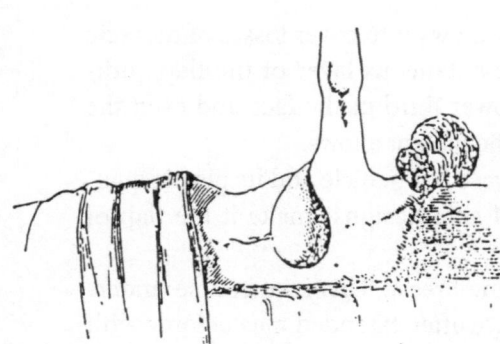

Fig. 204. Titles and diagram of reports by Tansini devoted to coverage of losses of thoracic substance after mastectomy:

left: 1896, coverage by skin flap

right: 1906, modification of procedure by inclusion of thoracodorsal and circumflex pedicles and the latissimus dorsi muscle (this is therefore a latissimus dorsi flap benefiting from reinforcement by a parascapular flap)

Anatomy

The latissimus dorsi muscle (fig. 205) has its origin posteriorly from the spinous processes of the six lower dorsal vertebrae, the last three or four ribs, and the lumbosacral aponeurosis attached to the lumbar and sacral vertebrae as far as the posterior third of the iliac crest. It is also attached to the last four ribs, its fibers mingling here with those of the external abdominal oblique muscle. From here, the fan formed by the sheet of muscle fibers narrows above and outwards, skirts the inferior angle of the scapula and the inferior border of the teres major muscle, passes in front of it, and ends in the depth of the bicipital sulcus between the insertion of the pectoralis major in front and that of the teres major behind.

The latissimus is the largest muscle in the body and has a long course. To ensure its blood-supply and follow its course, its main vascular pedicle —which is also the surgical pedicle— is long and of large caliber, which allows the construction of pedicled island flaps, muscular or even entirely vascular, easily covering every loss of thoracic substance.

The maximal course of this widely spread and thin muscle is situated along its free border, at the level of the lateral thoracic skin. Its minimal course is in the lumbar region. These features explain the orientation, course and length of its main pedicle and its cutaneous vascular distribution at the level of the muscle and in front of it, towards the anterior thoracic region.

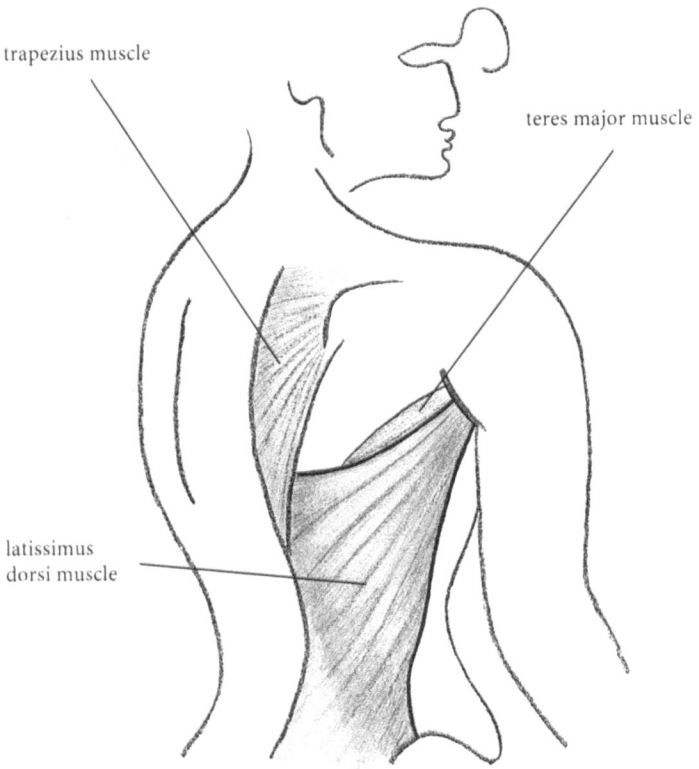

trapezius muscle

teres major muscle

latissimus
dorsi muscle

Fig. 205. The latissimus dorsi muscle

The chief vascular pedicle is the subscapular (fig. 206), the lumbar pedicles being accessory; it is of V type according to Mathes and Nahai. The subscapular (inferior scapular) artery arises from the axillary artery between the lateral thoracic artery (the former external mammary) and the posterior circumflex humeral artery. The subscapular vessel gives off a scapular branch, the circumflex scapular, then a thoracic branch, the thoracodorsal artery, which subsequently divides into two more or equal branches opposite the fourth rib: one dorsal, the artery of the latissimus dorsi, and the other thoracic, the artery of the serratus anterior.

The nerve to the latissimus arises from the secondary posterior trunk of the brachial plexus, between the subscapular nerve and the nerve to teres major; it often arises from a common trunk with the latter as the thoracodorsal nerve. At its origin, in the upper part of the axillary fossa, it forms a triangle with the vascular pedicle, which is lateral to it with its base above, and rejoins it at a variable distance before entering with into the muscle and branching therein.

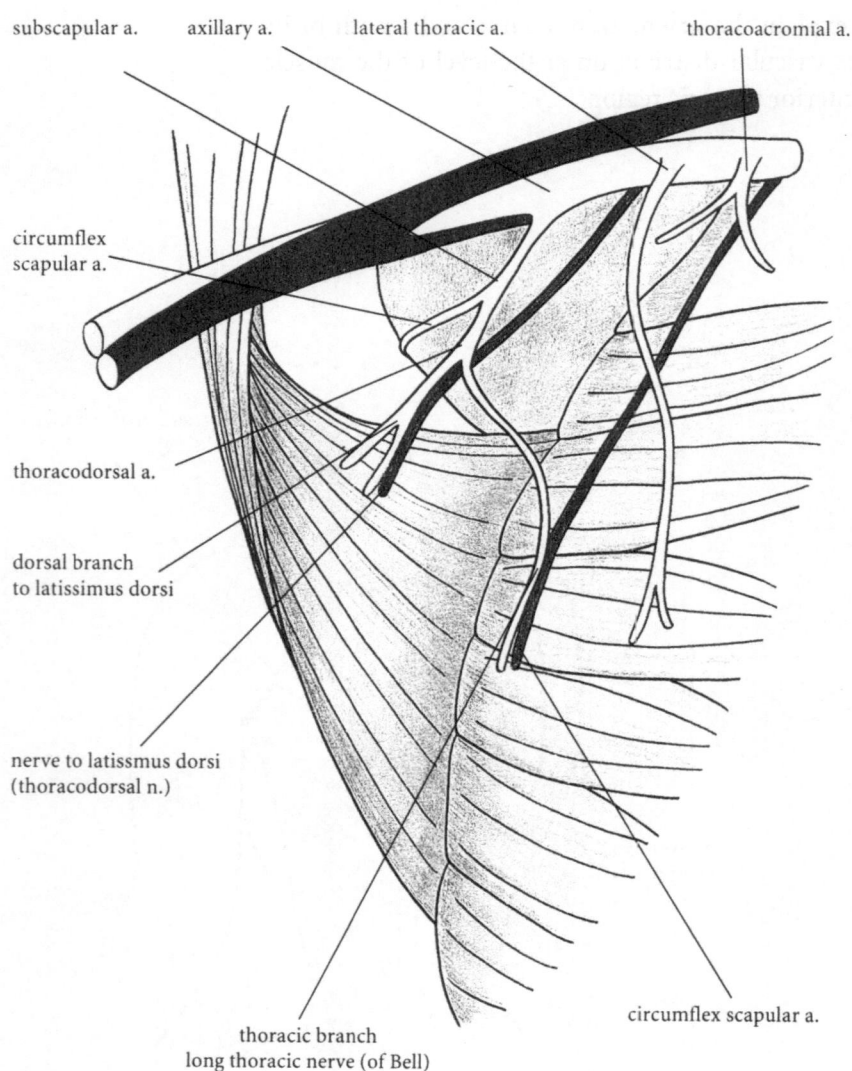

subscapular a.

axillary a.

lateral thoracic a.

thoracoacromial a.

circumflex
scapular a.

thoracodorsal a.

dorsal branch
to latissimus dorsi

nerve to latissmus dorsi
(thoracodorsal n.)

thoracic branch
long thoracic nerve (of Bell)

circumflex scapular a.

Fig. 206. Diagram of chief vascular pedicle

The pedicle as isolated surgically represents an average length of some ten cm; the longer the pedicle, the greater the arc of rotation of the flap, and — when isolated in an island flap, and provided all the collateral branches are ligated as far as the axillary vein (including the circumflex scapular) — the more it will permit the attainment of a distant point such as the face, where it may reach the middle third if the patient's build permits. In breast reconstruction the flap need not be isolated solely on its vascular pedicle to reach the zone of application; it is pointless and even risky in cases of sclerosis due to the dissection during nodal clearance, which may be associated with subsequent irradiation, to take the dissection too far into the axillary fossa, and the muscular pedicle can be preserved since it does not restrict placement of the flap in the breast area. Preservation of the muscle pedicle, at least at the first operative stage, is of course of supplementary assistance, and therefore a safeguard, in the venous drainage of the flap.

The caliber of the subscapular artery at its origin is around 5 mm and that of the thoracodorsal artery 3 mm. The single thoracodorsal vein follows a parallel course to the artery and only diverges slightly at its termination to open into the axillary vein.

After having entered the muscle, the thoracodorsal artery divides into two branches, of which the outer is the larger; it runs within the muscle fibers along the anterior border of the muscle, forming an axial vascular plexus parallel to the muscle fibers. The most posterior part of the muscle, close to its vertebral attachments, is supplied by the perforating branches of the intercostal and lumbar arteries, only slightly anastomosed with the main plexus.

Vascularisation of the skin is effected in two ways (fig. 207):
– in the posterior and lumbar region, where the skin is not very mobile because of the limited muscular excursion, the perforating branches from the lumbar vessels traverse the muscle directly without branching therein and are dis-

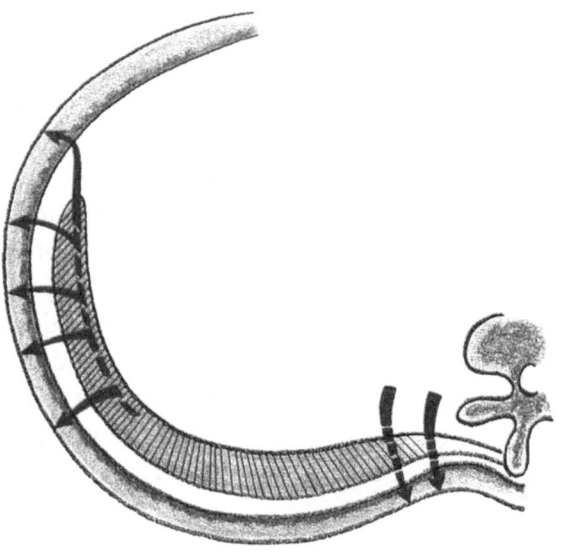

Fig. 207. Skin vascularisation at level of muscle

tributed to the skin; survival of the skin at the muscle level is ensured by this direct perforating plexus and not by the ramifying intramuscular plexus;

– the closer to the free anterior border of the muscle, the greater the muscle excursion and the mobility of the skin on the deep plane, particularly in front of the free muscle border in the antero-lateral thoracic region. Here, the skin is not supplied by direct cutaneous arteries from the depth, but on the contrary by branching of the axial muscular plexus which provides numerous small myocutaneous arteries emerging from the surface of the muscle and its anterior border, supplying the subcutaneous and dermal plexus by branches parallel to the surface and capable of following movements of the skin and muscle during contraction.

Thus, if it is desired to raise a large skin island safely, the largest and safest island will not be that raised entirely level with the muscle but one staggered forward astride the anterior border, excluding the posterior and lumbar skin. The anterior skin extension behaves like a random flap based on the myocutaneous segment situated behind it. However, it should be noted that, in the special field of breast reconstruction, where the skin layer does not usually need to be very large, various designs of skin islands can be safely employed, and that the method of raising the flap astride the anterior border is no longer the most favorable one for the morphologic result in the reconstructed breast, as will be seen.

Action, test of function and viability

Taking its origins as the fixed point, the latissimus dorsi is a medial rotator, adductor and retroflexor of the arm. Further, it depresses the shoulder and flexes the trunk laterally. The latissimi play an important part in climbing, walking with crutches, parallel bar exercises, all activities where the body is lifted with the arms fixed, and in every exertion requiring very energetic use of the arms, as in swimming or rowing.

In daily life or during moderate physical exercise, transfer of the latissimus dorsi muscle accompanying the raising of a flap is not actually associated with appreciable functional impairment. The entire group of shoulder muscles, especially the teres major, compensate for loss of the latissimus.

The problem posed to the surgeon during preoperative examination is to know how to test the muscle in order to confirm the integrity of its pedicle (if it is paralysed the nerve has been damaged at axillary nodal clearance and the chief vascular pedicle also very probably divided at this stage) and especially to differentiate between its contraction and that of the teres major.

The contraction of the muscle at its anterior border can be confirmed very simply by asking the patient to press her fist against her hip.

In case of doubt, the latissimus is tested more precisely in the prone position, with the arm extended and slightly away from the body, asking the subject to perform adduction of the arm with retroflexon in medial rotation, while the examiner resists this movement by placing a hand against the inner aspect of the forearm and applying passive abduction and slight anteflexion of the arm.

The position of the patient is the same for testing the teres major, but the elbow is flexed, the hand placed on the iliac crest, and the examiner's hand exerts resistance on the back of the elbow in the direction of abduction and retroflexion.

The contraction of the two muscles is easily palpable and even visible in the thin subject, where the vertical cord of the anterior border of the latissimus is clearly visible and the muscle bulge is higher up and more horizontal and posterior than that of the contracted teres major. The problem is more difficult in the obese subject, where there is a risk of mistaking contraction of the teres major for that of the upper part of the latissimus.

In summary, it is therefore better:

– to look for the contraction of the latissimus at the middle and lower part of its anterior border, rather than at its upper and posterior part,

– to use the tests for both muscles,

– and in cases of serious doubt, to begin the operation by checking the pedicle. However, if section of the main pedicle has been high, and the thoracic branch preserved, the latissimus may be revascularised by counterflow through this pedicle (fig. 208), where the flow is reversed. An increase in the caliber of this pedicle (fig. 208) is evidence of suprajacent interruption of the thoracodorsal pedicle. The flap can still be used, but in this case involves a paralysed muscle (as the nerve has been divided at the same time as the vessels), very thin, and whose trophic qualities and importance are no longer the same, even if it can ensure survival of the skin island.

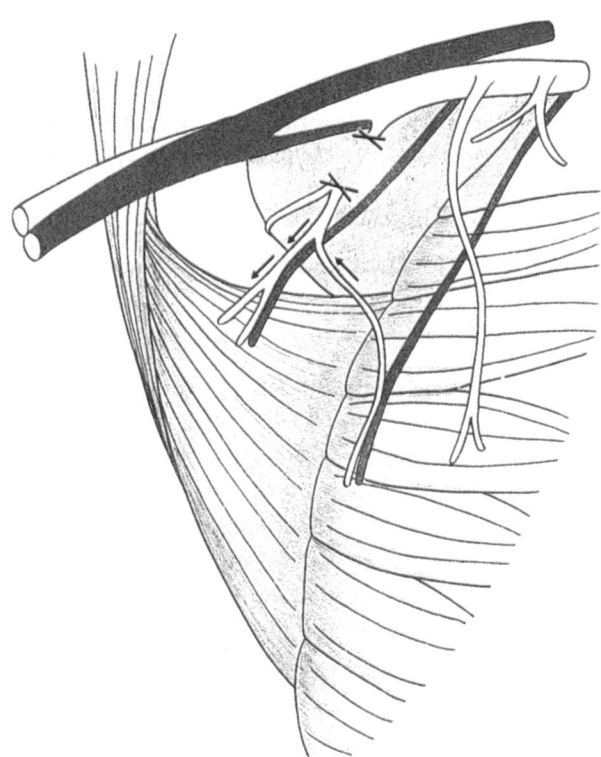

Fig. 208. In the event of high division of the pedicle, counterflow supply is possible via the thoracic branch

Findings at the preoperative examination

One should always attempt to obtain the records of the preceding mastectomy, in which it should be an invariable rule to respect and confirm the integrity of the pedicles and nerves of the latissimus and the serratus anterior. This is even more important when the previous operation was a long time ago and when it was a Halsted procedure. Actually, twenty years ago no particular care used to be taken with regard to these pedicles; reparative surgery in matters of breast cancer had few devotees, and the concept of a latissimus flap, initially described by Tansini in 1906, had been forgotten for many years to reappear only towards the end of the 1970s.

It will therefore be reassuring if the record clearly refers to respect of the neurovascular pedicle; often the nerve is not mentioned at all, but it is rare for the surgeon to have taken care to respect the nerve while neglecting the vessels. We have already mentioned that, in cases of section of the pedicle, the flap can still be raised on the thoracic branch or sometimes on an intercostal pedicle, but for safety reasons it will be more necessary and prudent not to divide the humeral attachments so as to preserve a muscle pedicle.

The clinical examination is completed by looking for telangiectases of the anterior thoracic region and axilla, as well as for any induration at this level, the sequelae to radiotherapy. In practice, and if the radiotherapy has been rather too energetic in the axillary fossa, the more so if the effects of sclerosis due to radiotherapy are added to those of the surgical dissection, and even if the flap pedicle is intact, its functional value may be diminished, not so much as regards arterial perfusion but in terms of venous return, since the fine and lax walls of the veins are more easily compressed by the adjacent sclerosed tissue than the arterial walls, which are thicker and more rigid and better resist the effects of irradiation. Thus, necrosis of flaps due to infarction of venous origin may be observed, the return circulation not being capable of ensuring drainage equivalent to the degree of arterial perfusion.

Design of the skin flap

We have seen that from the latissimus dorsi there emerge two kinds of perforating vessels, according to their direction, destined to supply the overlying and adjacent skin vascularisation. Over the whole surface of the muscle there emerge branches at right angles to it, which ramify in the subcutaneous tissue and ensure vascularisation of the overlying skin. Other perforating vessels emerge from the anterior border of the muscle and have a thoracic distribution in an anterior direction parallel to the skin plane, in which they terminate. This is explained by the course of the muscle, which is longer at this site, and by the skin mobility on the deep plane, which is also greater here; short vessels, derived directly from the depths and perpendicular to the surface, would not be compatible with such a course and with chest movements.

In consequence, two types of skin islands vascularised by the latissimus dorsi may be distinguished (fig. 209): islands situated entirely at the level of the muscle, and islands astride its anterior border and transgressing this widely. The choice of position and size of the skin island is conditioned by the intended usage and the relative or absolute importance of considerations of a cosmetic nature.

When it is desired to raise a very large flap (requiring closure of the donor area by graft), the largest and most reliable skin island is that raised astride the anterior border. This type of flap, raised as a vascular island with section of the muscle pedicle, may be transferred remotely, since the pivotal point becomes the origin of the vascular pedicle at the apex of the axillary fossa, and may even reach a point as far away as the middle third of the face.

In breast reconstruction there are several factors that condition the dimensions and position of the island:

– the dimensions of the skin island are restricted by the possibilities of direct closure of the donor zone, since this is a cosmetically aimed procedure and there is no question of grafting the loss of substance left by raising the flap. The size of the island will therefore depend in great part on the degree of skin laxity, which varies from one patient to another, and is particularly dependent on the thickness of the subcutaneous fatty layer but also on the site on the thorax where the island will be designed. The largest island will often be a posterior one, its main axis horizontal, as this is the one most remote from the zone of the mastectomy, and thus from the region where the greatest skin tension exists. The closer to the anterior axillary line, and the more vertical the axis of the flap, the lesser will become the dimensions of the skin island that permit direct closure of the zone at the donor site;

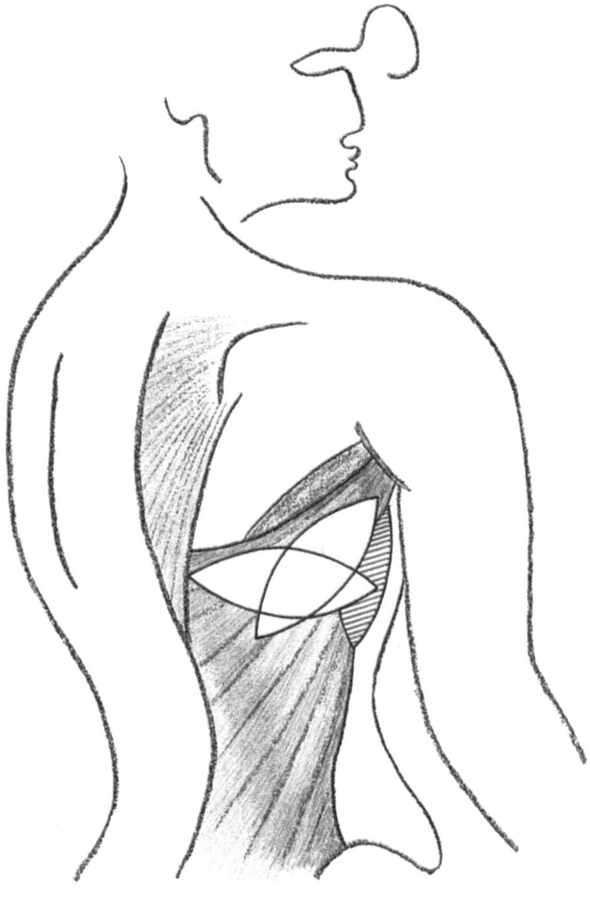

Fig. 209. Different types of available skin islands: white, with long axis oblique downward and inward or transverse; hatched, astride anterior border of the muscle (not very suitable in the particular case of breast reconstruction)

– the position of the skin island will thus be determined in terms of the necessary size and the choice of scar defect. An island astride the anterior edge of the muscle with its long axis vertical would be the one to give the most unobtrusive scar, but we feel that it is to be avoided in this precise use (except in the case of exceptional skin laxity) since the donor area of the skin flap is too close to the zone of transfer to the front of the chest, and the tension exerted on the margins to close the donor site is transmitted to the vicinity, especially at the region of the future inframammary crease, which becomes excessively deformed and horizontalised in its outer part, thus losing a great part of the benefit conferred by this tissue stock.

It remains to choose between two positions for the tracing of this skin island: oblique downward and backward, or the horizontal position. I prefer, whenever possible, to raise an island oblique downward and backward for two reasons: the scar is partly hidden under the arm at the upper part of the axillary fossa, and the wearing of a low-cut dress is less interfered with. Raising the island horizontally gives a more unpleasant scar in my opinion, as it crosses the back as much as the scar of the mastectomy crosses the front of the thorax, and it is not always easy to calculate its position so as to place it precisely within the brassiere. However, this design still has its indications in some cases, where a horizontally raised flap is the only one that can furnish an island of adequate size, and where closure of the donor site of an equivalent island with its main axis oblique cannot be performed immediately or will transmit excessive tension forward. This horizontal design is the only one generally usable in situations of immediate reconstruction where the provision of a flap is necessary;

– muscle overlap: the position of the skin island on the muscle also depends on the site where it is desired to place and utilise a muscle overlap of varying extent (fig. 210). If the residual anterior thoracic skin is very thinned and plastered against the ribs because of absence of the pectoralis major, and when one wishes to line it extensively by the latissimus after stripping, in this case too it will be useful to raise a horizontal skin island posteriorly, tangential to the upper border of the muscle. The muscle, raised integrally with the flap, is situated in anatomic position below and lateral to the skin island, but after rotation into the useful region and positioning of the skin island in the inferolateral quadrant of the breast to be reconstructed, the latissimus will form a large fan situated medially and above and will replace the absent pectoralis major. When the pectoralis major is preserved, the necessary anterior muscle overlap of the flap is less extensive, which is compatible with a skin island oblique downward and inward, the upper muscle overlap (in anatomic position) serving both to line the region of the inframammary crease and to fix it.

Preoperative design

This is made on the standing patient, before premedication. The inframammary crease is first designed, symmetrical with that of the opposite side, whatever the state of the remaining breast (normal, hypertrophic or ptosed) and above all at the same level in its middle portion (fig. 211).

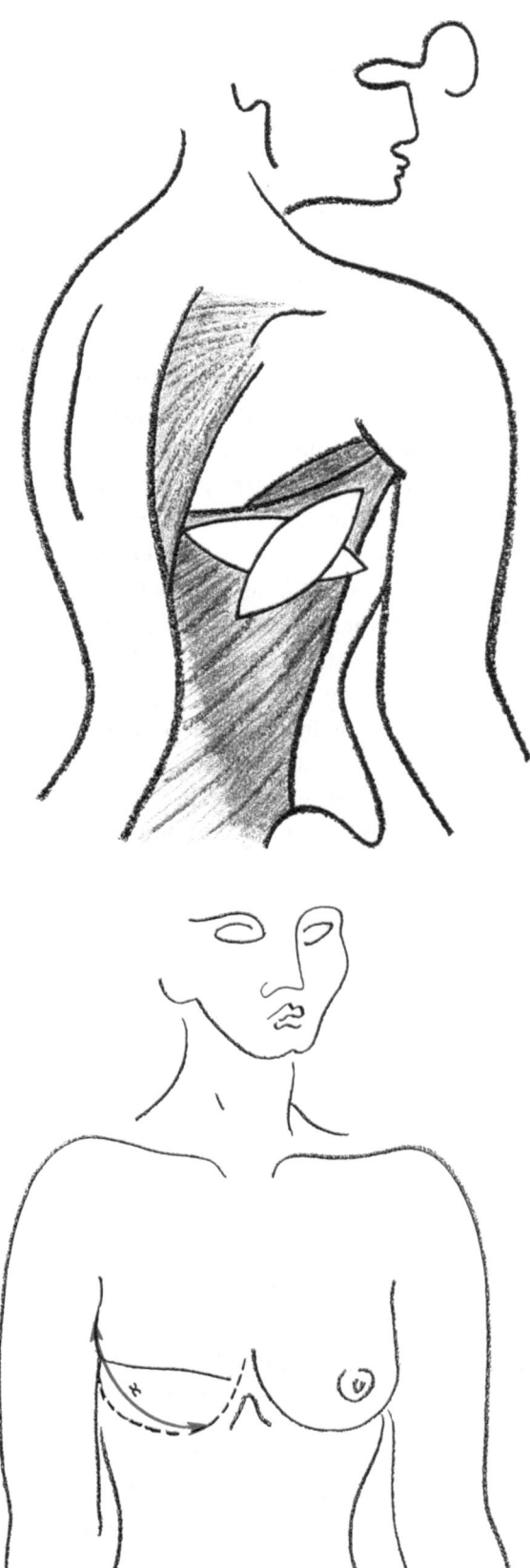

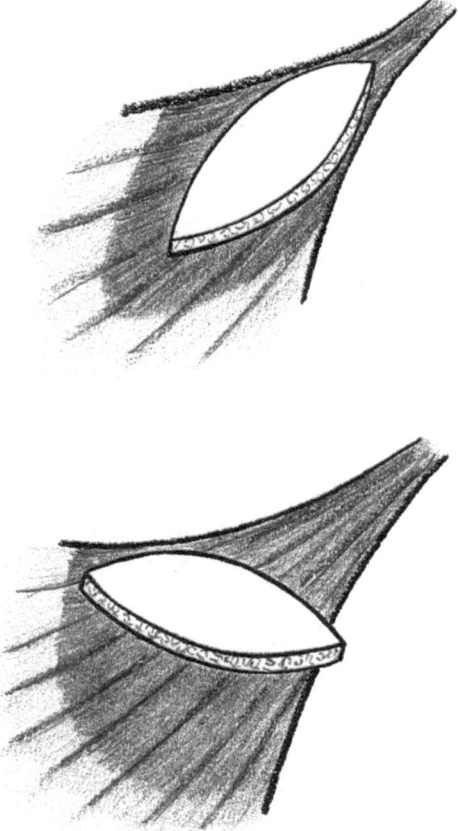

Fig. 210. Muscle overlap:
– when the island is oblique downward and inward: the muscle overlap is distributed all around the skin flap;
– when the island is transverse: the muscle overlap may be greater, but especially inferior (it will become anterior and medial once the flap is in place)

Fig. 211. Location of incision for placement of the flap and deciding its length (x)

A second line, which will allow measurement of the necessary length of the island, since it corresponds to its long axis, is drawn from the inferolateral border of the pectoralis major at the level of the anterior axillary line to join the inframammary crease in its medial third, making an asymptotic curve convex below and outward. This line is fundamental, since it corresponds to the zone of placement of the flap, but it does not necessarily have to correspond to the mastectomy scar and should not be too much influenced by it. If this scar is oblique downward and inward, the design very nearly corresponds to the mastectomy scar, which will be excised; if the scar is transverse, the flap is placed independently. The value of the myocutaneous latissimus flap is that it is thicker at the skin, subcutaneous and muscular levels than the residual anterior thoracic tissues, and therefore it can by itself reconstitute the relative excess of the inferolateral quadrant compared to the other quadrants, and therefore the natural curve of a normal breast, which is more important at this site. The implant, provision of which is nearly always necessary, will compensate for the overall lack of volume. Thus placed, the skin island may give a disagreable visual impression, especially if there is a difference of color between the skin of the back and that of the rest of the reconstructed skin (the skin is sometimes yellower at the back or, on the contrary, more pigmented in front after radiotherapy). But very often the reconstructed areola will be situated at the intersection of the scars and will attenuate this impression (fig. 213). On the other hand, if the flap is well placed, the scar of the inferolateral border is barely visible as it corresponds to the inframammary crease and to the outer limit of the breast. The axis of the skin island chosen is then designed (fig. 212), relating it to the length of the tracing of the anterior placement, the pivotal point of the axis of rotation of the flap. The skin island is designed as large as possible, while assessing the possibilities of direct closure by squeezing the skin together. This is more difficult in obese patients, as the thickness of the subcutaneous fat tends to lead to overestimation of the possibilites of closure.

Positioning

First stage

The first stage is performed in strict lateral decubitus, with the arm elevated to head level, slightly anteflexed and in no more than 90° of abduction so as to prevent hyperextension,which may lead to traction lesions of the brachial plexus. The forearm is immobilised horizontally on a support, the elbow flexed to 90°. The drapes are so placed as to expose the line of the spinous processes behind, the sternum in front, the iliac crest below and the clavicle, shoulder and axillary fossa above, enclosing the arm at is middle third. It is only in the raising of a latissimus flap astride the anterior border of the muscle — a situation not applicable in reconstruction apart from cases of previous expansion — that one can raise the flap in dorsal decubitus, with a rolled draw-sheet under the scapula in contact with the spine to elevate the lateral border of the thorax away from the plane of the table.

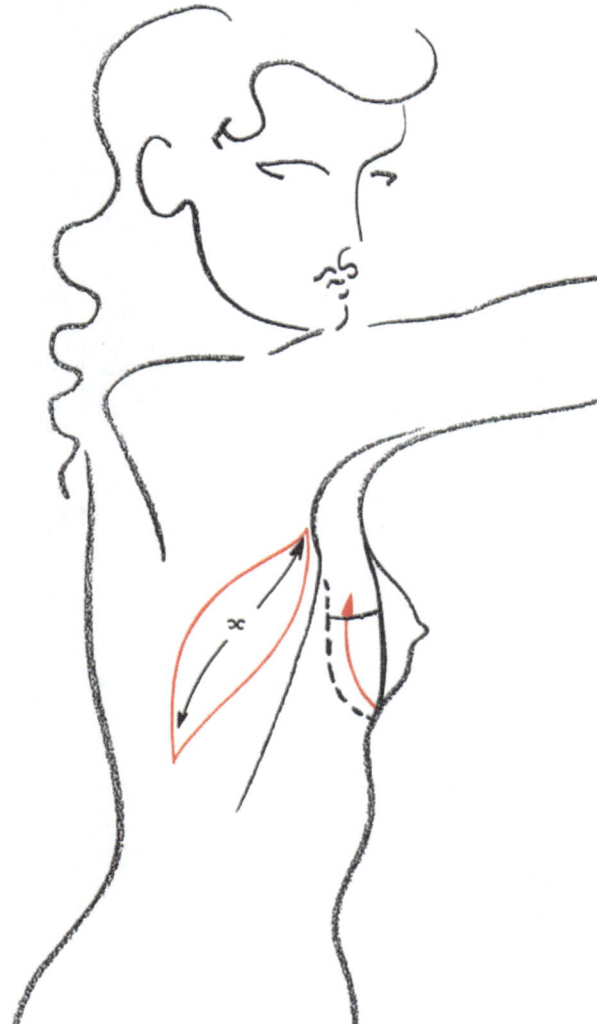

Fig. 212. This length x is carried to the axis of the skin island

Raising the flap

The incision is commenced at the outer end of the skin island when the design is horizontal, or at the upper part of the inferolateral border if the trace is oblique, in order first to expose the anterior border of the muscle and check the pedicle if there is any doubt as to its integrity. The skin incision is then completed all around the skin island, incising the skin and subcutaneous tissue as far as the perimysium, which must be carefully respected. The muscle is freed from the superficial planes at the lower border of the flap (the lower border will be stripped more extensively when it is desired to raise with the skin flap a large muscular overlap), then the anterior border of the muscle is freed at its middle portion. This anterior border is very thin, but is easily distinguished at this site by its mobility and its color is redder than the yellow type of fascia which joins it to the serratus anterior. After incision of this plane to where it contacts the anterior border of the muscle, the deep aspect of the muscle is then freed from the

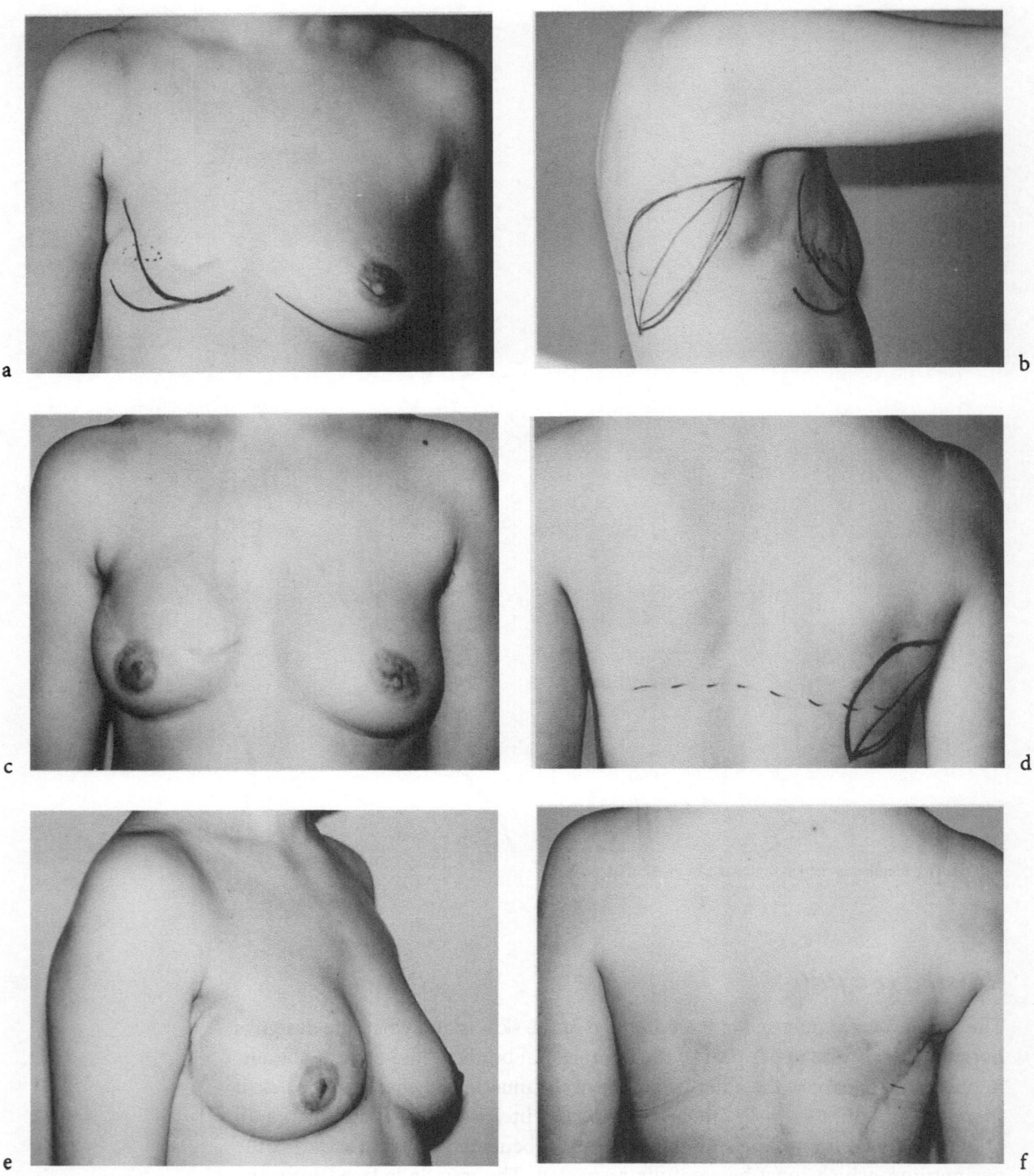

Fig. 213 a-f. Favorable position of the areola, placed at intersection of the scars. Flap skin 19 x 7 cm, smooth inflatable Sebbin implant of 150 ml inflated to 180 ml

thoracic plane, much of this stripping being performed atraumatically with the finger as this happens to be a zone of natural mobility. The dissection of the deep aspect is continued with scissors; the lower and more posterior the dissection, the more perforating vessels will be encountered where the latissimus is less mobile and where its fibers mingle with those of the adjacent muscles. After the entire deep aspect has been freed (except for the upper part of the muscle pedicle which is not easy to reach in this position at this stage), the dissection is continued by muscle section commencing at the distal end at the anterior border and progressing towards the spine, parallel to the skin island. When the medial extremity has been reached, the muscle section is continued towards the axillary fossa, progressively narrowing the muscle pedicle. By gradually elevating the flap, this allows monitoring of the position of the vascular pedicle. At the upper part of the dissection, elevation of the muscle exposes the teres major, which is connected to the latissimus by a sort of fibrous arch, perhaps the evidence of a common embryologic origin; these are all muscles of similar function and we have seen that it is not always easy to distinguish their contractions. In any case it is useful to split this fibrous arch as far as possible, almost to its humeral attachment, in order to separate the latissimus from the teres major. This procedure has two results: it facilitates anterior transfer of the flap without any need to divide the muscle pedicle, and the separation of the two muscles makes the dorsal "sabre cut" appearance often seen after use of this flap much less obvious. We prefer to keep the muscle pedicle intact whenever possible, and this is nearly always the case in breast reconstruction; it provides additional vascular security in cases of axillary irradiation, especially for the venous return (for the same reason the thoracic branch is preserved, which is no hindrance to forward positioning of the flap). Of course, keeping the muscle pedicle intact guarantees its better nutritional status; for the same reason we do not section the nerve to the latissimus, except in situations when the flaps are intended for the neck. The muscle wasting which results in part from the loss of function will then be less serious.

The anterior thoracic incision, whether it corresponds to the excision of the mastectomy scar or to a different design, will now permit the dissection of a tunnel for passage of the flap. This tunnel, situated at the lower and anterior part of the axillary fossa, is sufficiently large not to compress the pedicle, but the dissection must not be taken too low down at the level of the future inferolateral quadrant of the reconstructed breast; the risk is that during the immediate postoperative course, while the periprosthetic membrane is not yet formed, the prosthesis may migrate backward into the widely stripped zone where the flap has been raised.

After checking the hemostasis in the different zones of stripping, the flap is placed in temporary reserve in front and fixed by a few sutures while the zone where it was raised is closed. It is our habit, after insertion of a suction drain, to perform the closure in two planes with absorbable materal, using interrupted slowly-absorbed sutures: inverting deep dermal sutures, sometimes taking their support at a distance from the edges of the incision in the zone of greatest tension, and a superficial continuous rapidly-absorbed intradermal suture.

An adhesive sterile drape protects the flap while the patient is changed into a position of dorsal decubitus, the arms beside the body, and then into a semi-seated position with attention to leveling of the shoulders.

The flap can now be put in place and tacked down after having excised the tissues of very poor quality because of their lack of substance and suppleness. This hardly or at all concerns the upper margin of the incision for placement of the flap, as at this site the skin, even if thin, will be lined by the pectoralis major muscle and inferior muscle overlap of the flap, which, after a rotation maneuver, is found at the supero-medial part of the reconstructed breast.

On the other hand, the inferior margin of the incision is found in the inferolateral quadrant, in a region not padded by the pectoralis major, and where the skin cover is often thin and sclerosed. As far as possible, the skin coverings in this zone are excised and replaced by the skin layer of the flap, so as to place the inferolateral border of the flap in the inframammary crease at the outer limit of the reconstructed breast (fig. 214).

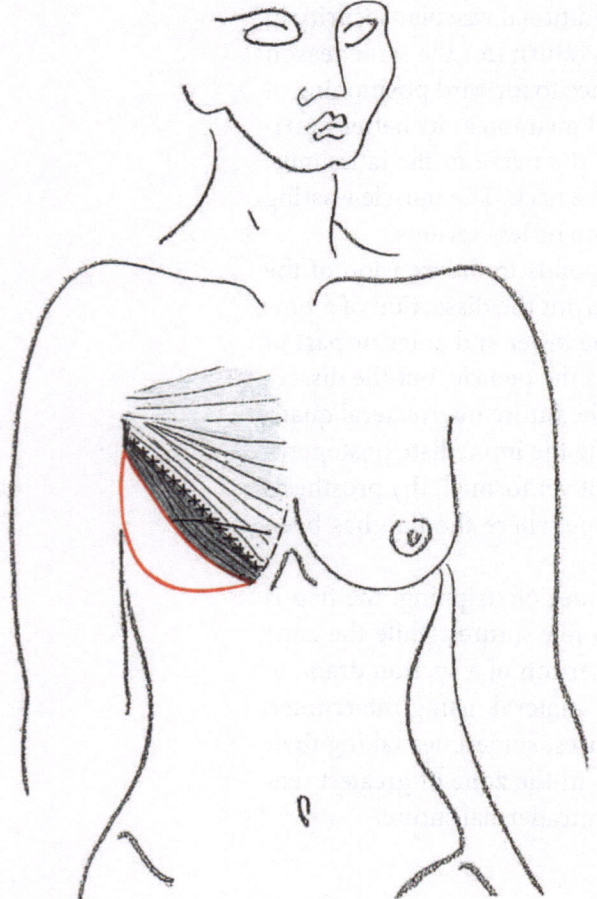

Fig. 214. The most favorable island is that placed (independently of the mastectomy scar) in the inferolateral quadrant of the breast under reconstruction, placing the lower suture line in the inframammary crease. The anterior muscle overlap of the latissimus dorsi (below when raising the flap) is sutured to the lower border of the pectoralis major to guarantee the prosthetic implant complete muscle cover, retropectoral above and retrodorsal below

After having sutured the inferior muscular border of the flap to the chest wall, and the deep dermis of the skin flap to the skin coverings at the inframammary crease, the deep aspect of the pectoralis major is stripped by detaching its lowest and innermost fibers to create the pocket intended to house the prosthesis. In practice, in the great majority of cases, the flap is not bulky enough to restore the breast volume by itself, even if virtually the entire muscle is raised. This prosthetic compartment is entirely retromuscular since its superolateral part is formed by the pectoralis major and its inferolateral part by the latissimus (fig. 215).

After checking the hemostasis, especially of the intercostal perforating vessels at the medial detachment of the pectoral fibers, a suction drain is inserted and then the free border of the pectoralis is sutured to the muscle overlap of the latissimus, contriving a central window for insertion of the prosthesis; in our practice this is always inflatable whether its wall is smooth or textured. In any case it is good practice, apart from ensuring the innocuousness of the content, to vary the amount of filling experimentally; theoretically, the anterior projection of the breast for a given base is determined by the volume indicated by the manufacturer, but in practice this is not the only factor since the entirety of the reconstructed volume is constituted in variable proportions by the thickness of the subcutaneous fatty layer and of the muscle, ie by the patient's tissues as well as by the prosthesis itself. With an eye to the relaxation of the tissues and the inevitable muscle wasting asociated with loss of function — even if minimised by preserving the nerve to the latissimus — it is better to complete the reconstruction with a volume apparently in excess of that desirable in the long term. This flap,which is of excellent trophicity, usually tolerates a slight degree of tension. The suture of the muscle plane (latissimus-pectoralis) is completed, with closure of the deep and superficial dermis in two layers, and the dressing is applied: tulle gras with or without corticoids, dry compresses, hypoallergenic adhesive strapping, modeling the reconstruction by compression at the site where the flap was raised but not at the axillary fossa, which must be free, and contriving a central observation window opposite the flap to monitor its color, warmth and time taken for restoration of normal color. The patient is returned to bed in dorsal decubitus and for the first few days the arm should be kept slightly away from the body to prevent any compression of the pedicle. The dressing is retained until removal of the suction drains, which usually requires 4 to 6 days of postoperative surveillance. The patient is then discharged with the sole instruction to wear a brassière that is not underwired, but preferably elastic with preformed cups, day and night for two weeks; the sutures are protected by adhesive strips, and she is allowed to shower after removal of the drains.

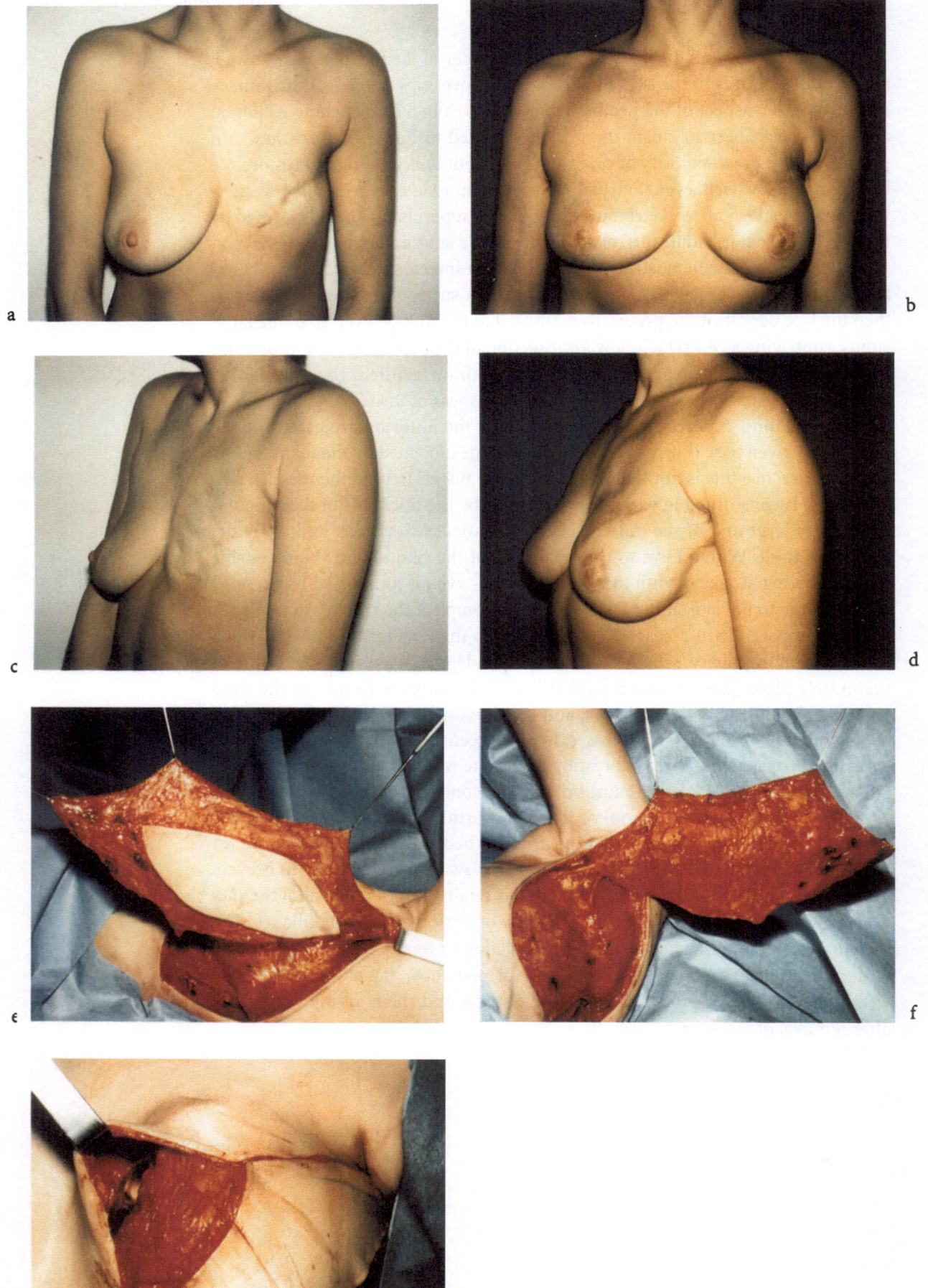

Fig. 215 a-g. Skin island 19 x 8 cm, wide muscle overlap, preservation of thoracic branch, suture of latissimus dorsi to pectoralis major, Sebbin LS20 inflatable implant of 175 ml filled to 220 ml

The fate of the flap

In the months following the procedure there is a more or less evident decrease in the apparent size of the reconstructed breast, linked to two phenomena: on the one hand, the loss of function of the transplanted latissimus produces wasting of the muscle, though less serious if the nerve has been saved, which ensures better trophicity; on the other hand, the skin component of the flap stretches under the thrust exerted by the bulk of the prosthesis (with some aid from gravity) and the reconstructed breast becomes convex in its lower quadrants while flattening at the upper quadrants, with an apparent decrease in size. This tissue relaxation may also be observed in the residual thoracic tissues, which regain better trophicity and often more flexibility because of the vascular reinforcement due to lining by the overlap of the latissimus dorsi muscle.

Also in the first few months it will be seen whether the prosthesis is well tolerated, or if unfortunately the foreign body reaction leads to visible and palpable periprosthetic contracture, the breast remaining too round, too firm and with an insufficiently spread implantation base. Placement of the prosthesis in an entirely retromuscular compartment does not prevent this phenomenon but makes it less evident because of muscle interposition between the integuments and the implant. Some workers even believe that periprosthetic contracture is less serious in this situation as the muscle exerts a permanent support comparable to massage of the implant.

The second operative stage is conducted after a delay of around four months, so that the muscle wasting and skin relaxation are stabilised, and when one can assess the possible periprosthetic contracture and its degree:

– the operation begins with minor adjustments, if necessary, of the modeling of the skin component of the flap and of the compartment of the prosthesis (fig. 216). In some rare cases, we have been led to divide the muscular pedicle at the lower part of the axillary fossa when it produced a cord-like appearance in raising the arm; but this procedure remains exceptional and we prefer to avoid it unless absolutely necessary, as it leads to atrophy of the remaining muscle fibers and thus to decreased thickness of the flap;

– then the future nipple-areolar plaque is designed;

– this is related to the position of the design employed for the mammoplasty of the opposite breast to produce symmetry, which is often necessary if only to correct a slight ptosis and to reduce the breast base;

– it is only after having performed this procedure on the opposite breast that placement of the nipple-areolar plaque will be definitively located, a visual compromise between the siting that would seem initially ideal in the reconstructed breast, ie at its apex, and the situation of the plaque on the opposite breast after correction. Rather than an exact symmetry as measured from the suprasternal notch and the midline, it is the visual impression that counts.

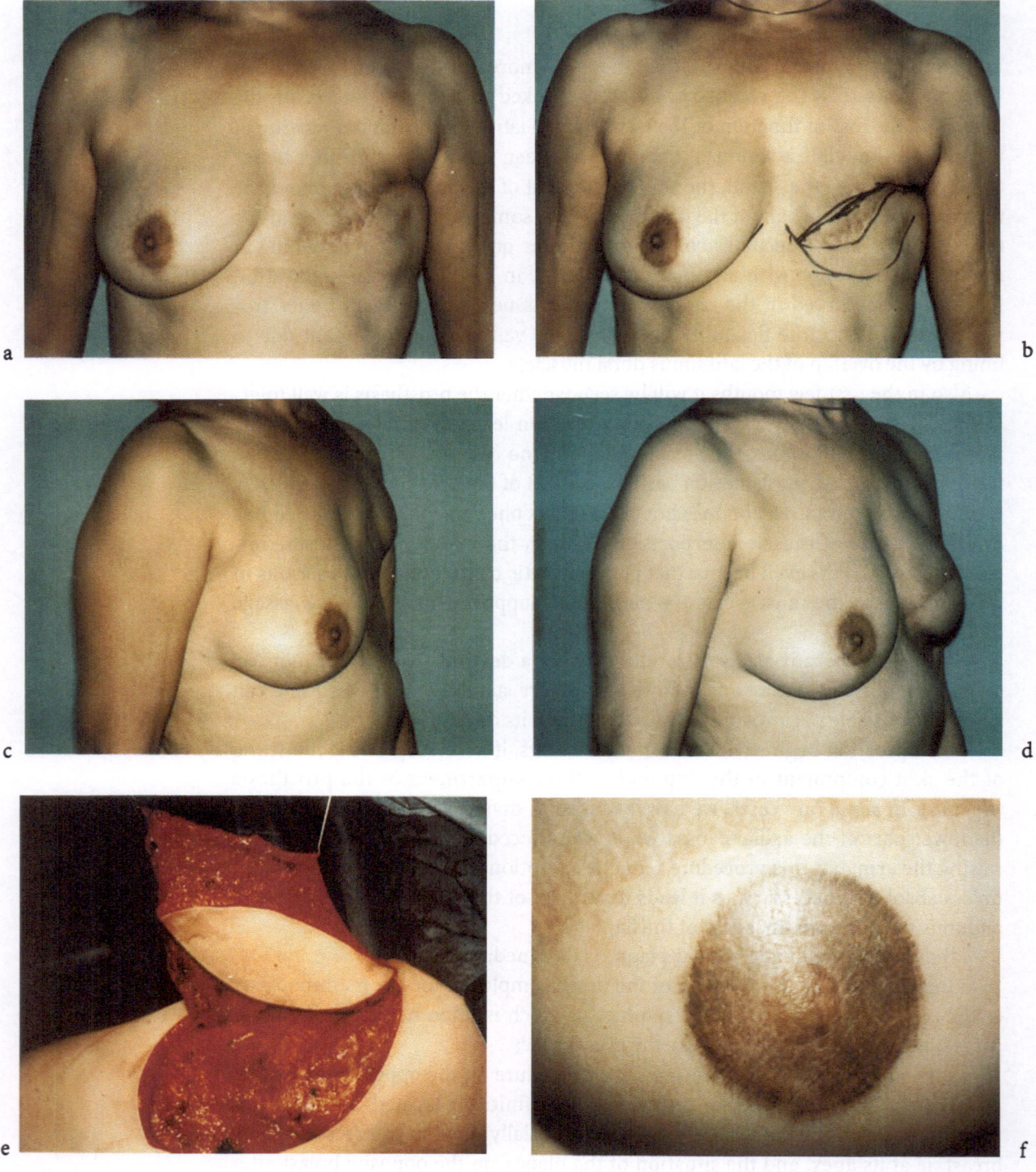

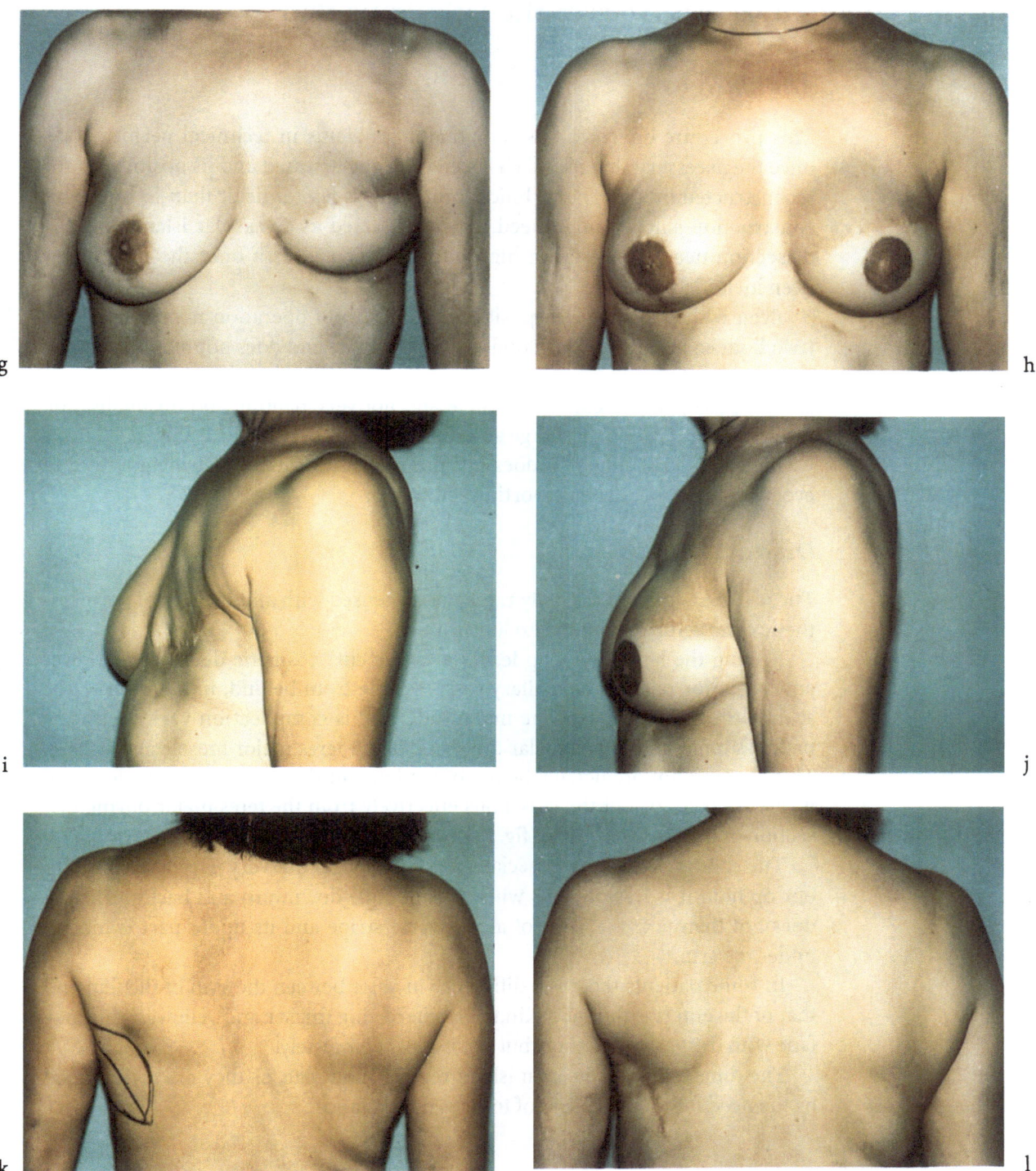

Fig. 216. a-c, i Loss of skin laxity, moderate irradiation sequelae, adherent and broadened scar to be excised, but whose direction is favorable to the placement of the latissimus dorsi flap; **e** the skin flap (15 x 9 cm) is raised with a wide muscle overlap to line the superomedial thoracic integuments; **g** after the first stage of reconstruction the inframammary crease is too high, the flap is not sufficiently spread out, and the volume of the implant (LS20, 175 ml filled to 200 ml) seems inadequate; **h, d, j, l** the compartment is revised and spread by incision of the periprosthetic membrane, which allows placement of a bigger implant: LS20 of 225 ml filled to 350 ml; **f** at the same time the opposite breast is reduced in size (reduction by 120 g and correction of ptosis) with areolar reconstruction by tattooing and graft of lower half of opposite nipple

Advantages and disadvantages of the latissimus flap

Advantages

This procedure does not pose any major problems in technical performance, once the necessary skin island has been correctly assessed and its position on the reconstructed breast. The technical procedure is less difficult than in breast reconstruction since the flap need not be dissected as a vascular island, and the dissection need not be taken high into the axillary fossa once the pedicle has been identified.

Even with the change in position, the length of operation is not very great (two hours on average); the blood-loss is moderate and does not require transfusion.

The postoperative course is simple and not very painful, and hospitalisation rarely exceeds a week, discharge accompanying removal of the drains.

Raising a latissimus flap does not produce functional impairment, either in everyday life or in amateur sporting activities.

Disadvantages

The use of an implant can only rarely be dispensed with and the risk of periprosthetic contracture cannot be excluded.

Raising the latissimus flap leaves a "sabre cut" cosmetic defect at the lower and posterior part of the axillary fossa, visible from behind, in addition to the scar of the skin removal. The magnitude of this complication varies with the patient's build and in particular the shape of the teres major muscle and its size. This factor is not predictable before operation, but the sabre cut can be lessened if care is taken to split the latissimus effectively from the teres major during dissection of the muscle pedicle (fig. 217).

The skin excision scar, especially if transverse, is not very easy to conceal. In our opinion it is less obvious when it is oblique downward and backward, as it does not then take the form of a transverse stripe and its upper part is hidden under the arm.

In some patients there is a difference in color beween the skin of the flap and that of the anterior thoracic skin,the former being thicker and yellower; this may fade with the passage of time, but not usually completely.

The dimensions of the skin island remain moderate, as they are conditioned by the need for direct closure of the loss of substance.

Fig. 217 a-h. Cleavage of latissimus dorsi from teres major to minimise the "sabre cut" defect. (Skin island of 18 x 10 cm placed in the opening of the excised scar. Smooth inflatable Sebbin implant of 175 ml filled with 200 ml of normal saline, reconstruction of areola by tattooing and graft of opposite nipple, placement at second stage procedure, on right, of an identical implant of 125 ml filled to 150 ml intended to augment the anterior projection while conserving the same base)

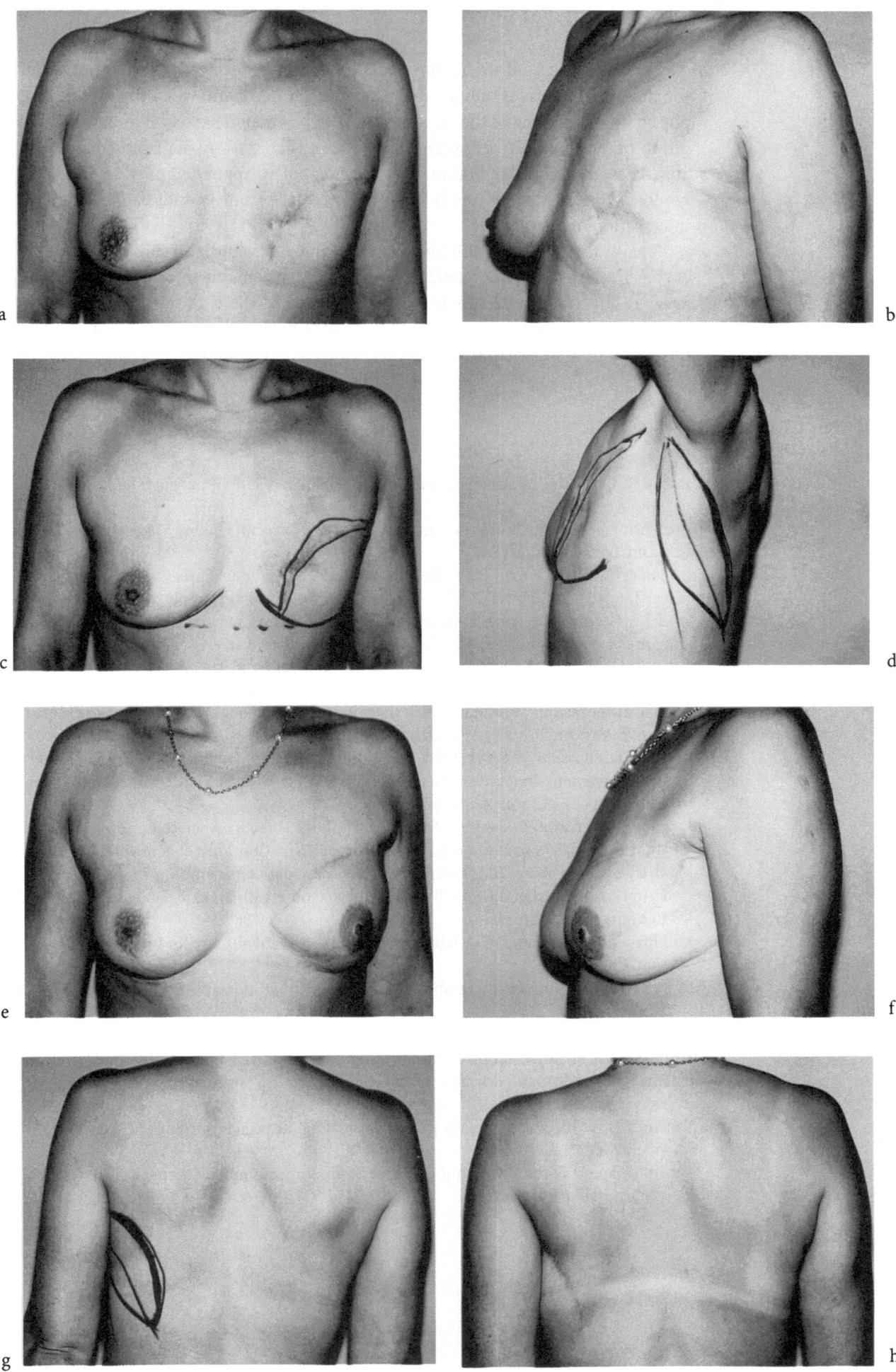

The scar defect on the reconstructed breast is reduced to a minimum when the mastectomy scar is oblique downward and inward, and when the skin island, placed in the opening of the excised scar, is large enough for its inferolateral margin to be placed in the inframammary crease (Fig. 218). Apart from such favorable cases, the skin island often gives the effect of an appended portion, especially if has a different color and if the nipple-areolar plaque cannot be placed at the intersection of the scars.

Finally, though it can still be performed in cases where the subscapular pedicle has been divided, but where a thoracic branch remains intact, there is a denervated flap which will supply only the volume of the skin island. The wasted muscle will be of less satisfactory trophicity and much less useful as regards the possible blood-supply to the remaining thoracic integuments.

References

Bostwick J, Nahai F, Wallace J G, Vascibez L (1979) Sixty latissimus dorsi flaps. Plast Rec Surg 63: 31-40

Bostwick J (1990) Plastic and Reconstructive. Breast Surgery, Quality Medical Publishing, Saint-Louis, Missouri

Brizon et Castaing (1967) Les Feuillets d'Anatomie, ed Maloine, Paris

Fisher J, Bostwick J, Powell R W (1983) Latissimus dorsi blood supply after thoraco-dorsal vessel division: the serratus collateral. Plast Rec Surg 72: 502

Gregoire et Oberlin (1967) Précis d'anatomie, éd. Baillière, Paris

Guedon C, Vu P, Gehanno P, Andreassian B, Soussaline M (1988) Transposition conjointe des muscles grand dorsal et grand dentelé en chirurgie reconstructrice cervicale et thoracique. Résultats de 40 dissections anatomiques et applications cliniques dans 21 cas. Ann Chir Plast et Esth vol. 33, n°4: 321-328

Legre R, Boghossian V, Servant JM, Magalon G, Bureau H (1990) Analyse des séquelles du prélèvement du lambeau de grand dorsal. A propos de 44 cas revus et testés. Ann Chir Plast et Esth, vol. 35, n°6: 512-517

Lejour M, Alemanno P, De Mey A, Gerard Th, Eder H (1985) Analyse de 56 reconstructions mammaires par lambeau de grand dorsal, Ann Chir Plast et Esth vol. 30, n°1

Maxwell GP, Mc Gibbon BM, Hoopse JE (1979) Vascular considerations in the use of latissimus dorsi myocutaneous flap after mastectomy with an axillary dissection. Plast Rec Surg 64: 771

Muhlbauer, Olbrich (1977) The latissimus dorsi myocutaneous flap for breast reconstruction. Chir Plast: 4, 27

Muller GH (1986) Intérêt du lambeau antérieur de grand dorsal. Ann Chir Plast et Esth 31, n°4: 359-365

Olivari N (1976) The latissimus dorsi flap. Brit J Plast Surg 29: 126-128

Talmant J Cl Reconstruction mammaire après amputation pour cancer par lambeau myo-cutané de grand dorsal. A propos de 45 cas avec 9 ans de recul. Ann Chir Plast et Esth (à paraitre)

Tansini I (1906) Nuovo processo per l amputazione della mammella per cancro. La Riforma Medica 12: 3-5

Tansini I (1906) Sopra il mio nuovo processo di amputazione della mammella. Gazetta Medica Italiana: 141-142

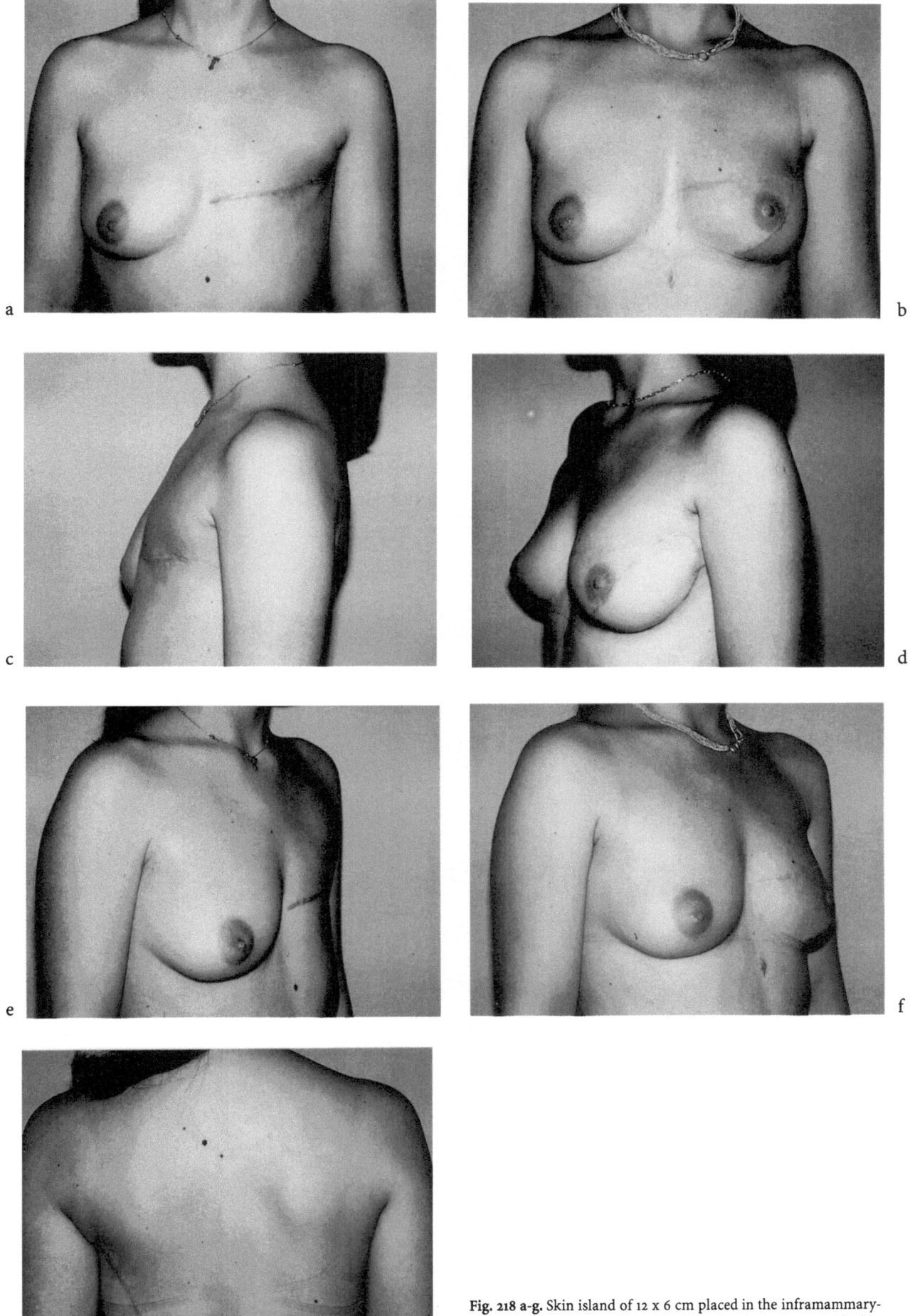

Fig. 218 a-g. Skin island of 12 x 6 cm placed in the inframammary-crease. Textured inflatable Sebbin LS21 implant of 175 ml filled to 200 ml. Reconstruction of areola by tattooing and graft of lower half of opposite nipple

The rectus abdominis flap

Since its description in 1982 by Hartrampf, this technique of reconstruction has gained great popularity, due mainly to its major advantage: the possibility of reconstructing a breast of satisfactory size and natural consistency without the help of supplementary prosthetic material.

It is, in a way, "the art of using the left-overs", as the principle of this operation is based on the use of excess subumbilical skin and fatty tissue to restore the lost substance and volume, the skin island being represented by the cutaneo-adipose triangle which is ordinarily sacrificed in an abdominal plasty (fig. 219).

Unlike the latissimus flap, the volume represented by the muscle is negligible, and it is the muscle itself which serves as the vascular pedicle. It does in fact contain the anastomotic plexus between the superior and inferior epigastric arteries, still called the epigastric arch.

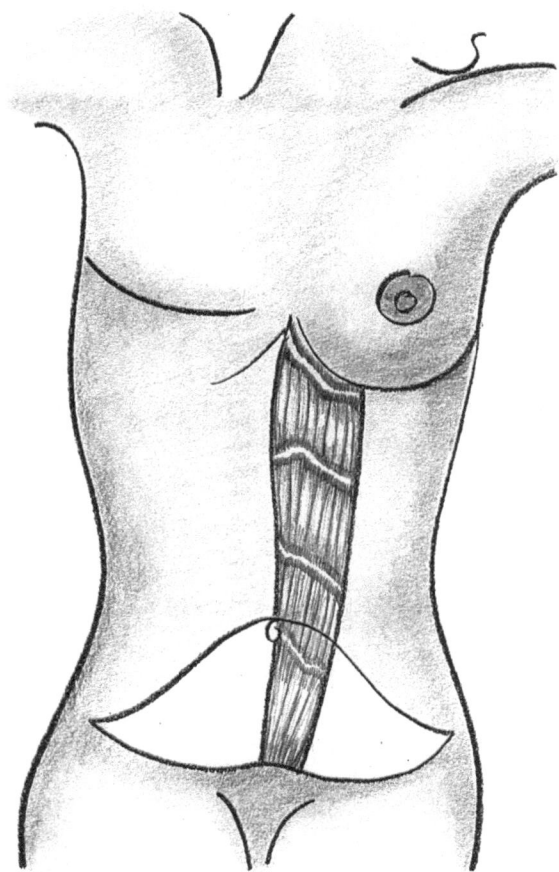

Fig. 219. The myocutaneous flap of the rectus abdominis is based on utilisation of the excess subumbilical skin and fatty tissue

It must be stressed at the outset that, to benefit from this fine intramuscular vascular plexus, it is necessary to raise the muscle throughout its extent.

While this is a technique that gives excellent results, it requires — apart from the proper indications — a degree of experience as regards both the dissection of the pedicle and the stage of assessment of the vitality of the skin component and of its modeling, and should not in our view be performed in inexpert hands.

Anatomy

The muscle belly and its sheath

The rectus abdominis muscle (fig. 220) originates from the inner end of the 5th rib, the costal cartilages of the 5th, 6th and 7th ribs, and the xiphoid process. From here the muscle bundles travel vertically towards the pubis, the muscle belly becoming more compact and narrower below the umbilicus. The muscle ends as a short flattened tendon inserted on the pubis, from the pubic spine to the symphysis, and on the symphysis itself.

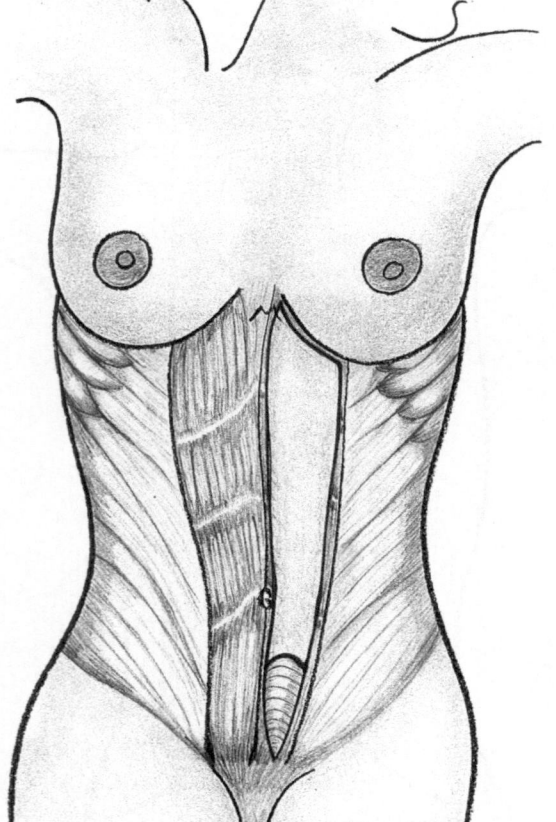

Fig. 220. Muscular anatomy: *left* the anterior surface of the muscle with its tendinous intersecton; *right* the posterior aspect of the sheath

Fig. 221. Structure of the rectus sheath.
above: in the supraumbilical region the aponeurosis of the external abdominal oblique forms the anterior layer of the sheath, which is lined by the internal abdominal oblique. The posterior layer, equally firm, is formed by the posterior layer of the aponeurosis of the internal abdominal oblique and the middle of the transversus aponeurosis. The muscle is firmly adherent to the sheath opposite the intersections.
below: below the arcuate line, the aponeurosis of the flat muscles of the abdomen (external and internal oblique and transversus) pass in front of the muscle belly

The fleshy belly is divided transversely by tendinous intersections firmly adherent to the anterior part of the sheath (figs. 220 and 221). These vary in number from two to five, but three are most often found. The two supra-umbilical intersections are practically transverse. The third, situated at umbilical level, is rather more oblique downward and outward. When there are supplementary intersections, at least one will be found below the umbilicus. These intersections do not involve the entire thickness of the muscle and do not interrupt the muscle fibers at the posterior aspect of the muscle. The muscle belly therefore forms a continuous posterior ribbon from origin to insertion, only slightly adherent to the posterior layer of the sheath, and easily freed from it, unlike the situation at its anterior aspect.

The structure of the rectus sheath changes from above downward (fig. 221):

– above the arcuate line (of Douglas) the aponeurosis of the internal abdominal oblique muscle is duplicated in two sheets; its anterior sheet fuses with the aponeurosis of the external abdominal oblique to form the anterior lamina of the sheath of the rectus abdominis, while its posterior sheet fuses with the aponeurosis of the transversus abdominis to form the posterior lamina of the sheath of the rectus. From the xiphoid process to the arcuate line, situated at the upper third of the sub-umbilical portion of the rectus, the sheath is therefore fibrous, thick and firm on both aspects;

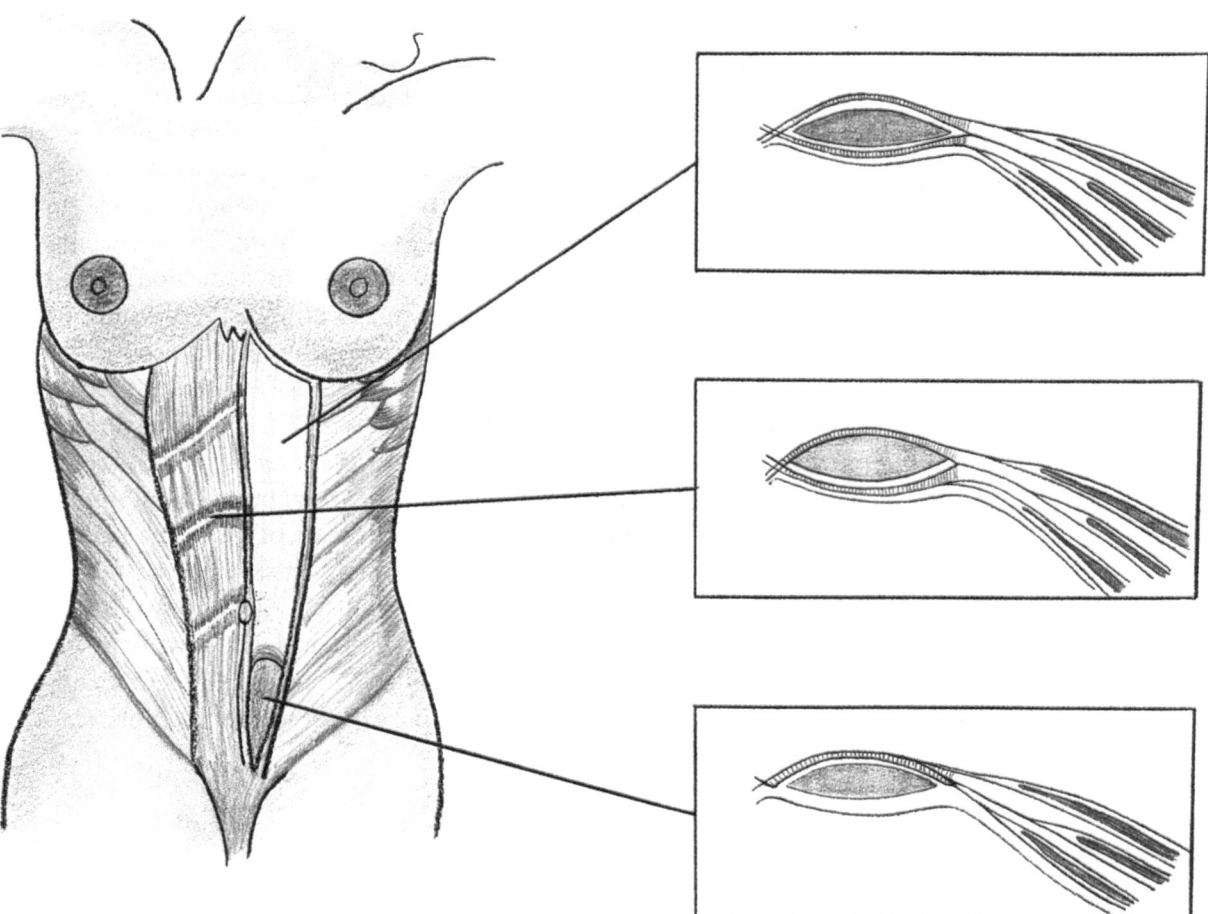

– below the arcuate line and and down to the pubis, the aponeurosis of the internal abdominal oblique no longer divides into two layers and the aponeuroses of all three muscles join to form the anterior lamina of the rectus sheath, all three now passing in front of the muscle belly. Behind, the muscle is separated from the peritoneum only by a rather thin cellular layer, the transversalis fascia. The practical outcome of this is that after raising the flap the abdominal wall at this level must be carefully and firmly repaired to prevent subsequent dehiscence.

Vascularisation

The epigastric vessels (fig. 222)

The inferior epigastric artery arises from the inner border of the external iliac artery, to describe a curve concave medially behind the deep orifice of the inguinal canal, below and then medial to the round ligament. It reaches the outer border of the rectus 5-6 cm from the pubis and then passes to the deep aspect of the muscle while remaining in front of the transversalis fascia. It approaches the midline, passes in front of the arcuate line, and then travels applied to the posterior aspect of the muscle, usually remaining at the junction of the middle and inner third of the muscle, before entering the thickness of the muscle below the umbilicus. But besides this arrangement, which remains the most common, we have observed a number of anatomic variations related to the course of the artery and its site of penetration of the muscle. It is not uncommon to see the artery remain attached to the outer third of the muscle without more closely approaching the midline before entering the muscle belly. This argues against certain dissection techniques, which, for theoretic reasons of partial preservation of rectus function — though these have been refuted — aim precisely to leave the outer third of the muscle in place. By so doing, there is a risk of damaging the vascular pedicle. It is also not rare to find the artery traveling entirely at the deep aspect of the muscle and giving off perforating branches to it, its short course keeping it at the deep aspect without ever penetrating the muscle. The dissection of the deep aspect of the muscle must therefore be particularly atraumatic so as not to risk injuring the inferior epigastric vessels and their branches, which are particularly at risk before they enter the muscle belly.

The superior epigastric artery is the medial terminal branch of the medial thoracic (internal mammary) artery. It arises at the level of the 6th intercostal space, passes through the sternocostal hiatus (of Larrey) between the sternal and costal portions of the diaphragm, and enters the sheath of the rectus muscle. After having given off a branch which is often seen to follow the costal margin downward and outward before entering the muscle, it divides into several branches in the thickness of the muscle belly. These anastomose with the homologous terminal branches of the inferior epigastric artery to form a complex intramuscular plexus in which the inferior epigastric system predominates.

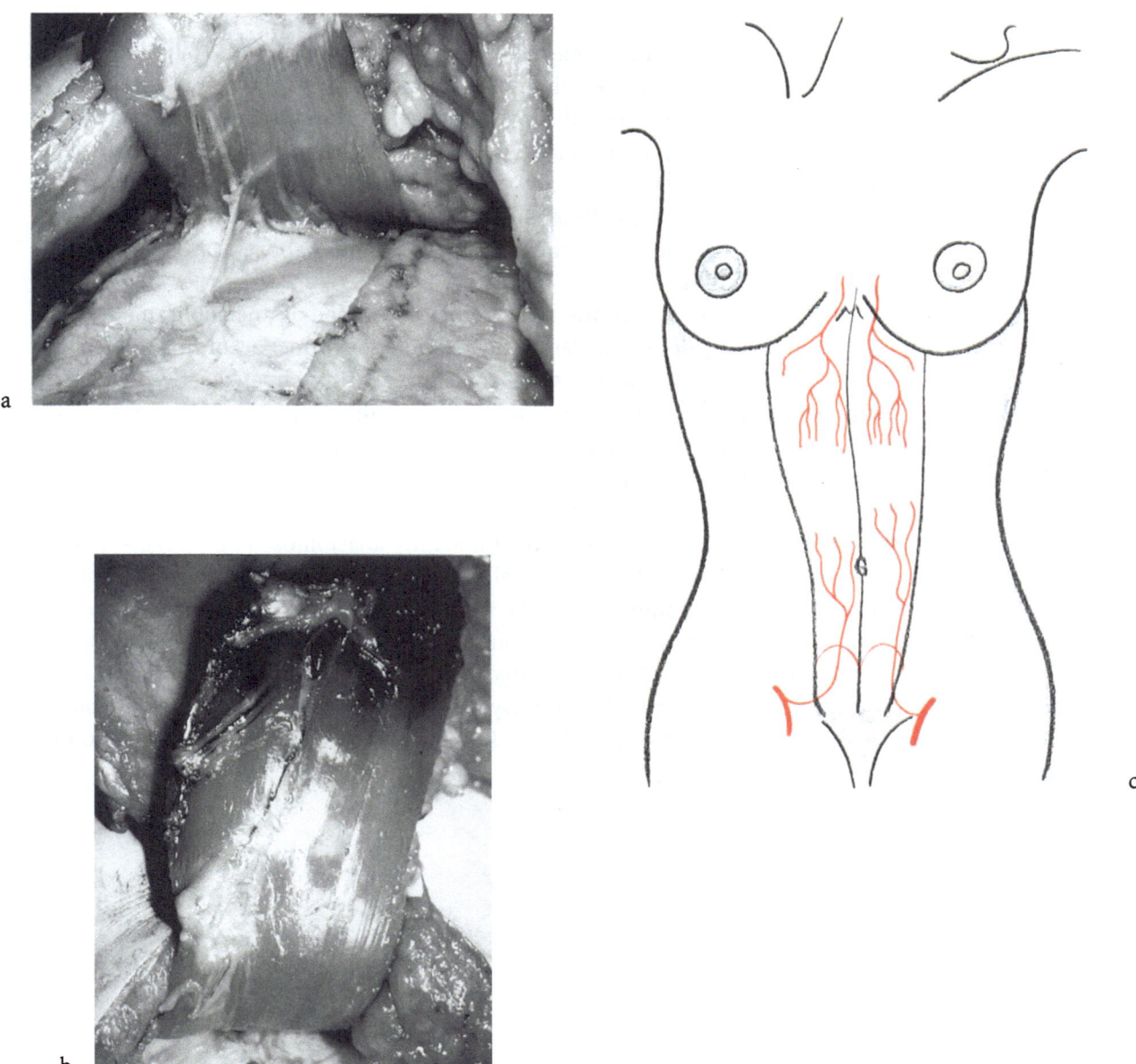

Fig. 222 a-c. Arterial vascularisation. **a** The superior epigastric artery penetrates the muscle quite close to the costal margin; **b** *(left)* the inferior epigastric artery classically crosses the deep aspect of the muscle to enter it below the umbilicus, but **b** *(right)* it is not uncommon to see it plastered against the outer third of the muscle, which it enters late, which also justifies raising the entire breadth of the muscle belly (**c**)

Cutaneous vascularisation (fig. 223)

The epigastric anastomotic plexus plays a dominant role in the blood-supply of the abdominal wall. In the subumbilical zone, which is the site where the skin portion of the flap is raised, the myocutaneous perforating vessels appear sparse and small in relation to the flap utilisable. The larger vessels, usually three or four in number to the naked eye, are situated near the midline and mostly in the upper third of the space between umbilicus and pubis. These perforators traverse the superficial fascia and branch transversely, more above than below, before passing to the skin.

The vascularisation of the skin therefore depends on the subdermal plexus. The skin portion of the flap can be divided into four zones according to the quality of the vascularisation. The safest zone is clearly that situated above the muscle chosen for the pedicle (I); then comes the equivalent contralateral zone (II); a little less abundantly vascularised is the outer half on the side of the pedicle (III); and finally, the zone which is most subject to possible damage is the outer half of the side opposite the pedicle (IV).

The subdermal plexus is more abundantly anastomosed and larger than the plexus situated under the superficial fascia, which accounts for the development of certain cytosteatonecroses on the side opposite the pedicle even when the skin has survived. This anatomic distribution will allow in some cases partial de-fatting of the flap. Indeed, if a dye is injected into the inferior epigastric artery in vivo after having stripped the skin layer of the wall except in the zone of contact with the relevant rectus muscle, the first phenomenon is staining of the parame-

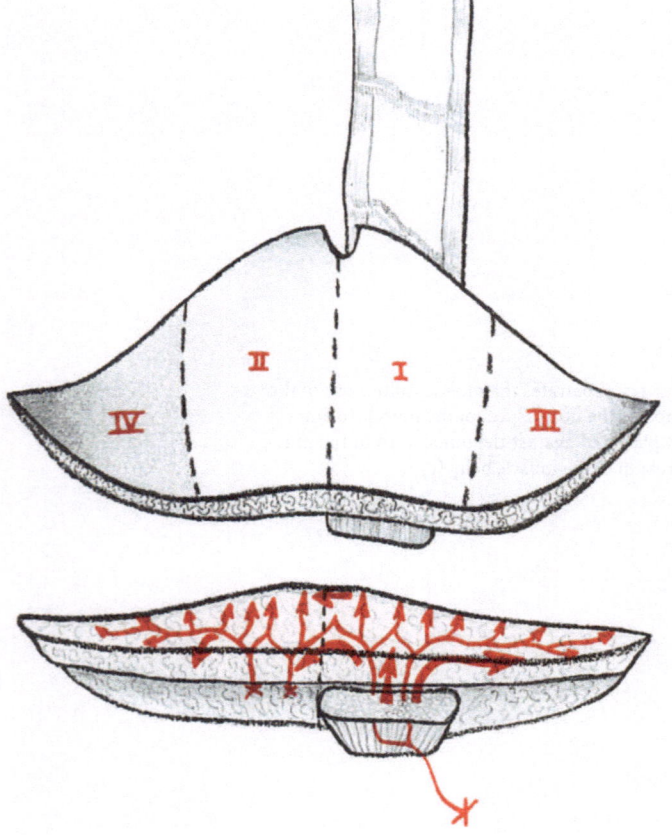

Fig. 223. Skin vascularisation:
above: arterial supply; the perfusion pressure and thus the quality of venous return are better the nearer to the pedicle. In I there is no problem, nor in II, with a minor exception for the immediately lateral umbilical zone where minor venous stasis is sometimes seen, rarely resulting in a narrow band of necrosis of the cutaneous border of the flap, which does not usually require excision, merely dressing with tulle gras. In III and IV the extent of the peroperative excision of the lateral extremities of the skin island depends on their color and is more extensive in IV then in III
below: the arterial perforators arriving from the muscle belly, and situated mainly near the linea alba, branch and anastomose chiefly above the superficial fascia. The fatty tissue least well vascularised is therefore that situated under the superficial fascia on the side opposite the pedicle, since it is at the end of the vascular plexus

dian skin plexus on the side of the pedicle and then of the outer zone of the flap. The color then crosses the midzone superficially, ultimately to reach the opposite plexus situated in the deep fatty layer under the transversalis fascia. It is therefore possible, if the flap is too bulky, but when one wants to retain more skin than fat, to eliminate the layer of fatty tissue situated under the superficial fascia on the side opposite the pedicle,

Venous return

In the medial region, the venous return is ensured by satellite veins of tbe perforating arteries and by a periumbilical plexus, the whole joining the inferior epigastric plexus. Laterally, the venous return from the abdominal wall occurs preferentially by quite large superficial veins which drain towards the low pressure region in the inguinal crease, but these veins are divided when the flap is raised. This lateral plexus anastomoses with the median plexus; as this does not represent the preferential drainage plexus, this partly explains the difficulties of venous drainage of the skin island at its extremities, which may lead to necrosis. This is why it is preferable during the procedure to sacrifice as much as may be required of the extremities of the island until it regains a normal color, so as to prevent distal damage from impairment of venous return.

Innervation

The rectus abdominis is innervated by the terminal branches of the lower intercostal nerves (D5-D12), which pass with the terminal branches of the intercostal arteries between the oblique and transverse muscles and enter the muscle sheath at its outer border. These branches travel on the deep aspect of the muscle before entering it some 3 cm from its outer border. This confirms that it is pointless, during the dissection of the muscle, to leave in place an outer or inner band, as these denervated and nonfunctional muscle fibers are doomed to atrophy and fibrous degeneration, as a recent study confirms.

Action, tests of function

Contraction of the rectus muscles produces forward flexion of the trunk with increase in the dorsal kyphosis and straightening of the lumbar lordosis. If the fixed point is the pelvis, the recti approximate the pelvis to the thorax. Muscle impairment leads to reduced possibility of forward flexion of the trunk; in dorsal decubitus, the subject has more difficulty in lifting the thorax toward the pelvis, and therefore in lifting the head and upper part of the trunk from their supporting surface. In the standing position, the deficit accentuates the lumbar lordosis.

Clinical examination

The findings at clinical examination allow assessment of the conditions of making the flap, its limitations and contraindications. Apart from examination of the mastectomy region and of the sequelae of previous treatment, it comprises essentially a study of the morphology of the patient and the presence of abdominal scars and striae. Numerous striae are evidence of deterioration of the dermis and suggest that the dermal and subdermal vascular plexus may be itself be affected. Some authors consider the presence of numerous major striae to be a contraindication.

History

Enquiry will also relate to the general health, to the amount of smoking (because of its effect on the micro-vascularisation), the patient's mental state and any medication, especially of aspirin and antidepressants (risk of hemorrhage with the former, and of mental instablity in the latter).

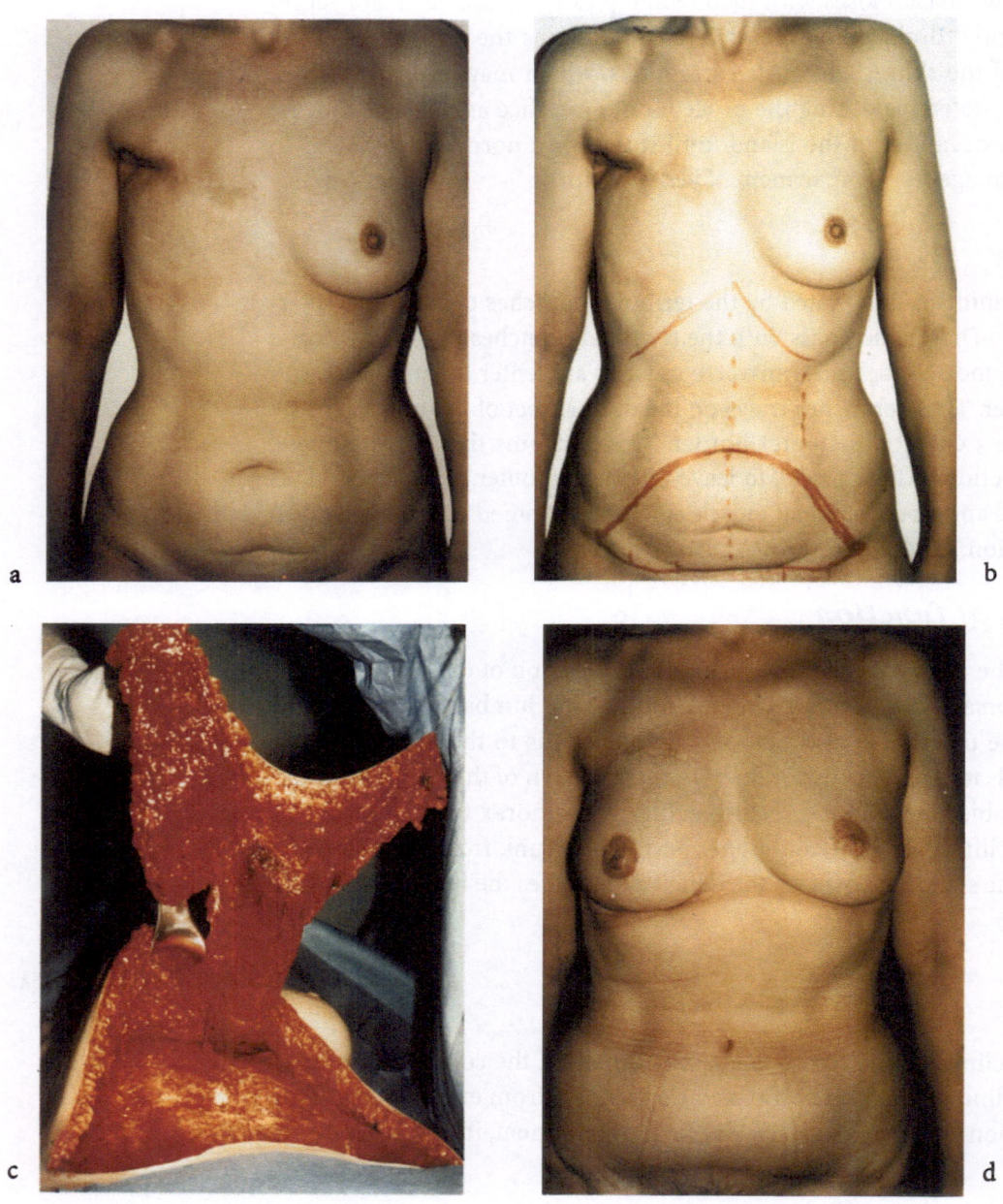

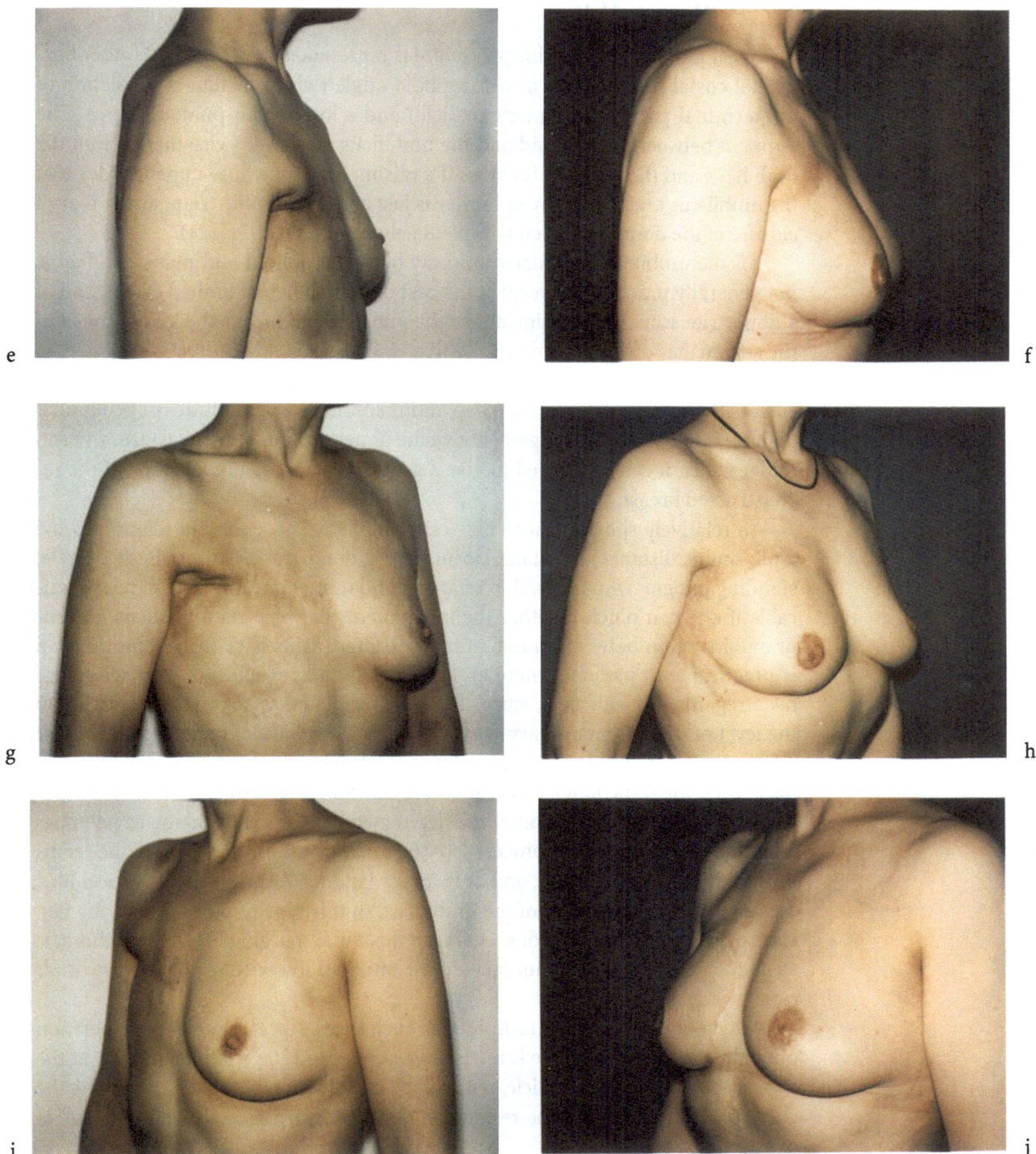

Fig. 224 a-j. a Preoperative appearance; **b** design of skin island; **c** freeing of the deep aspect of the muscle is taken up as far as the costal margin; **d** lack of skin laxity and afer-effects of radiotherapy, high scar, favorable longilinear morphology compatible with volume of remaining breast; the transverse subumbilical crease is not due to a scar; **e, g** preoperative appearances; **f, h, j** after areolar reconstruction by inguinal graft and graft of half of the opposite nipple

Morphologic study

The ideal morphology for this procedure is represented by a high and rather horizontal costal margin with a wide xiphoid angle (which facilitates dissection of the terminal part of the muscle pedicle) and a long xipho-pubic distance. The segment between the xiphoid and the umbilicus measures twice that betwen the umbilicus and the pubis (this allows the raising of a flap whose upper border is at the umbilicus and whose lower border is just above the pubic triangle, the scar of closure of the donor zone being immediately suprapubic (fig. 224).

- If the umbilicus is situated midway between xiphoid and pubis, the flap is not generally practicable except at the cost of a small flap of limited extent, and of a donor site scar situated high above the pubis, which means the loss of much of the advantages of this technique;

- a widely splayed rib-cage associated with a long xipho-pubic distance increases the arc of rotation of the flap and therefore the possibilities of bringing it high up into the thoracic region, above the upper margin of the mastectomy scar, under which it can be slipped to give a gentle curve to the upper slope of the reconstructed breast;

- a relatively short distance between umbilicus and pubis (in relation to the xipho-pubic distance) facilitates closure of the donor zone. This is checked in the standing patient, who is asked to relax her abdominal muscles. The flap is practicable if one can pinch together the integuments between the umbilicus and suprapubic region between thumb and index finger. This is evidence that this flap is practicable in patients where an abdominal plasty would not otherwise have been regarded as indicated, since closure is facilitated by taking the stripping to the level of the inframammary crease. One must be wary of patients who exhibit relatively minor skin laxity in relation to the thickness of the subcutaneous adipose layer, for if the latter is considerable one may overestimate the possibilities of closure. The arc of rotation of the flap may be identified by taking as its upper landmark, not the xiphoid process, but the middle of the attachment of the rectus muscle to the costal margin, and as its lower landmark, on the same vertical line, a point situated at the level of the umbilicus. In this type of morphology, the flap risks not ascending high enough to reach the upper margin of the loss of thoracic sustance, with an inframammary crease situated lower than that of the other side;

- we prefer to avoid this technique in such cases, since an unduly low position of the inframammary crease is retrievable at a second stage procedure only at the cost of severance of the pedicle, with ascent and fixation of the new crease on the chest wall, provided that the residual abdominal laxity allows such a movement of ascension.

Preexisting scars

The presence of a subcostal scar (such as a cholecystectomy scar) is an absolute contraindication, not as regards the vitality of the flap that can be raised on the left rectus muscle but because of the risk of necrosis of the upper margin of the stripped abdominal wall, a phenomenon that has been observed after performance of a classic abdominal plasty.

Other abdominal scars constitute relative contraindications:

– a midline supra-umbilical scar, if it is fine, supple and not restricted,will not hinder lowering of the upper margin for closure of the abdominal plasty;

– a midline subumbilical scar will necessitate a bipedicled flap if it is desired to preserve the skin island of the other wide of the midline;

– the problems posed by a Pfannenstiel scar vary, and the information supplied by the operative record, which is not always available, is often insufficient. If the rectus muscle has been divided parallel to the skin incision and at the same level, the flap may be made without anxiety; indeed, this procedure may even have resulted in a stage of pre-established autonomy if the inferior epigastric pedicle has been divided. If the skin incision is transverse and the stripping has been vertical, the problem is identical whether the stripping was over or under the aponeurosis: the perforators risk being damaged if the stripping is taken high up and extended laterally. It is important to know how far the stripping had been taken, which will only be discovered at operative exploration. The length of the scar may give some clue; if it is long, and relates to a hysterectomy, the stripping was probably major; if it only related to an ovariectomy and the scar is short, the stripping was probably taken no higher than the lower third of the pubic-umbilical distance, and therefore before the zone of the larger perforating vessels. If it is found that the fibrosis does not go beyond the lower third, the flap may be performed immediately without worry. If it ascends beyond this, it is certainly wiser to perform a first stage of autonomisation; the flap margins are incised, and the skin island stripped to the outer border of the muscle on the side of the pedicle and as far as the midline of the side opposite the pedicle. The quality of the arterial perfusion may be monitored before complete stripping of this half-island by an injection of methylene blue into the inferior epigastric pedicle, the perforators being essentially symmetrical. The margins are sutured, if only to prevent retraction of the skin island, and the flap may be put in place a week later.

Operative technique

Designing the flap (fig. 225)

The skin island is outlined on the standing patient, before she is premedicated, with careful checking of symmetry in relation to the abdomen so that the final scar at the donor area will be harmonious. Although the tracing often shown in the literature is an elliptical one, we have always preferred the classic "cocked hat" outline of an abdominal plasty. The outline is made first on one side, after having drawn the midline from xiphoid to umbilicus; first the lower border is drawn, as close to the pubic triangle as the skin laxity allows. This line is slightly curved, which helps compensate for the excess in length of the upper margin. One should try not to go beyond the anterior superior iliac spine, or not too far, so as not to add unnecessarily to the length of the scar; the zones situated beyond the spine usually correspond to the zones sacrificed at the vascular level. Then the upper line is drawn tangential to the upper border of the umbilicus, first convex upward and then concave more laterally, to finally join the ends of the lower line, and completed after having made vertical markings every 5 cm. At the thorax only the inframammary crease of the side to be reconstructed is marked out, also designed in symmetry with the opposite breast. The design used for the skin island is entirely comparable to that used for an abdominal plasty, but its upper

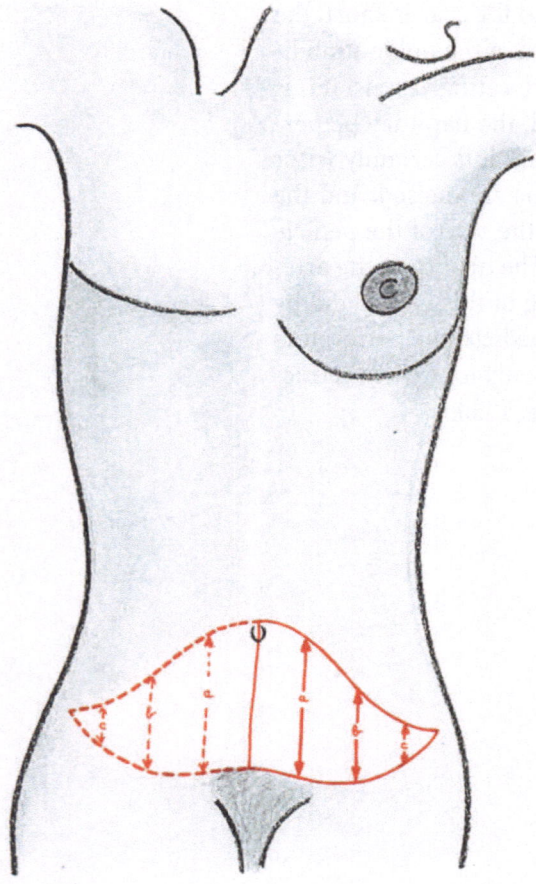

Fig. 225. Design of skin island of flap

border will have a greater slope when the patient has a moderate excess of sub-umbilical skin and fatty tissue. The advantage of this type of design is that it brings the scar of the donor zone of the flap as low as possible, and therefore lessens the cosmetic defect by making it easily concealable.

Positioning

The operation is performed on a table which allows change from dorsal decubitus to a semi-seated position, checking that the break of the table corresponds to the gluteal fold. It begins in dorsal decubitus, the arms beside the body, for dissection of the flap and parietal repair. The table is broken, with the legs slightly elevated and the trunk in the semi-seated position for the stage of placing and modeling of the flap, this position also facilitating closure of the superficial planes at the donor region.

Dissection technique

First stage: freeing of the integuments

The two margins of the skin island are first incised down to the aponeurotic plane. Hemostasis is important only as concerns the satellite veins of the superficial iliac circumflex, superficial epigastric and subcutaneous abdominal arteries, which are divided at the lower and outer part of the flap as they drain into the arch of the great saphenous vein or directly into the femoral vein. The umbilicus is also incised and freed to the aponeurotic plane, while retaining a little fatty tissue around it to better preserve its blood-supply. The skin island is not stripped from the parietal plane at this stage to prevent any risk of its being lacerated.

The skin and subcutaneous tissue of the upper margin are then widely stripped from the aponeurotic plane, ascending on either side to the inframammary crease. Then the mastectomy scar is excised and the stripping is completed by this incision towards the future inframammary crease to join the inferior stripping, constructing an adequately sized tunnel between the xiphoid and the middle part of the costal margin for passage of the pedicle of the flap. This tunnel must be wide enough to pass the flap from the abdomen to the thorax without compression of the muscular pedicle, but yet not so wide as to over-mobilise the region of the future inframammary crease and lead to its depression once the breast has been reconstructed. This is why the dissection does not strip the outer half of the abdominal integuments at the level of the future crease. Hemostasis at this stage must be particularly careful because of the possible section of some perforating branches derived from the intercostal arteries and emerging at the inner ends of the intercostal spaces and in the xiphoid region.

The upper margin of the mastectomy incision is also freed from the parietal plane upward, symmetrically ascending the upper pole of the opposite breast but remaining in front of the muscle plane. In practice, in this type of reconstruction, unlike the procedures that require provision of support behind the pectoral plane, whether by a simple prosthesis or a latissimus flap, the flap is interposed between the integuments and the muscle plane in a physiologic situation for the breast tissue. When this stage of freeing is completed, the loss of substance associated with the skin sacrifice of the mastectomy has been almost completely re-created.

Often the flap can be put in place without much supplementary skin incision, especially if resort to this technique has been decided on for lack of substance and not because of dystrophic or sclerosed tissues, which would require a wider excision to be replaced by the skin of the flap. The commonest excision is that of the band situtated between the lower margin of the mastectomy and the future inframammary crease, in order to place the lower scar of the flap in the fold and to better demarcate this. It will be more extensive when the residual tissues are sclerosed, as the resulting loss of elasticity prevents the margins of the mastectomy incision from regaining their initial position after freeing.

Though one may predict the necessary excision at this stage of the dissection, it is is not actually performed until the stage of placement of the flap, when the patient is in the semi-seated position.

Second stage: isolation of the muscular pedicle

When only one pedicle is used, the flap is isolated preferentially on the muscle of the side opposite the mastectomy for two reasons:

– the muscle pedicle, after rotation of the flap, describes a more harmonious and unkinked curve, facilitating venous return;

– after irradiation of the chest wall. and more particularly of the medial thoracic nodal chain, the functional quality of the homolateral medial thoracic pedicle, the origin of the superior epigastric pedicle, may be diminished, less as concerns the arteries than the veins, whose thinner walls are more sensitive to irradiation.

First, using an ink tracing (fig. 226), the linea alba and the outer border of the relevant rectus muscle are defined from the xiphoid and lower costal margin to the upper border of the flap. The breadth of the muscle varies greatly in different patients. Two other lines are drawn so as to respect a central aponeurotic band representing about two-thirds of the sheath.

After having incised the sheath along these two landmarks, it is stripped from each side to the edge of the muscle. The dissection must be very cautious opposite the tendinous intersections, for at these sites the sheath is very adherent to the thinned muscle and care must be taken not to perforate it for fear of damaging the intramuscular anastomotic plexus, the sole pedicle of the flap in this part of the muscle.

The earlier accounts of this technique used only a single central landmark, incising the sheath at its middle and opening its two layers. Leaving the middle part of the sheath in place on the muscle has the advantage of simplifying the dissection by minimising the tricky stage at the intersections and also allows preservation of the major part of the immediately subaponeurotic vascular plexus. The aponeurosis is then incised transversely at the upper border of the skin island, stopping at the outer border of the muscle. The same procedure is performed below, at the lower border of the skin island, which allows determination of its breadth, markedly less here than above.

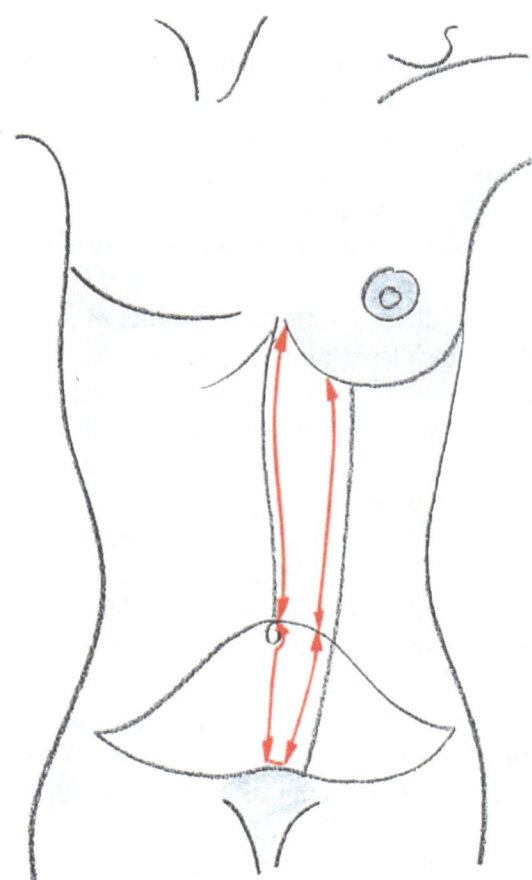

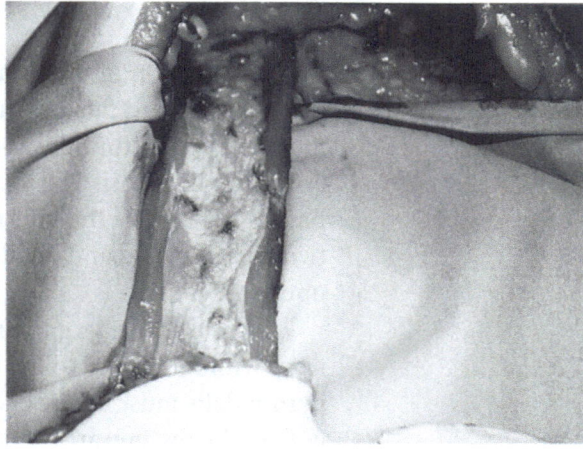

b

a

Fig. 226 a,b. The aponeurotic incisions

Third stage: freeing of the skin island

The undermining of the skin island is begun on the side opposite the pedicle. Dissection is easy with the scalpel and made from without inward, remaining flush with the aponeurotic plane and seeing to hemostasis of the perforators, even if small, before they retract under the aponeurosis. Thus, on the deep aspect of the flap, a thin fascia is contrived which contains a fine vascular plexus. The dissection is pursued on this side as far as the intersection of the fibers at the linea alba, location of which is facilitated by the position of the base of the umbilicus, which has already been freed.

Beginning the dissection on the side opposite to the pedicle has the advantage, in the performance of a unipedicled flap, of satisfactorily defining the position and direction of the lateral border of the muscle, which is more or less oblique downward and outward, as well as the number and position of the perforating vessels, the more important of which are situated near the midline in the upper third of the interval between umbilicus and pubis.

The dissection of the skin island is then pursued on the side of the pedicle, where the stripping must be halted as soon it arrives in contact with the larger perforating vessels; this allows the dissection to be carried to about 2 or 3 cm medial to the outer border of the muscle.

Fourth stage: raising the flap

When dissection of the skin island is completed, the aponeurosis is incised from above downward flush with the deep face of the flap. The anterior aspect of the muscle is freed from the aponeurosis up to its outer border. Preservation of this strip of aponeurosis will facilitate subsequent repair of the parietes. At the lower part of the muscle the inferior epigastric pedicle is located; it is isolated between two ligatures, tied and divided at this level without seeking to tie it more medially under the muscle.

The muscle belly of the rectus is then divided at the lower border of the flap, from without inward to the linea alba, which leads to simultaneous section of the pyramidalis muscle. The deep aspect of the muscle can now be freed progressively from below upward, while dividing at the same time the inner border of the aponeurosis at the linea alba. Preservation of the linea alba, which is always possible in a unipedicled flap, reinforces the firmness of the parietal repair; but section of the aponeurosis must be made very close to the linea alba, especially at its upper part, since the useful perforators are very close to the midline. To avoid any risk of shearing between the muscle and the cutaneo-fatty island during manipulation of the flap, the lower cut edge of the muscle may be temporarily anchored to the dermis or superficial fascia by a few sutures.

The muscle is very easily separated from the deep plane as adhesions are loose, and it is easy to distinguish the inferior epigastric pedicle which, after having reached its outer border, penetrates the muscle after some delay, usually a little below the umbilicus after having neared the midline.

Quite near the umbilicus a branch of the inferior epigastric pedicle is often seen which perforates the posterior aponeurosis to travel deeply and needs to be ligated to pursue elevation of the flap. This dissection must be done atraumatically, using scissors with their convexity turned downward and without any avulsion maneuvers, working at the level of the posterior plane to better deal with the pedicle.

The freeing is pursued up to the costal margin, dividing laterally the lateral neurovascular pedicles derived from the terminal branches of the last intercostal pedicles which penetrate the muscle just within its outer border. A major pedicle is usually identified for each muscle belly. Their section is necessary to elevation of the flap, and we have already seen that there is no point in preserving a lateral strip of muscle since the penetration of these pedicles occurs more medially, so that such a strip would be denervated and doomed to fibrous degeneration.

Up against the costal margin, it is often possible to identify the superior epigastric pedicle, emerging from the thorax near the xiphoid and dividing into two main branches, one vertical and rapidly entering the muscle, the other following a course parallel to the costal margin and a few mm from it before branching and embedding itself in the muscle. It is best to be very cautious at this part of the dissection, and not to extend it once the costal margin is seen. On the other hand, it is quite safe to divide the most lateral attachments of the latissimus at the upper aspect of the costal cartilages above and beyond the costal margin to facilitate rotation of the muscular pedicle and avoid supplementary traction during placement of the flap.

Fifth stage: temporary placement of the flap

After verifying hemostasis of the whole abdominal wall, particularly at the xiphoid region before this becomes inaccessible, the flap is slid upward under the zone of stripping to the thoracic loss of substance and fixed temporarily to the skin margins by a few sutures.

Placing the flap at the thorax at this stage will allow monitoring of its viability while the parietal repair is done, this latent period allowing better assessment of the sacrifices necessary at its extremities as determined by the color assumed by the flap, sacrifices that will be made a little later when the patient is the semiseated position and the abdominal wall repaired.

At the start of our series, we placed the flap either by a translation movement (umbilical zone above) or by a rotation movement of 180° (umbilical zone below).This latter position now seems preferable for two reasons:

– the muscular pedicle describes a more harmonious curve and spreads out better, thus promoting venous return, whereas simple upward transference is accompanied by folding of the muscle which is more prejudicial to arterial perfusion and venous drainage, and which also creates a more visible prominence under the abdominal wall even if the muscle does undergo subsequent atrophy;

– in rotation, the umbilical zone may be placed on the meridian of the reconstructed breast as a vertical subareolar scar, and this acts as a cutaneous "squeeze" which allows reduction of the mammary base of the flap and improves the convexity of the lower quadrants.

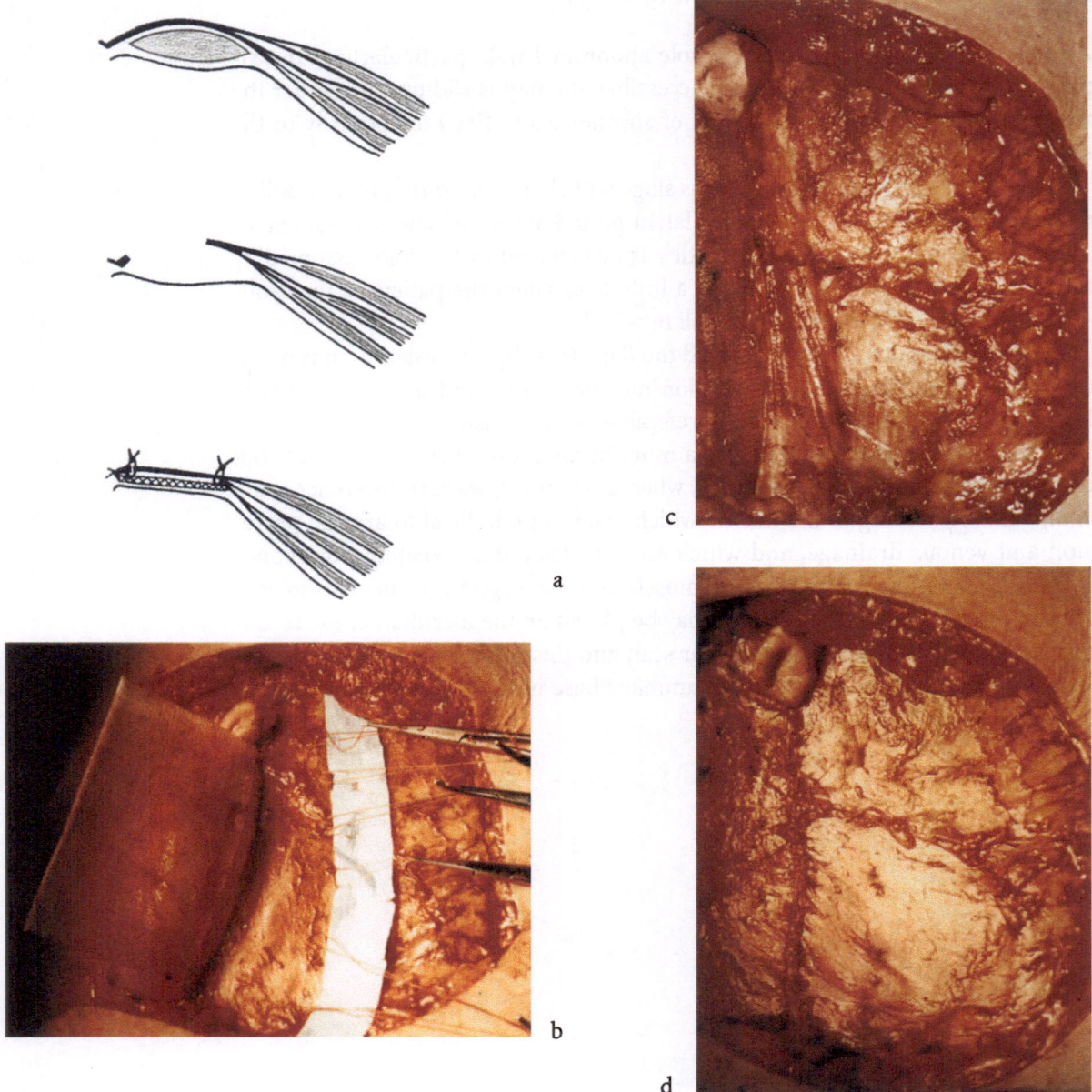

Fig. 227. Repair of the rectus sheath from umbilicus to pubis:

a *above:* below the arcuate line the three aponeuroses of the external oblique, internal oblique and transversus fuse and pass in front of the muscle belly

middle: after raising the rectus muscle: in this region the posterior wall is not firm because it is formed solely by the transversalis fascia

below: repair is made with a plaque from umbilicus to pubis (at least in the unipedicled flaps), sutured medially to the linea alba, laterally to the sheath at its angle of reflection; the residue of anterior aponeurosis which has been preserved is turned down over the plaque and sutured to the linea alba

b the sutures are passed under the remainder of the external oblique aponeurosis; the plaque is shown

c the plaque is then sutured under moderate tension to the midline, the external oblique residue is turned down

d the outer border of the aponeurosis has been sutured to the midline, completely covering the plaque

Sixth stage: repair of the parietes (fig. 227)

This is done after the anesthetist has produced very good muscular relaxation.

In the case of a unipedicled flap, despite the raising of a band of aponeurosis with the muscular pedicle, the repair in the segment comprised between the xiphoid and the umbilicus may be made by direct suture of the aponeurotic margins, but stopping some cm before the xiphoid so as not to risk strangulation of the pedicle.

In the region lateral to and below the umbilicus, we routinely reinforce the closure by a plaque, even if the suture seem to have been performed edge to edge. We use a mesh of nonabsorbable material, 5 cm wide, which extends from the lateral border of the umbilicus to the suprapubic region.

This plaque is first sutured under the outer border of the remaining aponeurosis at the limit of reflection of the sheath, under the inner border of the internal abdominal oblique muscle, then with moderate tension to the linea alba and the umbilicus, and finally under the suprapubic border of the lower cut edge of the aponeurosis. Minimal tension is important at this stage to prevent any subsequent dehiscence of the wall below the arcuate line.

Once this suture is made, the overlying aponeurosis can be brought down above the plaque and nearly always sutured directly to the linea alba. It is only when the muscle is very broad that the aponeurotic suture will leave a strip of plaque visible over one or two cm. It seems preferable to place the plaque under the aponeurosis, and so well isolated from the superficial planes, rather than to place it in front. The interposition of this material acts to reinforce the aponeurotic suture line, favoring the process of fibrous healing of the deep plane, and if there is any problem with healing of the abdominal scar the plaque will be well away from it. After having checked the hemostasis of the vast abdominal stripping for one last time, and ensured drainage by two long suction drains, the patient is placed in the semi-seated position to facilitate closure of the superficial layers, which will be done as in a classical abdominal plasty.

Seventh stage: shaping the flap

It is first necessary to proceed to resection of the lateral extremities of the flap, but this resection is made as required, depending on the changes in color and the bleeding from the skin island.

The necessary resection will be more extensive when the flap is thick, and more extensive on the side opposite the pedicle. When the flap is thin, there is usually no problem of viability, and we have even sometimes preserved the whole of the skin island without any subsequent problems.

It is relatively easy to assess the extent of the necessary resection on the basis of the color assumed by the skin island as a whole after its placement in thoracic position and during the latent period while the parietal repair and abdominal closure are being done. Shortly after its temporary fixation in thoracic position, and while the patient is still in dorsal decubitus, it is often congested. After installation of the patient in the semi-seated posture, which promotes venous return by the effect of gravity, several possibilities exist:

– if the entire skin island is bluish, with pallor of the cut fatty surface and no bleeding, the arterial supply is insufficient to ensure perfusion of the entire flap. The bluish hue indicates venous stasis due to pressure. Resection is then performed cautiously and gradually, allowing several minutes at each stage so as not to sacrifice too much tissue at the lateral extremities. First, dark venous bleeding reappears, while the fat remains pale. Then, when the resection is adequate. the venous bleeding brightens and the raw surface and the skin palette resume a satisfactorily pink color;

– if the entire skin island tends to remain cyanosed, though the bleeding from the cut surface seems satisfactory and the subcutaneous tissue is pink or even congested, one must check that there is no compression of the pedicle and that the tunnelisation in the latero-xiphoid region is adequate;

– if there is no mechanical obstacle to the venous return, a supplementary resection is necessary, the bluish color being due to venous stasis with insufficient functional return despite adequate arterial perfusion, and this venous stasis may itself lead to necrosis.

It often suffices to sacrifice only a few cm at the extremities for the flap to restore perfectly satisfactory color and warmth. This discordance between arterial flow and venous return is due to the normally preferential drainage of the extremities of the skin island by the superficial epigastric and subcutaneous abdominal veins that have been divided, and a rapid and sometimes difficult adaptation to the new circulatory conditions, all the venous return now having to pass via the satellite veins of the median perforating epigastric vessels.

Once the color of the flap is satisfactory, the shaping stage proper can be done (figs. 228 and 229).

The lower border of the skin island is symmetrically tacked to the opposite inframammary crease, if need be at the cost of supplementary excision of the inferior margin of the thoracic incision, usually of minor extent. This suture is performed by taking more tissue on the side of the flap than on the thoracic wall. The tissue excess will be greater at the middle, on either side of the umbilical zone, than at the two extremities. This procedure rounds off the lower segment of the breast and helps to project its central portion1, contributing to give it a natural appearance.

The margins of the umbilical zone are sutured together to form a cutaneous "-dart" — in dressmaking terms — which also contributes to the projection when it is correctly placed along the meridian of the breast, the inferior slope of the reconstructed breast.

The upper border of the flap is slid under the upper margin of the thoracic incision and tacked to the pectoral plane, or to the parietal plane if the pectoral no longer exists, at the level of the upper pole of the opposite breast; then the remaining integuments are redraped on top in order to assess the size of the upper part of the flap to be de-epithelialised. This procedure assures the upper side a gentle curve without a sabre-cut at the scar. The margins will be of equal length.

All the sutures are made in two layers: deep dermal inverting sutures of fine slowly-absorbed material and a continuous superficial rapidly-absorbed intradermal suture.

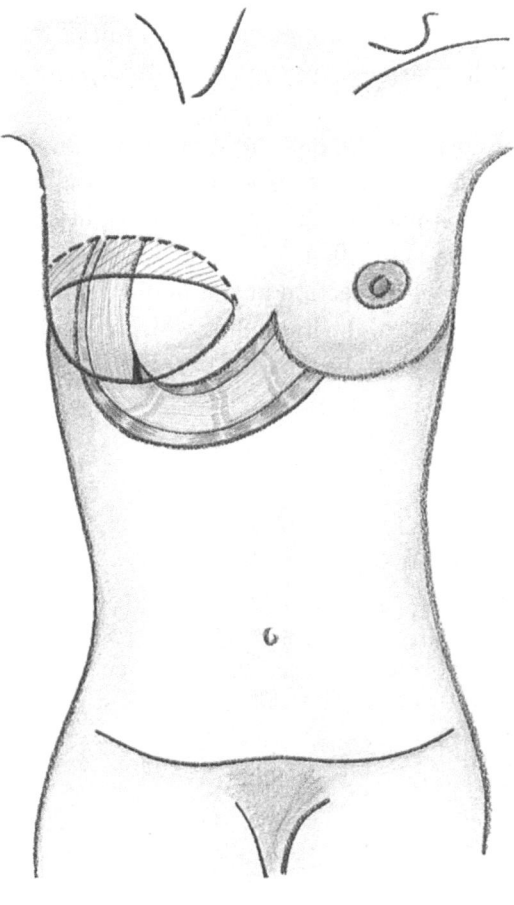

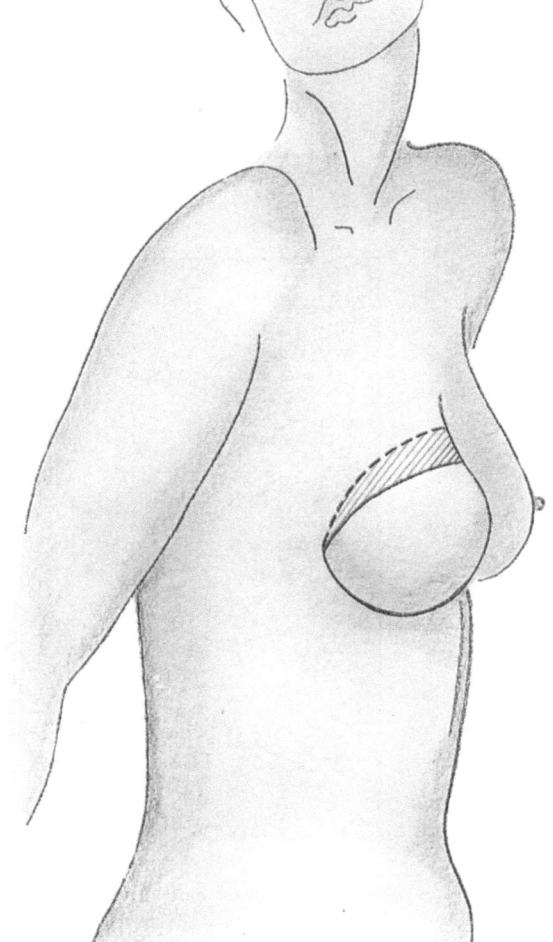

Fig. 228. Placement of the flap, frontal view. The flap is placed after a rotation movement which locates the umbilical zone below, closure of which forms a skin "dart" contributing to the curve of the flap. The upper part of the flap is de-epithelialised very superficially to preserve the dermal plexus, and slid under the upper margin of the mastectomy incision to give the reconstructed breast a gently sloping curvature

Fig. 229. Placement of flap: lateral view

Features of a bipedicled flap

– The identification of the perforators and therefore of the inner limit of the zone of stripping of the skin island from the parietess is rather more tricky, since both sides must be respected;

– as the vascularisation is greater, almost the whole of the skin island can be preserved, even when the flap is a thick one. This is of course the preferential indication for a bipedicled flap: the need, in a patient with gross overweight and with relatively major subumbilical excess, for a large flap;

– during elevation of the flap and the deep dissection at the midline, an attempt should be made to preserve the deep part of the linea alba, which provides a landmark for suture of the plaque, which may also be tethered over it;

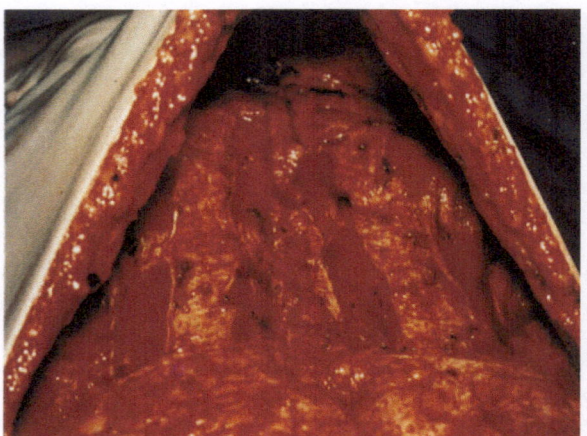

a

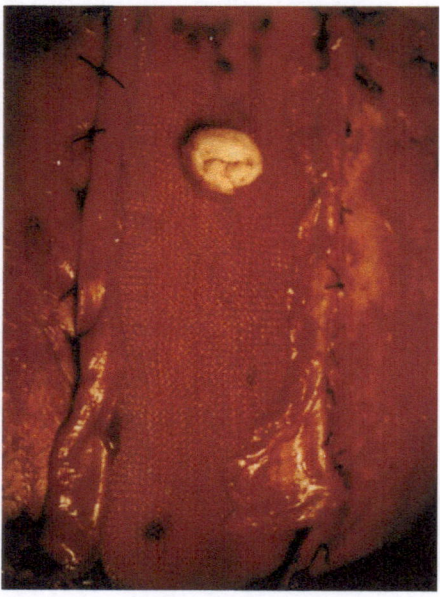

b

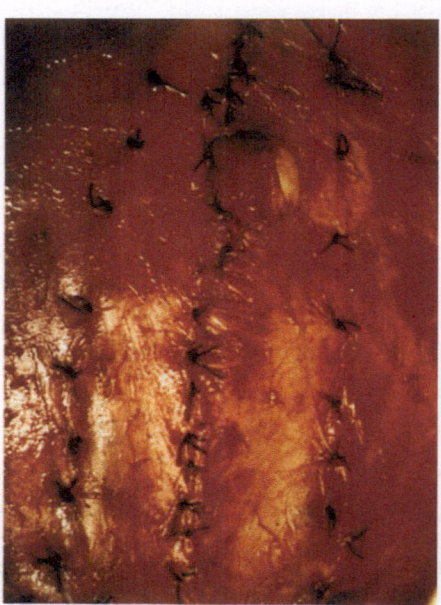

c

Fig. 230 a-c. Parietal repair of a bipedicled flap. **a** The two muscle bellies dissected with preservation of 2/3 of the sheath at the anterior aspect of the muscle; **b** suture of the plaque to the outer line of reflection of the sheath; **c** in this case the residual sheath has been completely turned down over the plaque above and below the umbilicus

– the plaque is placed under tension and sutured symmetrically in relation to the midline. The loss of aponeurotic substance being doubled, at both the supra- and subumbilical levels, it is usually difficult to suture the two aponeurotic margins edge-to-edge without excessive tension. With double or bipedicled flaps we prefer to interpose a plaque over the entire length of the sheath from the zone of passage of the pedicle to the suprapubic region. But it is sutured in the same way, within the sheath and under its outer borders, reflecting down over it what remain of the former layers. In this way the plaque is maximally covered and isolated from the superficial layers (fig. 230);

– the epigastric arch associated with the presence of the muscle pedicles is bigger since the muscle volume is doubled. If atrophy is not marked during the following months, it will more often be necessary than in the case of a unipedicled flap to sever and excise one or both pedicles at the second operative stage.

Dressings

These are made with tulle gras over the sutures, dry compresses and adhesive strapping. They should not be compressive at the upper part of the abdomen (zone of the pedicle) or at the flap, leaving a central opening for monitoring the color and warmth of the skin island. In the subumbical zone wide bands of elastic strapping may be used for support.

Postoperative positioning

Proper positioning in the bed is essential after leaving the recovery room, so as to avoid compression of the pedicle and facilitate venous return. At the end of the operation (and thus during the recovery period) the patient is positioned in a semi-seated posture, the knees slightly bent, but avoiding a dorsal kyphosis.

This position relaxes the abdominal wall, particularly the epigastric region, prevents compression of the pedicle by the wall, and promotes downward drainage from the flap. The color and warmth of the flap are regularly monitored via the window in the dressing.

The ideal is to have a bed with a double break, which can be bent at two places, under the buttocks and behind the knees. Positioning on a horizontal bed simply with the aid of pillows and bolsters is to be avoided, since these become bunched up and the patient gradually slides toward the foot of the bed and may end up in dorsal hyperextension, an altogether harmful position.

Maintenance of this position during the first week is in our view one of the most important factors — together with extremely careful dissection — in avoiding necrosis due to failure of venous return while the circulatory state of the flap is still in jeopardy.

Postoperative course

The drains are usually left in for 6 to 8 days; hospitalisation is usually for some ten days.

The blood-loss only rarely nowadays requires transfusion in cases of a unipedicled flap; this is due partly to the shorter duration of the procedure (three to three and a half hours in experienced hands), and partly to the use of controlled hypotension throughout the dissection stage.

The construction of a bipedicled flap is of course longer and somewhat more hemorrhagic, and in this case autotransfusion may be indicated and, if available, helps to diminish postoperative fatigue.

We advise the patient to wear a light support girdle after removal of the dressing for the next six months, the object of which is not so much to ensure moderate abdominal restraint as to remind her to avoid all abdominal exertion during the time that the fibrous scar tissue is supplementing and stabilising the immediate support afforded by the plaque. It is not uncommon for the patient to complain at the outset of feelings of cramp at the level of the muscular pedicle, but this discomfort disappears spontaneously after a few weeks.

The fate of the flap

Volume

Unlike what is seen with the latissimus flap, especially when the muscle is thick and the skin layer thin, the inferior abdominal rectus flap does not decrease in volume in the subsequent months. The muscle certainly becomes nonfunctional, as it is denervated and deprived of its distal attachments and therefore of any function, but as it does not participate to any great extent in the reconstructed volume compared with the size of the cutaneo-fatty layer, this factor is negligible. The muscle atrophy is especially visible, and palpable, at the epigastric arch created by passage of the muscle pedicle.

Shape

The reconstructed breast follows a course comparable to that expected in a mammoplasty. Under the same constraints of gravity and skin relaxation, it tends to undergo slight ptosis, the lower segment becoming a little more convex and the upper segment a little more flattened, the more so if the flap is bulky. This factor contributes to the natural appearance of the reconstruction.

Second operative stage

If readjustments are necessary, either of the abdominal or thoracic scar or as regards the shape, these are done 4 to 6 months later, at the same time as the reconstruction of the nipple-areolar plaque and any plasty of the opposite breast that may be required for symmetry. A delay of 4 months seems necessary to assess the stability of the reconstructed breast. As this second procedure is a relatively fatiguing one, it is also an interval that seems sensible to suggest to the patient. The muscle pedicle can be preserved if it does not create an obvious prominence, as is observable in the majority of cases.

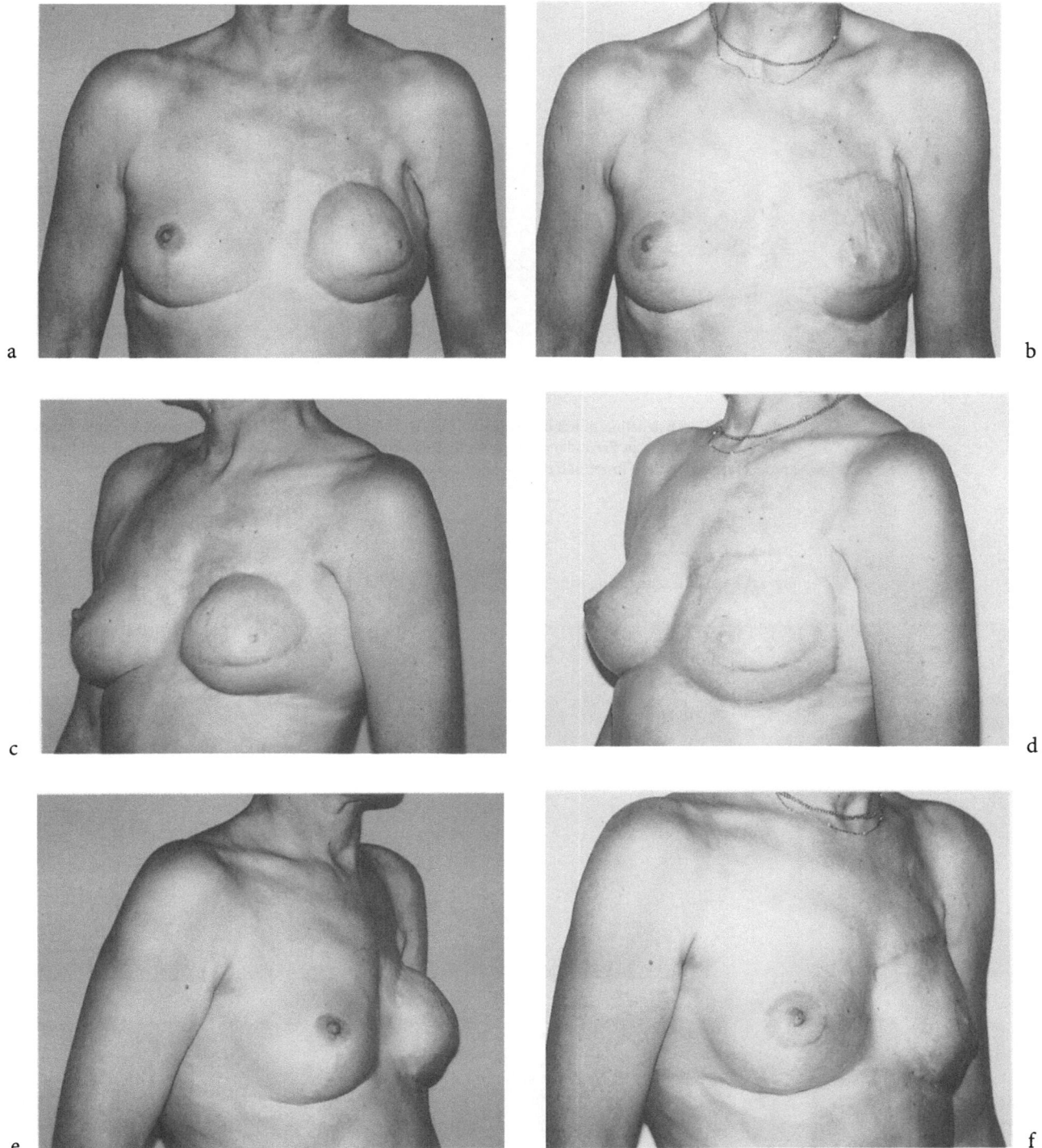

Fig. 231 a-f. Revision of reconstruction performed with latissimus flap and prefilled gel implant: use of a uni-pedicled and completely de-epithelialised rectus abdominis flap, secondary revision of areolar reconstruction by tattooing and transplantation of nipple graft

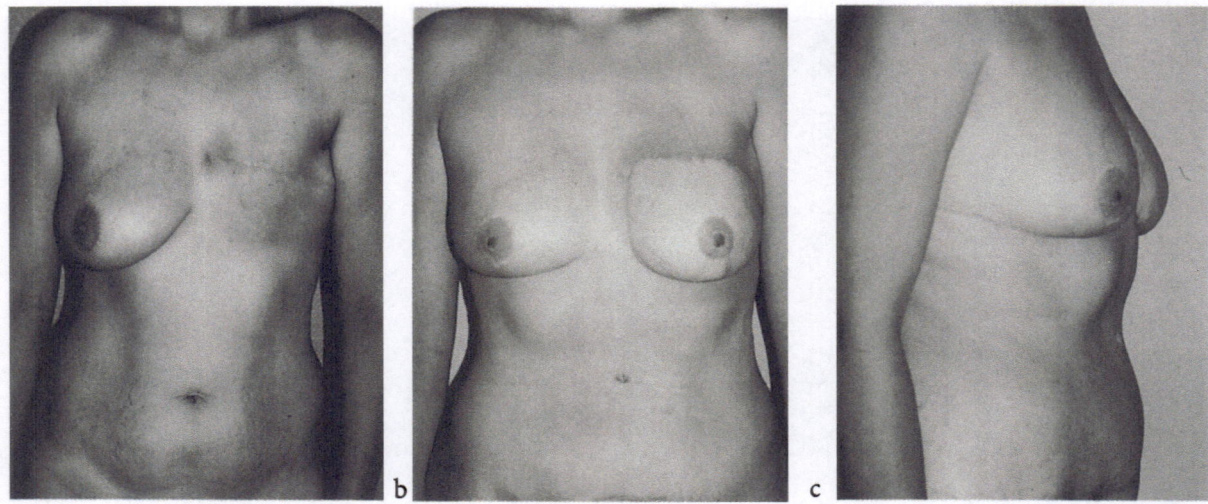

Fig. 232 a-c. Reconstruction of left breast (lack of laxity, trophic sequelae from radiotherapy) by unipedicled flap of rectus abdominis. Secondary reconstruction of areola at same time as plasty of opposite breast by inguinal graft and graft of lower half of opposite nipple

Fig. 233 a-d. See legend facing page

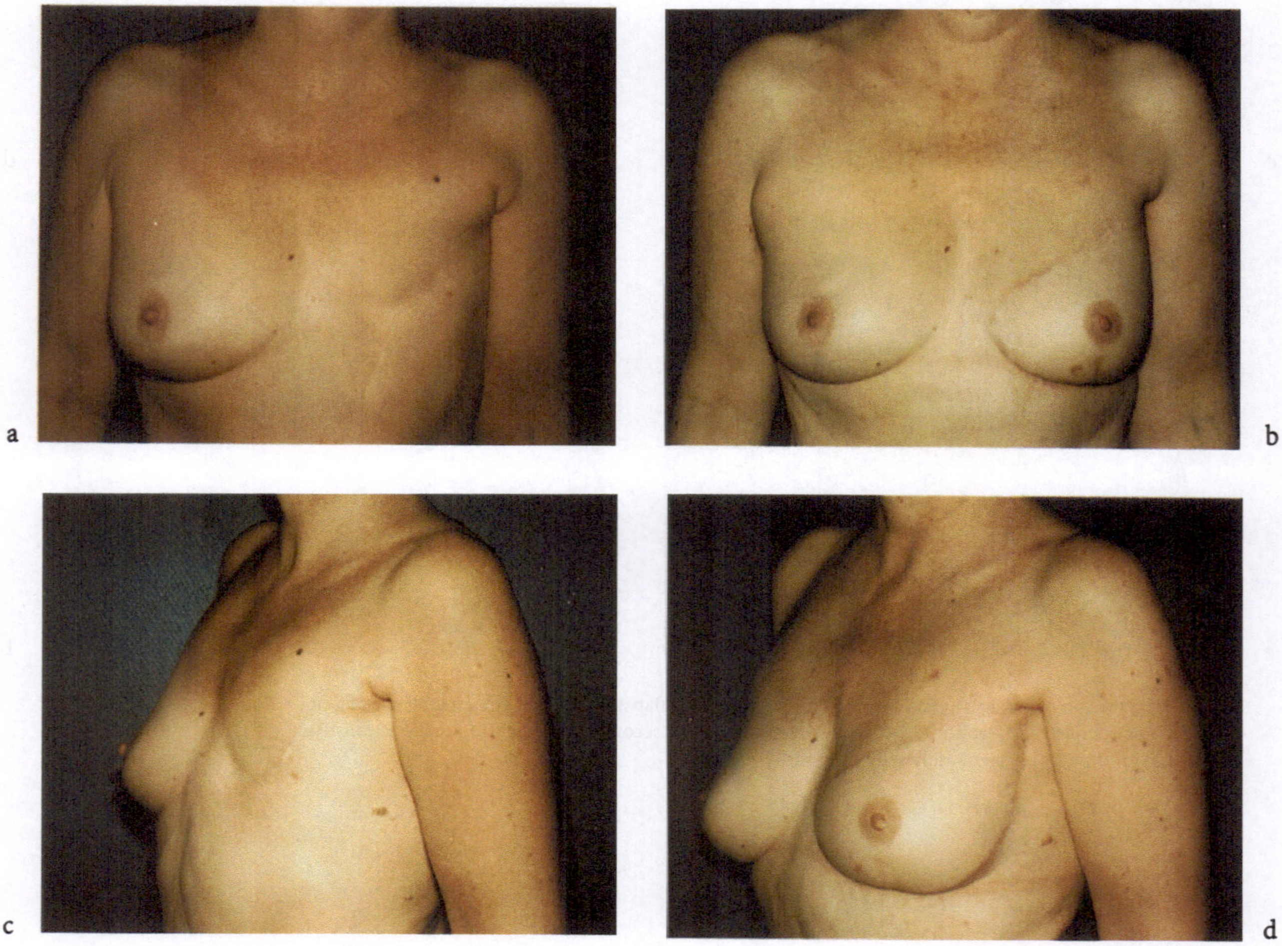

Advantages

When the indication is correctly defined, this is certainly the best and most satis-factory technique of breast reconstruction because of the quality and suppleness of the tissues supplied and the plastic possibilities it offers. The value of this flap relates to the following points:

– the modeling of the breast is done without the need for a supplementary prosthesis in the majority of cases, as the flap is realisable with a satisfactory vol-ume if there is a moderate subumbilical excess of skin and fatty tissue (fig. 231). In the two cases where we added an implant there was contralateral breast atro-phy and an implant was inserted on both sides;

– the reconstructed breast assumes a very natural appearance, which often makes a plasty of the opposite breast less necessary, though this is often required in cases of reconstruction by a simple prosthesis or by a latissimus flap with a prosthesis (figs. 232 and 233);

– the abdominal skin has a texture analogous to that of the thorax;

Fig. 233 e-h. Reconstruction of left breast by unipedicled flap of rectus abdominis. Secondary reconstruction of areola by tattooing and grafting of lower half of opposite nipple

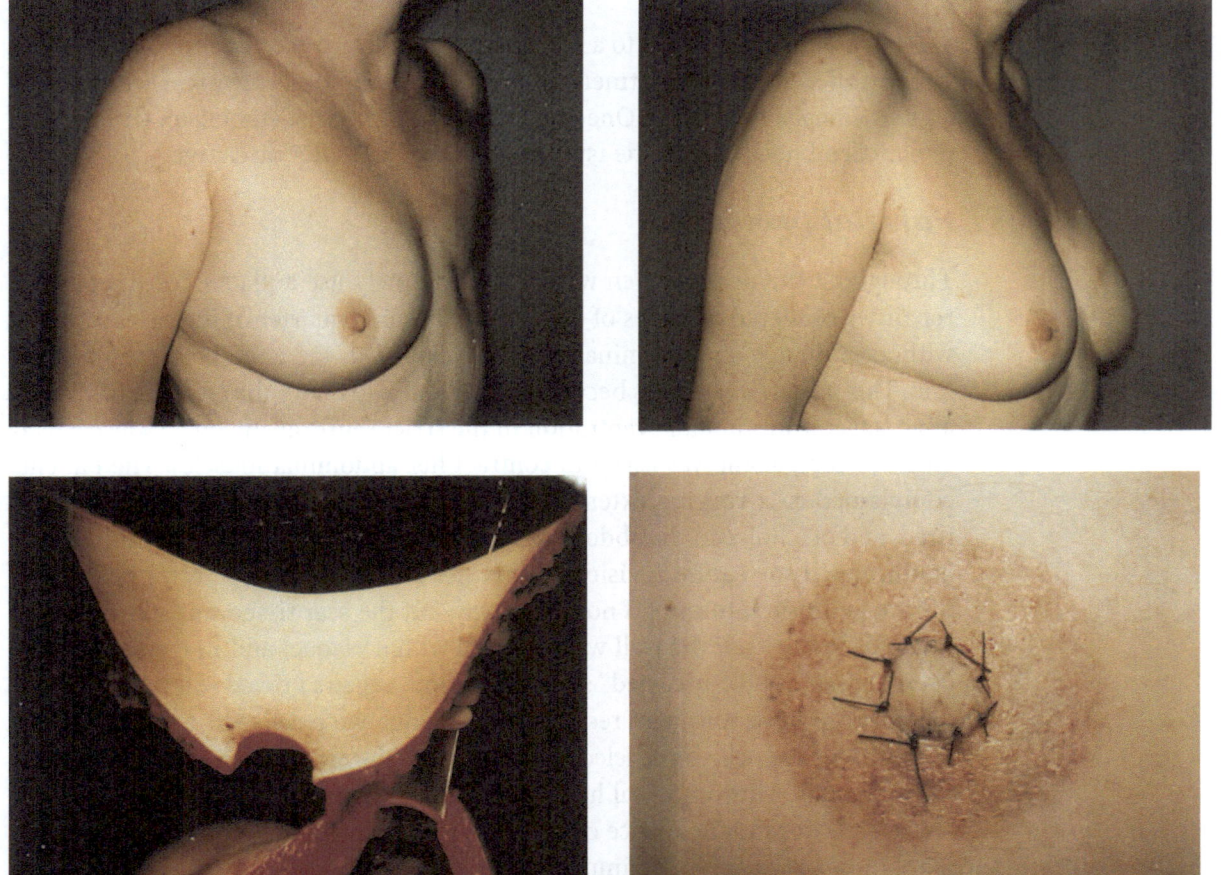

e

f

g

h

– the scar where the flap is raised is a long one, but quite easy to conceal as is is placed low down in the design we always employ;

– compared with a latissimus flap, the skin surface supplied is greater, which is useful if one wishes to close the donor region directly for cosmetic or other reasons (fig.234).

Disadvantages

Of all the techniques we employ, this is the one that is the most demanding and longest to perform; the discomfort of the first few days and the postoperative debility require a convalescence of around a month.

Immediate complications

The complications are few, and consist essentially of minor problems of healing, either at the medial part of the abdominal scar, which required surgical revision in two cases with perfect secondary healing, or, more often, a problem of parietal necrosis in the latero-umbilical zone on the side opposite the pedicle, a problem localised to the skin margin and cut surface of the under-lying fat. These are usually resolved by local management, and surgical revision was need only on two occasions, without compromising the volume of the flap by supplementary excisions.

One infection, localised to a hematoma of the latero-sternal region, was rapidly controlled by local treatment and suitable antibiotherapy, and without any sign of damage to the flap. One patient had a pulmonary embolism, without evidence of calf phlebitis, on the 15th postoperative day after discharge.

Parietal problems

Throughout the period when we did not routinely use a plaque for the parietal repair we observed no cases of dehiscence; but in a quarter of the cases repaired without a plaque an abdominal bulge developed in the zone below the arcuate line. This parietal weakness became manifest at 4 to 6 months after the first operative stage; it was not an eventration in the strict sense, as the bulge was corrected when the patient was asked to contract her abdominal muscles. The patients complained to a varying extent of pain at the end of the day, especially when tired, and of a bulge in the abdominal wall. Two of these patients were sufficiently handicapped to require revision at this site at the second operative procedure; the aponeurotic sutures had not given way, but the scar tissue was stretched and thinned. In one case the wall was repaired with a plaque, and in the other by an overlapping "double-breasted" suture, and both repairs proved solid.

Since we have routinely resorted to a plaque we have seen only one dehiscence, in the case of a bipedicled flap, not below the arcuate line but at the level of the umbilicus. This umbilical hernia was due to inadequate tethering of the base of the umbilicus to the orifice constructed at the center of the plaque for its passage, and was corrected by simple suture.

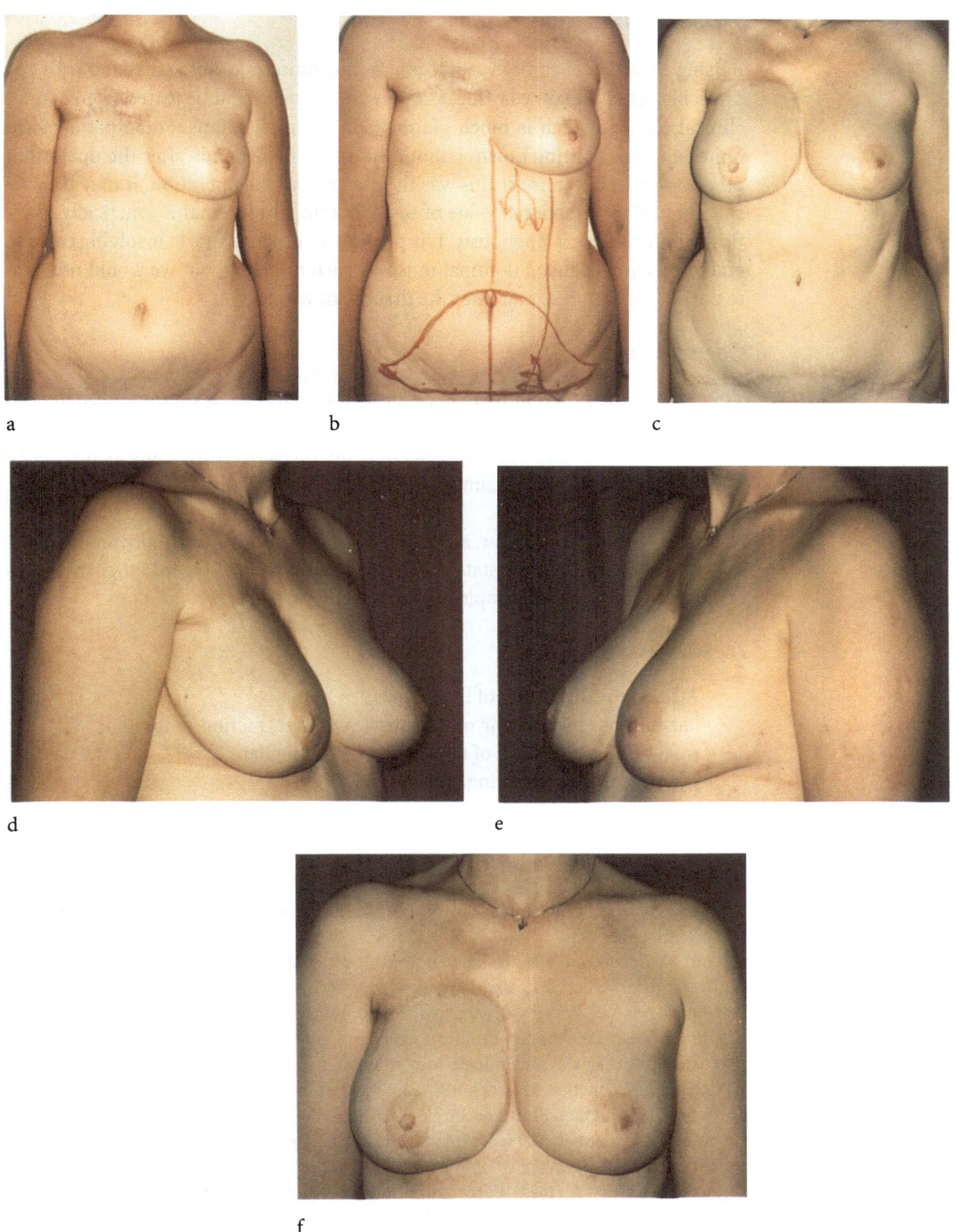

Fig. 234 a-f. Reconstruction of right breast (high scar, after-effects of irradiation, pectoral atrophy) by uni-pedicled rectus flap. Secondary reconstruction of areola by grafts from groin and lower half of opposite nipple

Muscle function

Raising of one or even both rectus abdominis muscles is not associated with appreciable deficit in everyday life, as opposed to what might be feared from careful clinical testing, which is much gloomier in its implications. Some patients are quite capable of sitting down without the aid of their hands after the operation; others are not, but in most this was the case before the operation. It may be considered that the functional value of the abdominal wall remains practically identical with what it was previously. It is possible to practise sports involving considerable exertion of the abdominal muscles, such as skiing, but we would not care to permit this before a year after the first operative stage.

Conclusion

Though this is undeniably a very fine reconstruction technique, perhaps the most satisfactory for the surgeon, and one allowing the reconstruction of breasts of a very natural shape and consistency, the operative procedure is obviously more demanding than the simple insertion of an implant, and the patient must be reminded of this.

This is why we have never, so far, proposed this technique simply on morphologic grounds, if the local state of the residual tissues as regards their quantity and quality allows of the simple provision of a prosthesis.

Important points

- Atraumatic dissection of the pedicle,
- harmonious positioning of the muscle without traction or torsion,
- resection "as required' of the extremities of the flap,
- postoperative positioning.

References

Bostwick J (1990) Plastic and reconstructive breast surgery. Quality Medical Publishing, St-Louis, Missouri

Bricout N, Banzet P (1986) Rectus abdominis myocutaneous flap of the lower type in breast reconstruction. Scan J Plast Surg 20: 93-96.

Bricout N (1987) Chirurgie de reconstruction du sein, Flammarion, Paris

Bricout N (1988) Le choix du lambeau dans la reconstruction mammaire. Bulletin de la société française de cancérologie privée, t.7, n° 21, pp 27-36

Hartrampf CR, Scheflan M, Black PW (1982) Breast reconstruction with a transverse abdominal island flap. Plast Rec Surg 69: 216-224

Hartrampf CR, Bennett GK (1987) Autogenous tissue reconstruction in the mastectomy patient. Ann Surg 205/5: 508-519

Lejour M, De Mey A (1983) Bases anatomiques et techniques des lambeaux musculo-cutanés de grand droit. Ann Chir Plast Esth, 28: 151-158

Lejour M, Dome M (1991) Abdominal wall function after rectus abdominis transfer. Plast Rec Surg 87/6: 1054-1068

Scheflan M, Dinner ML (1983) The transverse abdominal island flap: Indications, contra-indications, results and complications. Ann Plast Surg 10: 24

The opposite breast

Breast reconstruction, whether immediate or delayed, should not be limited to simple restoration of the size and shape of the missing breast.

For this reconstruction to be successful, it is also necessary to consider the appearance of the opposite breast and to know how to correct a ptosis or a hypertrophy, for it is undesirable and often impossible that the reconstructed breast should mimic the defects of the remaining breast if these go beyond the bounds of discretion and are not in conformity with the rest of the figure.

The difficulties of harmonisation of the opposite breast arise from the fact that the reconstructed breast represents an imposed model to which it must be adapted. This requires a precise study of the breast envelope in all its dimensions, and of course leads to readjustment of the breast for reasons of shape rather than size, modifications which would not have been made if both sides were natural and identical.

It is evident that it is the techniques without a preestablished design, apart from that for the areolar site, without predetermination of the skin excision, with reduction on a clamp, ie derivatives of the dermal vault technique such we use in the treatment of hypertrophy and ptosis, which allow the greatest variation and are most suitable.

The technique employed for reconstruction of the absent breast will also play a part in the extent of the procedure to be made at the opposite breast. A breast reconstructed by implant is rarely ptosed; the ptosis of a breast reconstructed by skin expansion is random and variable, and must remain unobtrusive in both these techniques, as also in reconstruction by a latissimus flap. It is more a matter of ensuring good definition of the inframammary fold, of spreading the breast base, and obtaining an upper slope longer and less convex than the lower slope, in a word of recreating a natural and harmonious breast rather than trying to recreate a ptosis.

On the other hand, it is undeniable that the plasticity of the "material" furnished by a rectus abdominis flap permits variations in shape at the width of the breast base, and in anterior projection and the shape of the more important segments II and III, rendering it less often necessary, or less important, to carry out a procedure on the opposite breast.

Nor should it be forgotten that this procedure takes place in a carcinologic context. The operation should modify the glandular architecture as little as possible, and all the breast tissue resected is, as always, sent for histologic examination. Sometimes the preoperative mammogram may show microcalcifications, a dystrophic zone, or an abnormal radiologic image which will suggest preferential excision in a particular zone during the plastic procedure. Sometimes even — though this takes us beyond the simple context of a procedure based on symmetry — a subcutaneous mastectomy or a classical mastectomy may be indicated.

Whenever the glandular architecture of the opposite breast has been modified, it should be routine to perform mammography at the 6th postoperative month (at this stage the phenomena of postoperative edema are resolved), which will serve as a reference study for subsequent surveillance. In experienced hands, this mammography poses hardly any problems of interpretation, and serves above all to detect radiological changes, subsequently stabilised, corresponding to healing of the modified gland.

Several situations may be observed:

The opposite breast is normal

This is not a common situation, but is more likely to occur in young and thin women; the opposite breast is normal, not ptosed, of satisfactory and not excessive size, with a harmonious distribution of the glandular tissue. Segment II contains such tissue and is slightly convex, and segment III rather more so.

No supplementary procedure is necessary in this breast; all the difficulty lies in trying to imitate it when reconstructing the missing breast.

To reproduce the same volume is not the most difficult thing; the real problem is to copy as well as possible the spread of the breast base without producing excessive anterior projection, while achieving good definition of the inframammary crease. This is a difficult situation when the base of the remaining breast is very spread for a small volume, when the fatty panniculus lacks substance, and when the implant required to obtain the same anterior projection has a markedly inferior base (fig. 235).

It is in this type of case that inflatable implants with a relatively spread base such as we have used for some years find one of their best applications, not forgetting to fill them sufficiently to avoid the formation of creases or waves.

In some cases, study of the opposite breast base, which there is no question of reducing, shows that it is clear that the necessary implant will have a greater volume and projection than the existing breast, or that, if an attempt is made to reproduce the same volume, the base of the reconstructed breast will be too narrow. This is often the case in longilinear women, with a thorax that is wide but flattened in the anteroposterior direction.

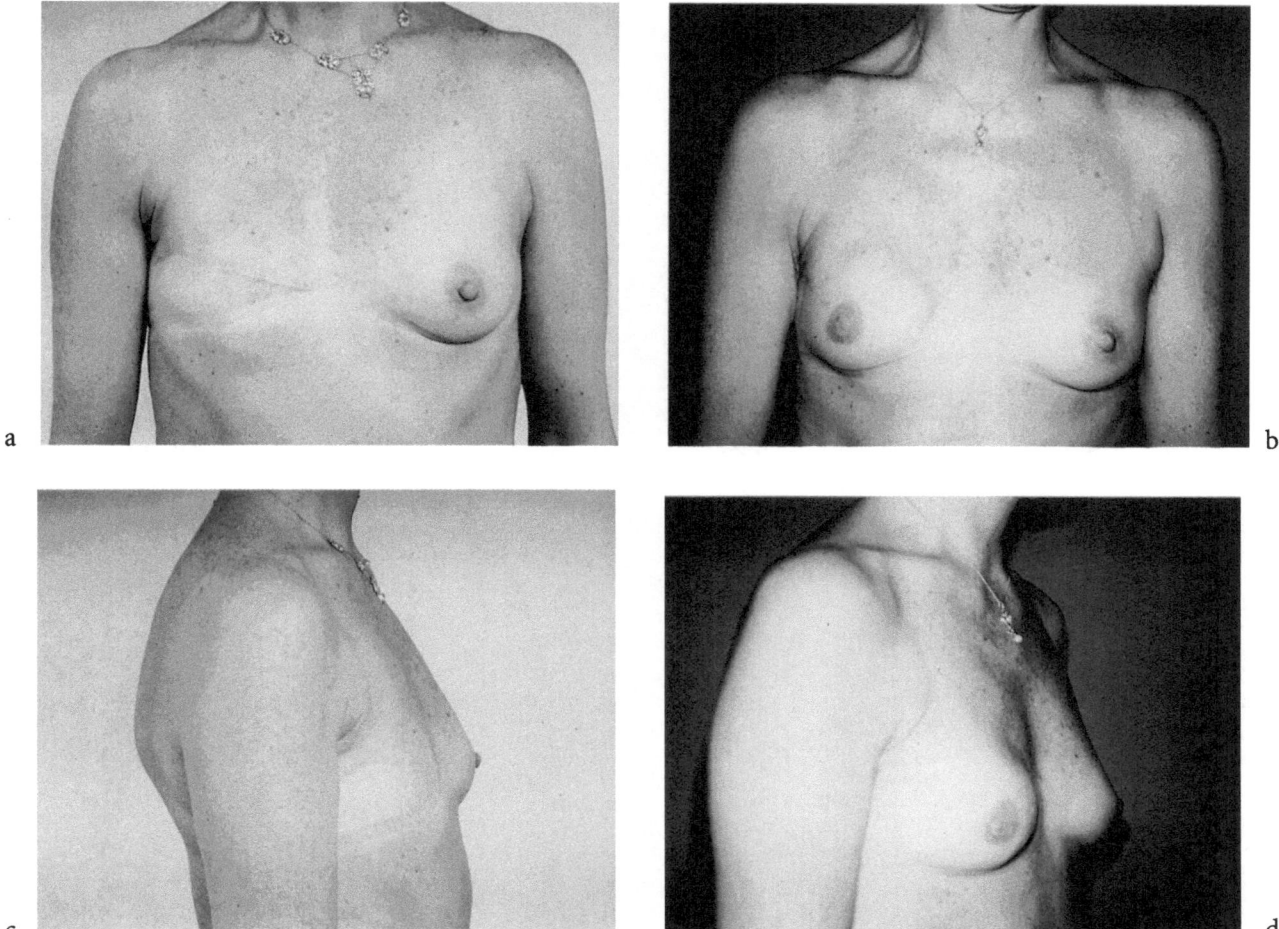

Fig. 235 a-d. Reconstruction by AHS implant of 125ml, filled to 130 ml with normal saline; base too narrow and spread insufficient for proper anterior projection; defect particularly obvious in the inner quadrants

The only way to resolve this problem is to insert on the healthy side a small implant, designed solely to produce a proportional augmentation of the global volume and anterior projection (fig. 236). This implant will necessarily have a smaller base, but this is unimportant since the contours of the base are obscured by the existing gland. For reasons of symmetry of the upper quadrants, and to facilitate radiologic surveillance, it is likewise better to place this implant in retropectoral position. It is to be recalled that one of the advantages of implants inflated with normal saline is their good radiotransparency, which, in particular, does not hinder surveillance of the peripheral limits of the gland.

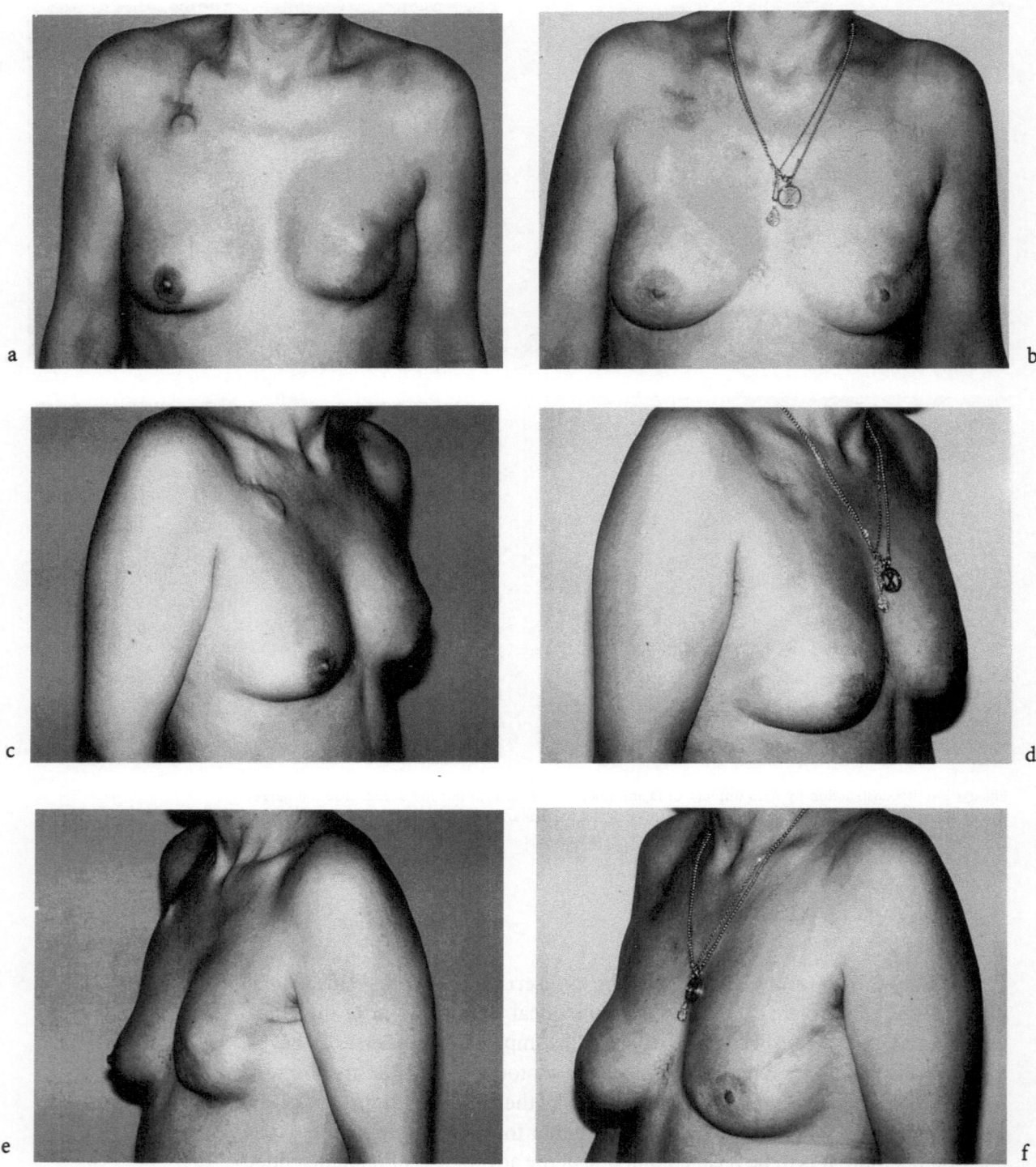

Fig. 236 a-f. Immediate mastectomy-reconstruction by prefilled implant followed by radiotherapy. *Left:* removal of implant (200 g), replacement by Sebbin LS20 smooth inflatable implant of 200 ml, filled to 230 ml *Right:* insertion of identical implant of 100 ml filled to 100 ml, reconstruction of areola by tattooing and graft from opposite nipple

The opposite breast is hypertrophic and ptosed

This situation is often encountered, both defects being combined in proportions that vary with the shape of the breast, the general build, and the interaction of different factors (fig. 237).

It may be that anterior glandular wasting due to pregnancies has occurred before the discovery of the breast lesion. Further, some forms of chemotherapy are often associated with a gain in weight of several kg, one that is fixed and very difficult to overcome. As much as we may insist on loss of weight before the correction of breast hypertrophy in a young girl, nevertheless in this particular situation we may have to accept the existing weight. These patients have undergone difficult times, where compensatory oral gratification does not account for all the weight gain; to insist on return to the previous state may be quite unrealistic, or even upset a precarious equilibrium.

The reduction of the hypertrophy and ptosis is made with skin reduction related to the reduction in size, which will be more extensive when the opposite breast is round, ie when the tissues are relatively unstretched in front of the implant.

Tactics and timing

Except in the case of very considerable contralateral hypertrophy, and more with the object of comforting the patient than obtaining good symmetry at the outset, we prefer to perform the mammoplasty at the second operative stage, at the same time as reconstruction of the nipple-areolar plaque.

The reasons for this policy are as follows:
– assessment of the necessary glandular excision and skin reduction is easier when the skin envelope is relaxed in front of the implant and when the shape of the reconstructed breast has stabilised;
– it is only after several months that it is possible to determine the proper siting of the areola on the reconstructed breast, a position which will also depend on the level of the opposite areola, since one of the necessary conditions for a successful reconstruction is not only that the areola be situated at the apex of the reconstructed volume but also for it to be symmetrical with the opposite areola;
– performance of the reconstruction in two stages is more suitable for possible readjustments of the implant compartment, or even a modification of its filling, or sometimes an actual change of implant if there has been a major error concerning the volume of the breast base;
– it is equally important not to interfere with the opposite areola before reconstruction of the missing areola if it is large, and preferable to use the peripheral part of the graft rather than to perform tattooing (which we have found the method of choice since its introduction). In practice, areolae which have been transplanted twice (nipple-bearing flap of the mammoplasty, then a free graft at the receptor site) have an unfortunate tendency to become depigmented even more considerably after a variable interval. The only resort then is to secondary tattooing!

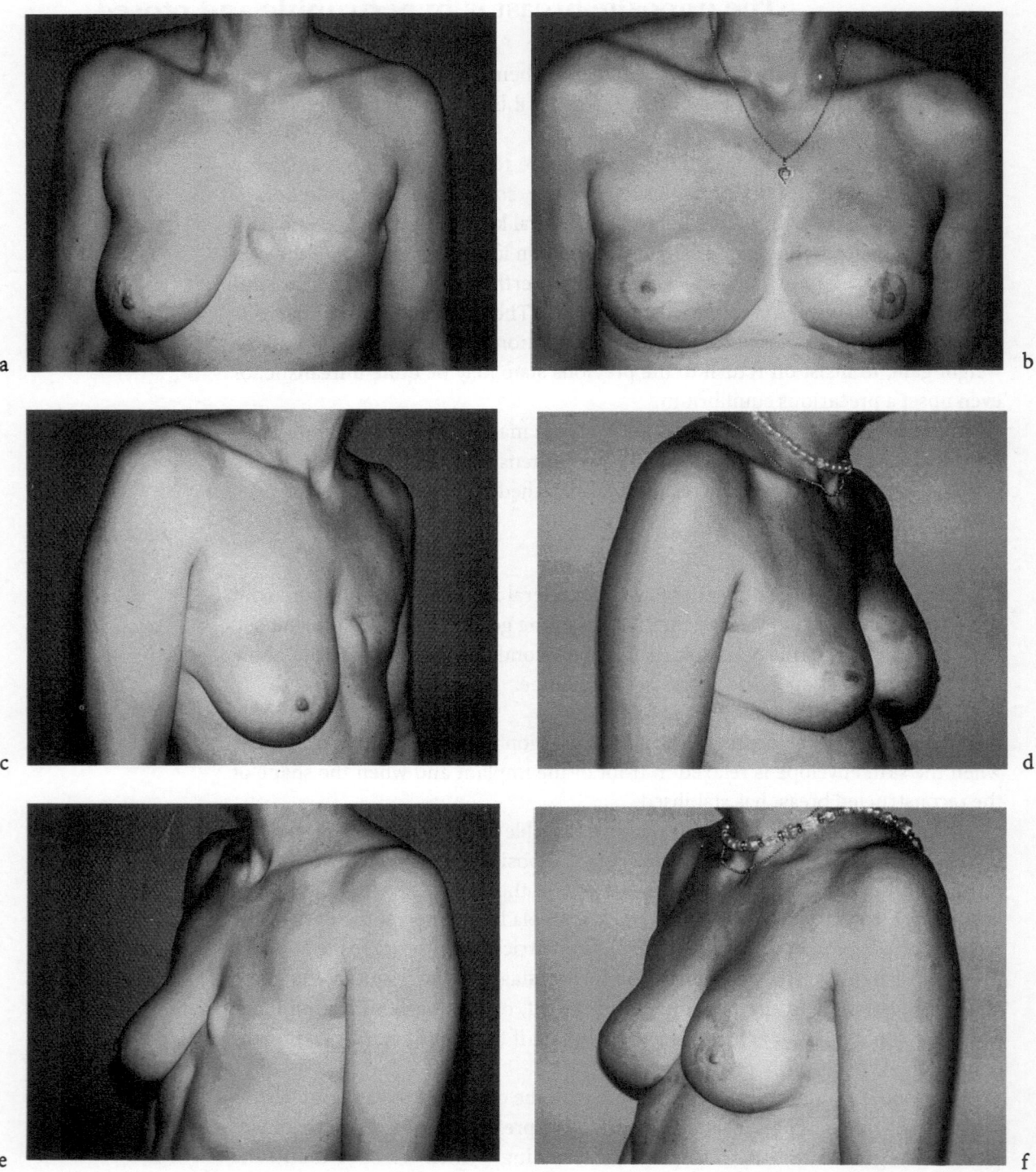

Fig. 237. Reconstruction by smooth inflatable Sebbin LS20 implant of 200 ml filled to 270 ml. Reduction mammoplasty of opposite breast; second stage reconstruction of areola by groin graft and graft of lower half of opposite nipple

Operative technique

The entire procedure is performed in the semi-seated position. The siting of the future areola and its approximate size are identified and drawn with a closed Dufourmentel ring. The distances measured and recorded are:

– from the suprasternal notch, or a point situated 5 cm laterally on a horizontal line through it, to the upper border of the areolar design,

– from the medial tangent to the same design to the midline,

– finally, from the lower border of the design to the inframammary crease.

The axis of the opposite breast is drawn in the same way, from a point 5 cm lateral to the supra-sternal notch on a horizontal through it. The superior areolar point is referred to this axis, in principle 1 cm lower than the other side; it is important to be wary of ascension of this point after the skin has been relieved of the weight of the excess glandular tissue. If its elasticity seems excellent, this point can even be placed as much as 2 cm lower than the opposite side, even if this entails completing the mammoplasty by a supplementary de-epithelialisation if it is still rather too low.

The tangent to the inner border of the areolar design is referred symmetrically in relation to the midline.

The same Durfourmentel ring, now closed, is applied within these limits, with variable divergence of its limbs as related to the size of the skin envelope. When ptosis and hypertrophy are not very considerable, the limbs of the ring are opened out just enough not to infringe on the areola. On the other hand, when there is hypertrophy, the spread of the ring is comparable to the design used in a mammoplasty, ie between 7 and 9 cm.

The size of the areola is reduced using a ring of slightly smaller diameter (0.5 cm less).

The mammoplasty is then carried out as usual, if need be with supplementary de-epithelialisation at the end of the reconstruction to reestablish symmetry with the opposite design as regards both the upper point and the distance to the midline or the inframammary crease. At the end of the procedure, the reduced breast must have a somewhat more concentrated appearance than the reconstructed breast to compensate for the inevitable secondary relaxation of the skin envelope.

It is only when the mammoplasty is completed that the definitive design of the areola to be reconstructed is determined, as a compromise between the initial design and the areola of the opposite breast.

The siting of the nipple is not modified in essence, but the size of the areola is settled at this time, often a little larger than the initial design. If tattooing is used, the size should be made a little larger than that of the opposite areola at the end of the procedure, as it will tend to spread slightly during the following weeks because of the centrifugal tension exerted on the areola by the skin envelope.

The opposite breast is atrophic

The placement of an implant is also necessary on this side, and may be made at the same time as the first stage of reconstruction, or at the second stage.

If the gland is virtually non-existent, the same size of implant can be used since its diameter will define the breast base, but simply a little less filled to compensate for the asymmetry associated with the very sparse amount of breast tissue.

If the glandular volume is not quite so negligible, and if it is of sufficient peripheral thickness to blur the peripheral outlines of the implant, whose chief role is no longer to define the breast base but to augment its global volume and anterior projection, a smaller implant can be used with a slightly lesser diameter (fig. 238).

The surgical approach is chosen in relation to the size of the areola and the nipple and the preferences of the surgeon. It may be useful to use an inframammary approach if it desired to perform tethering of the crease to obtain good symmetry with the other side. The position of the implant will again be retropectoral, and for the same reasons.

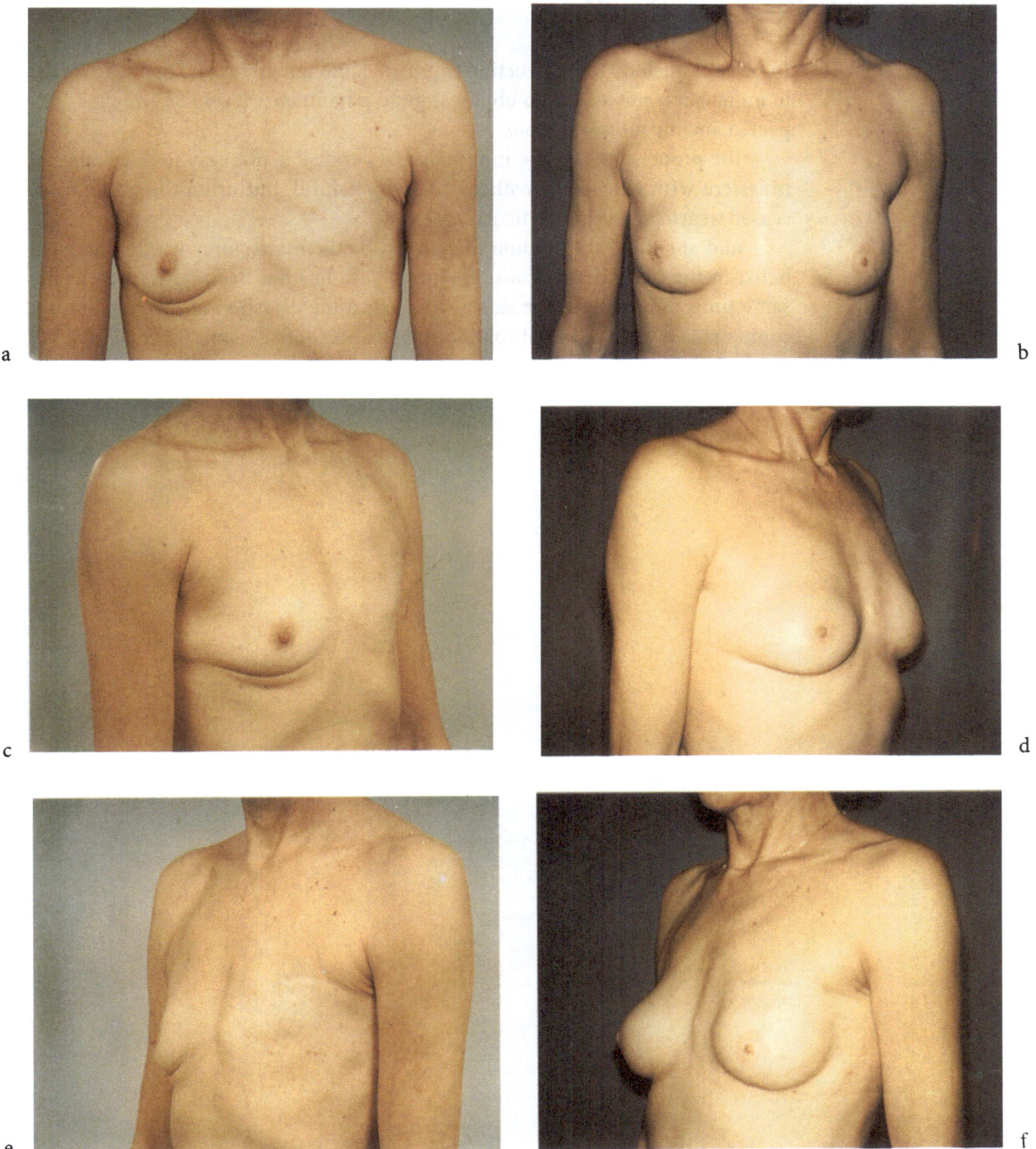

Fig. 238 a-f. Reconstruction of left breast by Sebbin implant of 125 ml filled to 130 ml, augmentation of right breast by Medilens implant of 80 ml filled to 80 ml

The opposite breast is absent

In cases of bilateral reconstruction (fig. 239), although there is no opposite model to imitate, it is not as easy to obtain as good a symmetrical result as might be expected, mainly for two reasons:

– the proper place of the inframammary crease is not easy to determine (a brassière with external prostheses may be helpful, but often the patient has ceased wearing it in this particular case);

– and above all, the amount of skin left by the mastectomy is often unequal between the two sides, because the procedure has not been performed at the same time, and because the skin sacrifice and the direction of the scar are not comparable due to the initial volume and position of the lesion.

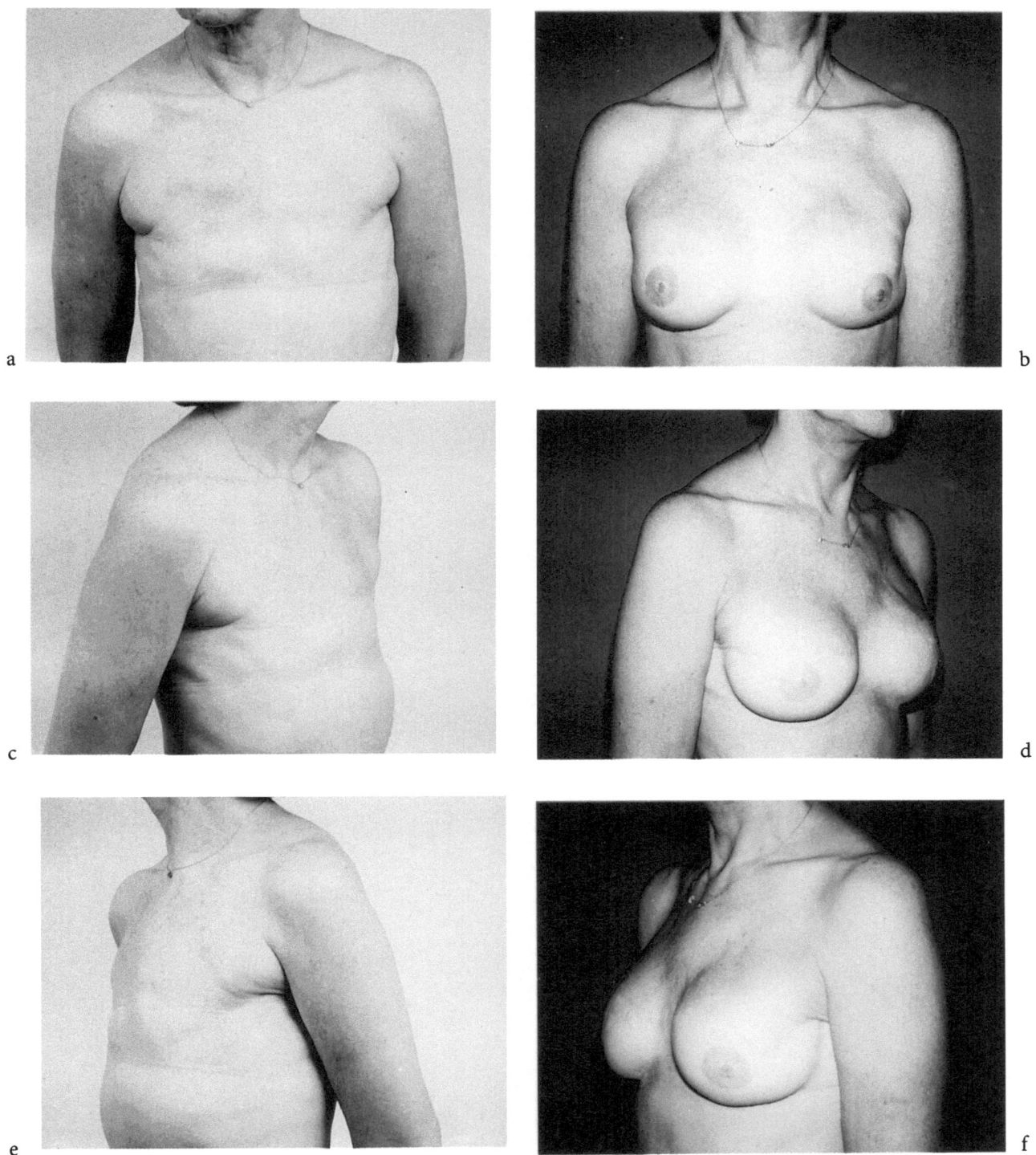

Fig. 239 a-f. Bilateral reconstruction: AHS implants of 250 ml filled with 275 ml, reconstruction of areolae by grafts from inguinal crease and local flaps, secondary tattooing

Reconstruction of the nipple-areolar plaque

Reconstruction of the nipple and areola is the final procedure in breast reconstruction, one that will make one forget that so far only a volume has been reconstructed, incapable in itself of representing a breast.

This new areola is insensitive, in fact only an attractive optical device to provide the onlooker with a visual target.

But it may also help, by acting as a focus, to distract attention from the scars of the mastectomy, and those which may have been added by provision of a flap.

For this simulation to best play its role, it is important for it to be well placed at the apex of a successful size, symmetric with the opposite side (the patients who do not ask for reconstruction of the areola are usually those for whom the reconstruction of shape has been disappointing).

The symmetry can only be considered once the reconstructed volume is stabilised, and also in relation to the volume and shape of the opposite breast.

This is why we do not recreate the areola at the first stage of the reconstruction procedure. We prefer to leave this to the second stage, wether as an isolated procedure, or combined with the finishing touches to the reconstructed breast or with any mammoplasty wich may have been performed on the opposite breast.

Reconstruction of the areola

Grafts

These may be taken from different parts of the body, selecting areas of similar coloration.

Grafts taken from the opposite breast:

– grafts taken superficially with a razor from the opposite areola are subject to two risks: that of obtaining a thinnish graft of unsatisfactory color, and that of its becoming depigmented with time like the donor site. This disadvantage applies to both the receptor and the donor sites; therefore we do not employ this technique;

– the "snail " method consists of coiling up a spiral strip on the opposite areola. We do not use this technique, the suture of which is very tedious, because it leads to an unattractive white scar which exactly reproduces the initial spiral;

– when the areola is averagely sized, and no reduction plasty or skin reduction is necessary (really a rare situation), the inner half of the areola may be taken, which conceals the scar around the nipple and makes it much less obvious, since the outer half of the nipple retains its contour;

– when the areola is large, an outer rim can be removed at the same time as the mammoplasty of the opposite breast (fig. 240). The result is two symmetrical areolae, but often rather too small, and still with the risk of depigmentation of the grafted areola after several years.

Grafts taken from another site

The most satisfactory color and texture are found at the inguinal fold. The donor site is chosen on the basis of the pigmentation desired, which is darker below the prominence of the adductor longus muscle than above. In all cases, the graft, which is of full thickness, is removed astride the sulcus and not at its larger lip which is too dark. It is carefully defatted on its deep aspect, taking care to get rid of the hair follicles. If, despite this, some hairs regrow on the areolar site, electrical depilation can be performed subsequently. This graft is sutured on the de-epithelialised site, and immobilised by a bolus tie-over dressing left in place for around four days, followed by tulle gras dressings for ten days.

Grafts of the lesser lip of the groin sulcus are usually too dark, but tend to become chestnut-colored with time. Their color cannot be controlled, so that in our opinion they have only one indication: bilateral reconstruction of the areola (the development will be symmetrical) when there is a deliberate intent to obtain a permanent brown color.

The fate of areolar grafts, of whatever origin, is variable. Some will tend to spread, notably on flaps, perhaps because of the good vascular quality of the substrate and its trophicity, while others tend to contract, under whatever tension they have been sutured, and in an unpredictable manner.

Thinness of the integuments is not always a contraindication to a graft; de-epithelialisation of the donor site is very superficial, and it may even be considered that the provision of a full-thickness skin graft may rather thicken this zone.

Tattooing

This recently developed technique is currently our preference for several reasons.

Since it has a wide range of available colors, a pure color may be chosen or a mixture of two or more tints.

This is a simple, rapid and easy technique which avoids the disadvantages of removing a graft (disadvantages that are immediately obvious and unpleasant when the graft is taken at the groin, rather than the supplementary scar defect which is usually unobtrusive). The result is stable and satisfactory, provided some precautions are taken:

– it is best to tattoo with a color that is possibly a little too light, which can always be revised subsequently, rather than the other way round;

– if the tattooing is done in the operating-room, one must be careful of the lighting, in particular of the scialytic light, which is often too yellow; it is best at the time of deciding on the color to use ambient light, especially the "daylight" neon light;

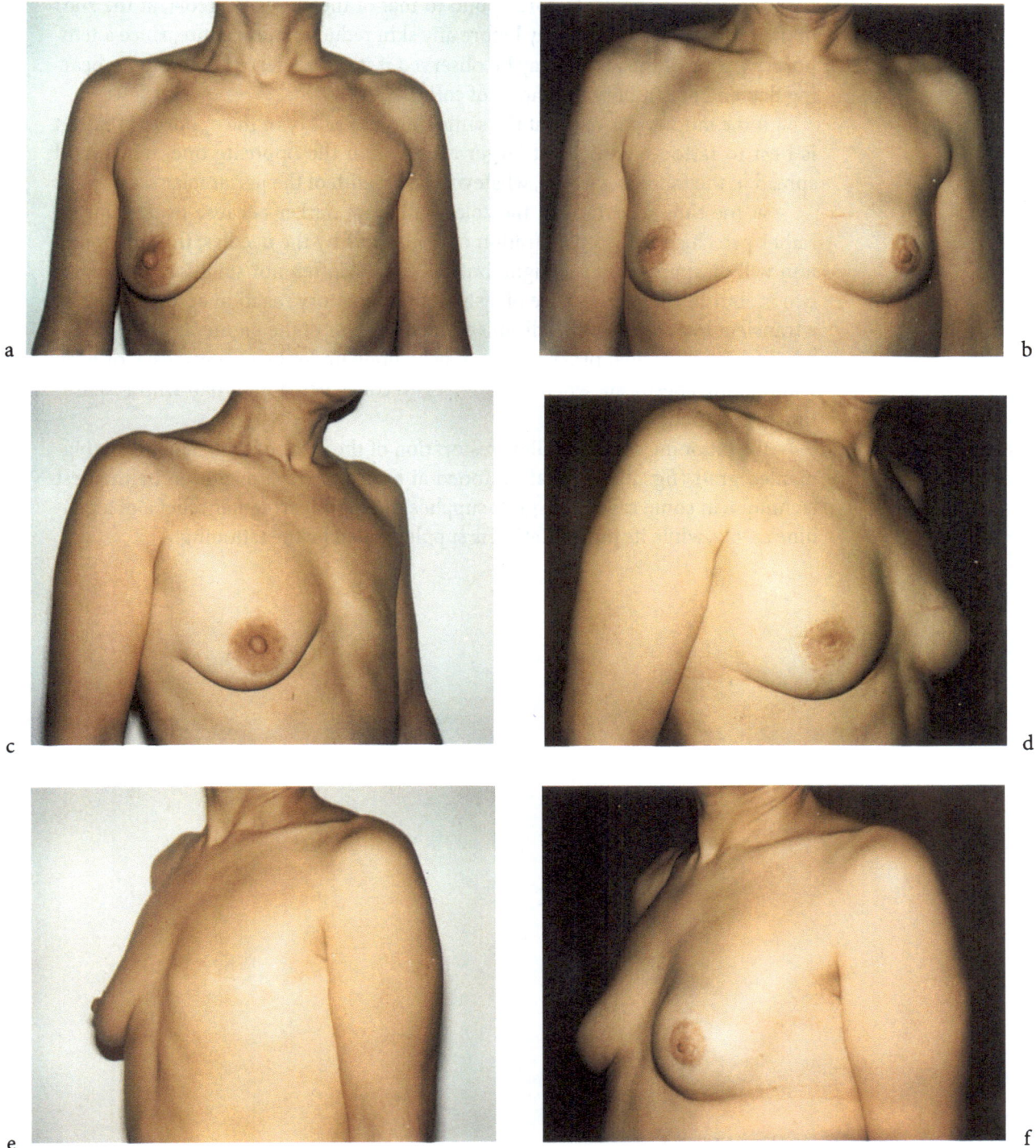

Fig. 240 a-f. Reconstruction of left breast by smooth inflatable Sebbin LS20 implant of 150 ml filled to 180 ml. Reconstruction of nipple-areolar plaque at second operative stage by graft of outer half of areola and free graft of lower half of nipple, at same time as correction of contralateral ptosis

– the color is chosen to correspond to that of the opposite areola, at the start of the procedure, and certainly before any skin reduction procedure, since a temporary pallor of the areola may be observed if it is transferred on a nipple-bearing flap and may nullify the choice of color;

– if the tattooing is made at the same time as a plasty of the opposite breast, it is best to tattoo a somewhat larger areola than the opposite one, which will spread in the following weeks, whatever the breadth of the periareolar scar;

– at the time of tattooing, the color will seem darker because of bruising or rather petechiae, due to penetration of the dermis by the needles; this phenomenon will disappear in a fortnight, but the color is often not stabilised until after two months, probably because of a slight inflammatory reaction accompanied by a transient hyperemia which disguises the true color of the pigment;

– if it is an isolated procedure, it may be done under local anesthesia, or even without any anesthesia when the areola is reconstructed on a flap whose sensation is impaired;

– the tattooing may also allow restoration of the color of an insufficiently pigmented graft (fig. 241). A graft tattooed at a second stage may even be the best technique in some cases. The graft supplies the slightly irregular relief a of a genuine areola, while its pigmentation is supplemented by the tattooing.

Fig. 241 a-h. Reconstruction of left breast by smooth inflatable Sebbin implant of 175 ml filled to 220 ml, and of nipple-areolar plaque by local flap and graft of lower half of opposite areola. Secondary depigmentation of both areolae and flattening of local flap. Tattooing of both areolae and cartilage graft (from ear) beneath the nipple

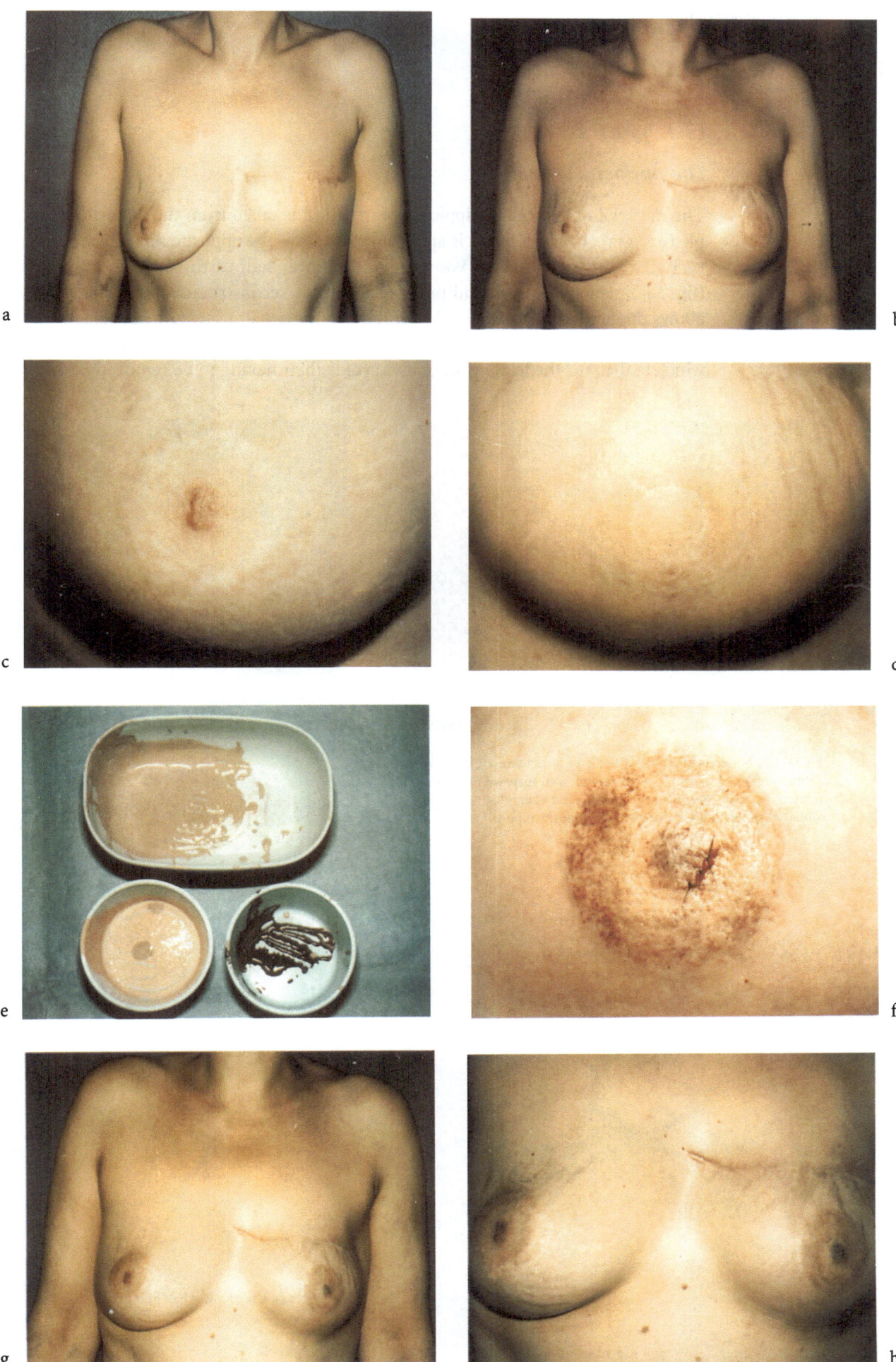

Reconstruction of the nipple

Free grafts

The opposite breast

The material of choice for nipple reconstruction is taken from the opposite nipple (fig. 242). This technique is applicable whenever the opposite nipple is of correct size and prominence. We remove the lower half of the opposite nipple (fig. 243), which ensures good prominence of the reconstructed nipple and also allows downward reflection of the remaining upper half to restore adequate and symmetric size. Suture is made with interrupted rapidly-absorbed stitches, which suffice for the healing stage and avoids their having to be removed in this

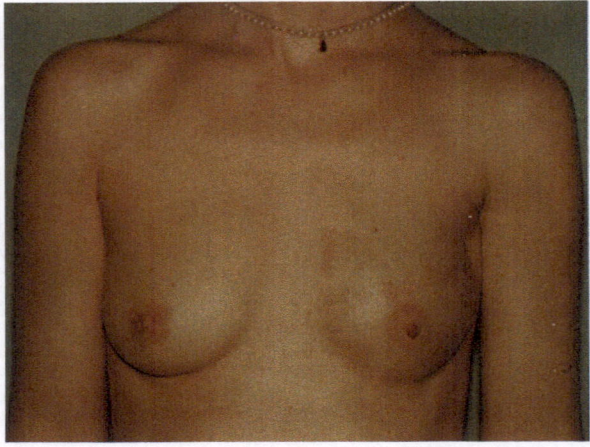

a

Fig. 242 a, b. Reconstruction of left breast by textured inflatable Sebbin implant of 175 ml filled to 200 ml, with suspension of inframammary crease. Secondary reconstruction of areola by tattooing and of nipple by graft of lower half of opposite nipple

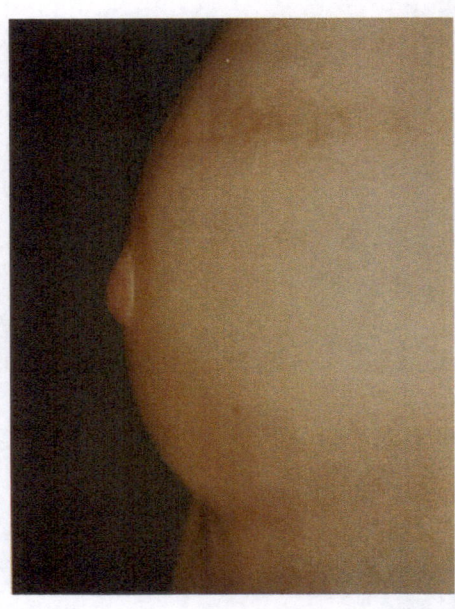

b

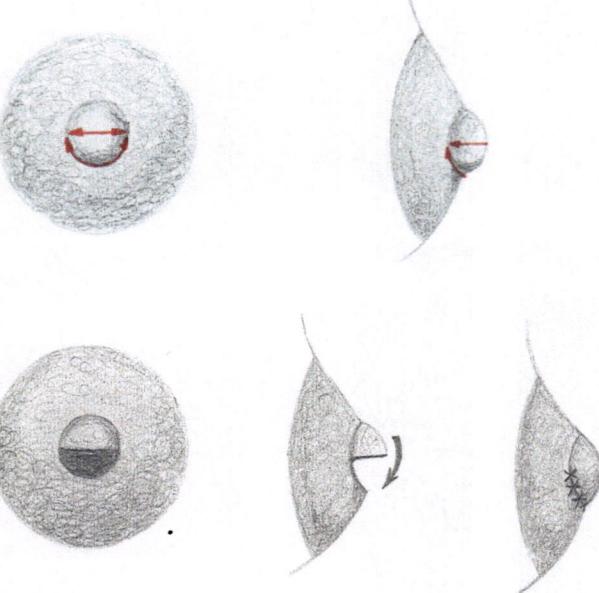

Fig. 243. Use of lower half of nipple

sensitive region. When the nipple is combined with a graft, the whole is immobilised under a bolus tie-over dressing. Probably because of its epithelial structure, this full-thickness fragment tolerates the transfer without any damage, and with rapid vascular repermeation. When the fragment is sutured after having been expressed gently in normal saline, it is pale. Very often, at the 4th day, it is purplish in color; it is likely that capillary arterial reperfusion occurs more quickly than venous return; then the color lightens and the nipple becomes pinker day by day, regaining a normal color around the 15th day. After removal of the initial dressing we allow showering, but for the rest of the time the graft is kept under a greasy dressing.

When the nipple graft is combined with tattooing, the central zone destined to receive the graft is not tattooed, to avoid traumatising the substrate and giving rise to microthrombi which might impair acceptance of the graft. In this case, since the graft is placed on a relatively restricted and virtally immobile region, we do not use a bolus tie-over but only a greasy dressing.

Other full-thickness grafts

The pulp of the toe

We have found grafts from the toe pulp rather disappointing. While the color is satisfactory, this is not true for the relief and there is a tendency to flattening with time. Moreover, the donor area is often painful during the healing period and walking is hindered.

The earlobe

Removal of a full-thickness triangle at the inner part of the earlobe, on the other hand, gives excellent results as regards both color and relief. Healing is rapid and the graft is pink at the 5th day, which is by no means always the case with grafts from the opposite nipple.

It is possible to remove a fragment of adequate size even when the lobe is not very large. There are no complications at the donor site, and the scar is unobtrusive since it is placed at the base of the attachment of the lobe against the cervical skin in a natural sulcus.

This is the technique we most often employ in bilateral reconstructions, taking an identical fragment from each ear.

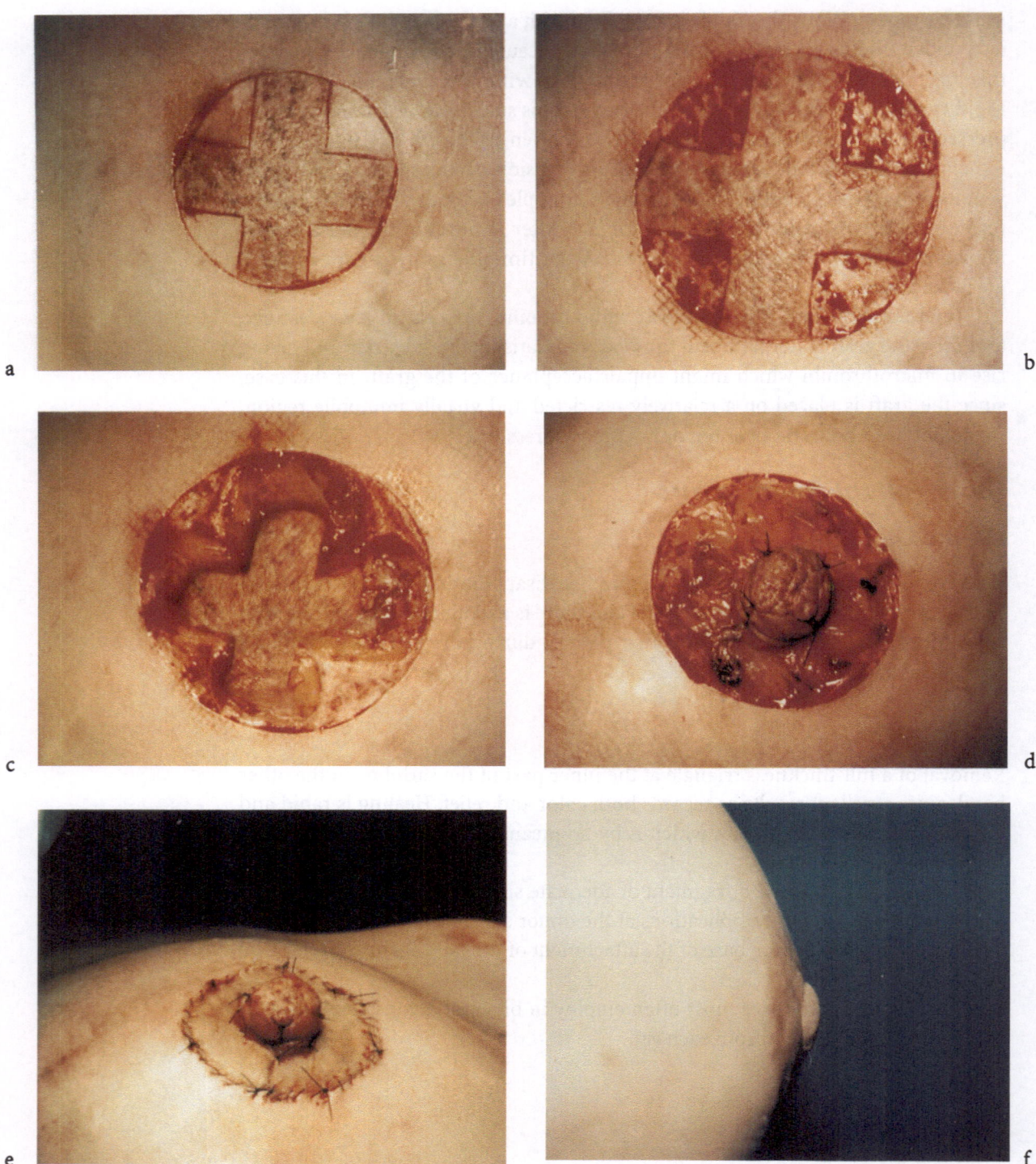

Fig. 244 a-f. Local "Maltese cross" flap. **a** Preliminary tattooing of four limbs; **b** de-epithelialisation of angles; **c** incision of the four limbs to their base; **d** suture of sides two by two; **e** areolar (inguinal) graft; **f** appearance at 2 years

Local flaps

The technique we have most often used is that of the "Maltese cross", with some variation from the technique as originally described. As this skin is white, we tattoo the four flaps before incising them, using a somewhat lighter color than that desired subsequently. Actually, after having been incised, the small flaps retract because of their skin elasticity and their optical density increases (fig. 244).

The nipple so reconstructed retains satisfactory size, provided one has taken the precaution to suture the flaps at their base in slightly concentric fashion, so that the nipple does not spread. Use of this technique requires the taking of a graft for the areolar reconstruction because of the raw areas left by raising the four flaps.

The limitation of this technique is probably represented by those quite common cases where a scar (mastectomy or junction of a latissimus flap) bars the zone of areolar reconstruction. For vascular reasons, we have not dared to cut flaps in full scar tissue.

Important points

Areola: the outcome of tattooing is promising, whether alone or combined with a graft.
Nipple: the best source is from the opposite side.

Timing

The nipple-areolar plaque should only be reconstructed at a second stage procedure (delay of 3 to 6 months), when the shape and size of the reconstructed breast are considered as stabilised.

The indications for breast reconstruction

The choice of the most appropriate technique depends essentially on the state of the tissues left after the mastectomy and the possible after-effects of radiotherapy, but also the build of the thorax and of the body as whole.

If the tissues are of good quality

When the integuments are supple, substantial and of adequate amount, with a uniform fatty panniculus under the entire skin envelope, which is in particular not thinned on either side of the scar, when the pectoralis major is present and of good quality over its whole extent and without atrophy of its lower heads, it is logical to perform the reconstruction by:

Placement of an implant
*   – in retropectoral position,*
*   – with revision of the mastectomy scar, which is variably excised,*
*   – with suspension of the inframammary creasewhenever possible,*
*   – using an inflatable implant with normal saline, for its flexibility in use and the harmlessness of its content,*
*   – the choice of the size of implant depending on the necessary breast base, but also on the opposite breast; if this needs to be reduced subsequently, whether for correction of hypertrophy or of ptosis, the base of the implant must be less than that of the opposite breast before correction, since the latter will also be reduced.*

If the local tissues are of good trophicity but obviously inadequate amount to admit

Here, the indication is to insert an implant immediately filled to its definive volume:
    – provided these tissues are of proper and especially uniform thickness, that there are no signs of unequally distributed tension (local reduction in thickness, local partial rigidity), and that there are no after-effects, however minimal or localised, of radiotherapy (a supplementary treatment which calls for great caution in this indication),

The reconstruction may be attempted by a first stage of expansion in situ:
  – with a hemispherical prosthesis
  – of the same base as the definitive implant,
  – a remote valve,
  – without suspension of the inframmary crease,
  – placing the new fold at the outset at the same level as the opposite crease,
  – without excessive overinflation.

If the tissues are insufficient in amount and/or of poor trophicity

Provision of a flap becomes necessary:
  – skin flaps are not to our liking as they do not give a lining effect in front of the implant with which they are necessarily combined;
  – myocutaneous flaps have transformed the possibilities of reconstruction since their development, once tissue provision is necessary.

The latissimus dorsi flap

  – Is employable provided its pedicle has been respected;
  – its property as a muscle lining is very useful provided the relative lack of skin is not great and that the local tissues do not require major excision;
  – it nearly always requires the insertion of an implant;
  – the skin island available depends on the dorsal laxity, which varies in different women and is not usually very great, unless a preliminary expansion is made under the donor site.

The rectus abdominis flap

  – Allows reconstruction of a very natural breast;
  – without the need for a prosthesis in the majority of cases;
  – so that plasty of the opposite breast is less often necessary, or less extensive;
  – but it is suited only to particular morphologic features, and when there is sufficient excess of subumbilical skin and fatty tissue;
  – it is relatively or absolutely contraindicated by the presence of certain scars;
  – the indication for a uni- or bipedicled flap depends on the need to preserve the largest skin island possible, and is certainly not routine;
  – it is a more demanding procedure than a latissimus flap.

Free flaps

These seem to be only rarely indicated in breast reconstruction.
  – If they take the form of a rectus flap in a free rather than a pedicled version, as proposed by some authors, for the quality of perfusion and because the procedure of abdominal repair is of less magnitude, and as an alternative to a bipedicled flap, the incidence of failure due to necrosis seems higher than with a pedicled flap, since any problem with the pedicle of a free flap means loss of the entire flap.

– We have no experience with a free flap of the gluteus maximus, which may cause unpleasant complications (gluteal depression and lesions of the sciatic nerve have been described), which are far from negligible.

In breast reconstruction, it is our belief that it must not be forgotten that these patients have already undergone a serious burden of illness, that this reconstruction is intended to give them a degree of hope, but that this must not be at the cost of further burdensome procedures carrying a high risk, as may be the case with microsurgical procedures.

The delay

A deferred reconstruction may be performed from the 6th month after a simple mastectomy without supplementary treatment, such an interval usually sufficing for stabilisation of the healing process, thus allowing assessment of the degree of relaxation of the tissues and choice of the best mode of reconstruction.

If supplementary treatment, whether by radiotherapy or chemotherapy or both, is necessary, it is also necessary to await the end of such treatment, whose programs must not be tampered with, and not to interfere with the general repercussions of chemotherapy or the local after-effects of radiotherapy.

Immediate reconstruction

As with delayed reconstruction, the technical methods are identical, but it may simply be remarked that skin expansion is certainly involved in a higher proportion of cases when the necessary skin excision does not allow placement of the definitive implant, even at the cost of an abdominal advancement, and if there is hesitation in raising a flap because of a relatively minor lack of skin substance.

The problem of the indication for an immediate reconstruction, in our view, rests more with the carcinologic and psychologic context:

If radiotherapy has to be given after operation, the results of implant-reconstruction seem of less quality than those of delayed reconstruction, with a higher incidence of immediate complications and periprosthetic contracture.

The technique chosen must be reliable, so as not to complicate the postoperative course, and must not cause significant delay to supplementary treatment, whether chemotherapy or radiotherapy.

The responsiblity for the psychological management of a patient desirous of an immediate reconstruction is a heavy one, and calls for the imparting of even more detailed information about the limitations and possibilities of the reconstruction. In effect, the patient does not see the situation clearly, and will not have experienced the intermediate stage of an absent breast and the inevitable presence of at least one chest scar. This woman will in fact leave for the operating room with her breast intact, even if diseased, and come round to find something that is inevitably different, not symmetric with the opposite side, and on which a secondary scar defect will often be imposed subsequently...

Partial reconstruction

The morphologic sequelae of so-called conservative treatment (which is no longer truly conservative once the breast is deformed to the point of necessitating a reparative procedure), raise difficult problems in treatment for which there is no routine solution.

However, some concepts may be singled out from an analysis of the problems encountered:

– the deformities are due to the combination of a loss of volume of the breast, global or partial (due to quadrantectomy) and to sclerosis after radiotherapy, often given in major dosage;

– not only is the breast deformed, but it has usually lost its plasticity;

– the severity of the residual scarring and of clinical and radiologic fibrosis demands the greatest caution if a plastic procedure using local tissues is contemplated, avoiding procedures of cutaneo-glandular cleavage as much as possible;

– the method of repair chosen should not hinder surveillance of a breast which has already been the site of a tumor. Some have suggested partial implants to repair the after-effects of a quadrantectomy; but such implants, if prefilled with gel, are radio-opaque and this makes monitoring of the residual gland at the margins of the implant difficult.

Several situations may be encountered:

– the treated breast is globally reduced in size, contracted and fixed, not so much because of the tumorectomy as of the radiotherapy. Without touching the irradiated breast, the operative indication may be for a mammoplasty of the opposite breast to restore balance betwen the two sides, at least as far as volume and ptosis are concerned (fig. 245);

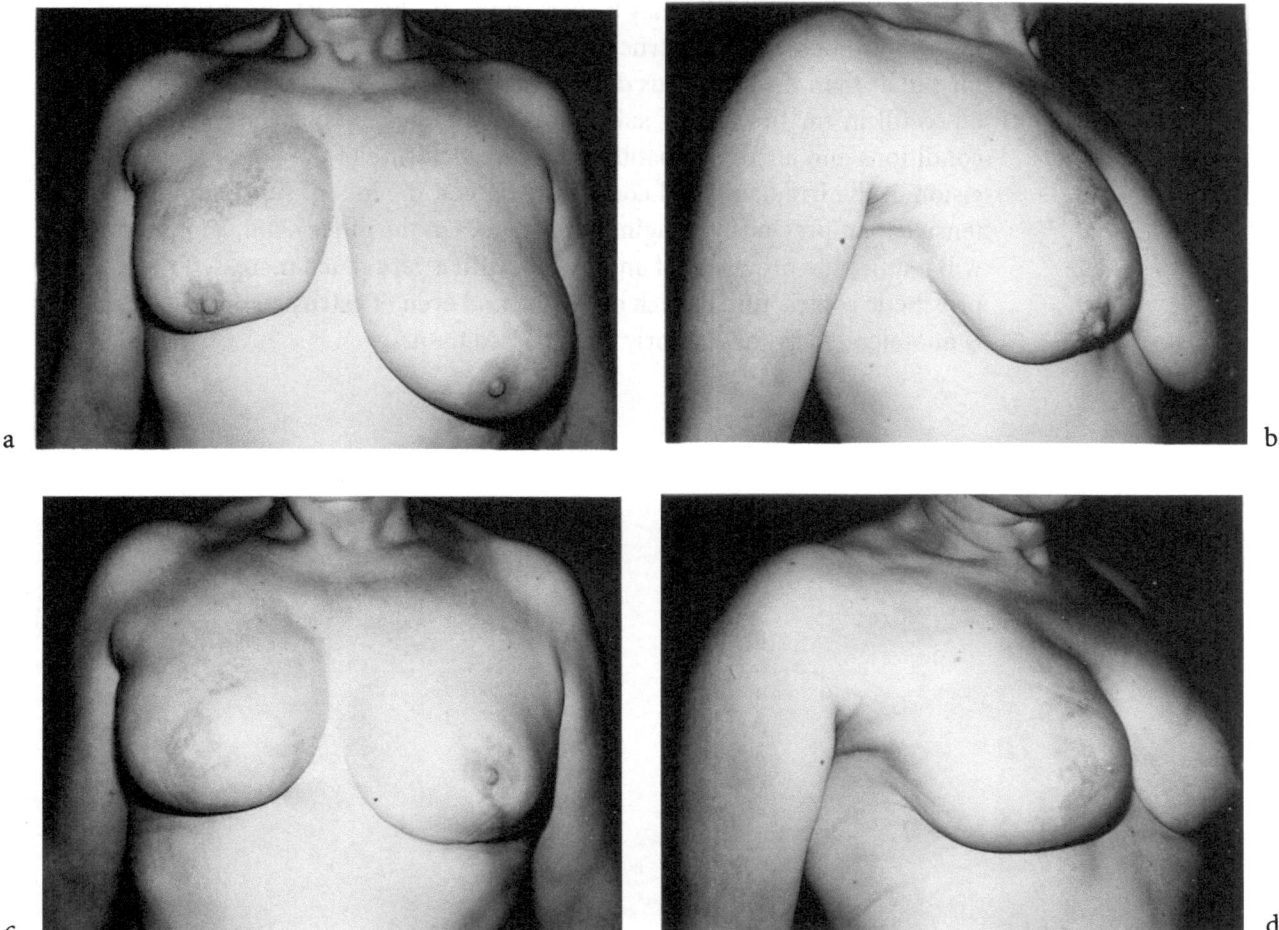

Fig. 245 a-d. "Conservative" treatment of right breast. **a, b** Rigid breast, glandular shrinkage and sclerosis; **c, d** reduction mammoplasty of opposite breast. The only procedure for which permission was granted at the right breast was simple transplantation of the nipple-areolar plaque by free graft, which underwent subsequent depigmentation

– no plastic procedure may be performed on this breast, other than mastectomy with immediate reconstruction by flap, usually one from the rectus abdominis rather than the latissimus dorsi, which does not possess the skin cover needed to fill in for the loss of substance engendered by mastectomy under such
conditions and is not compatible with direct closure of the donor area. After excision of the irradiated and contracted tissues, the loss of substance is more extensive than previously imagined (fig. 246). On the other hand, a latissimus flap
will require the provision of an implant, with a very much increased risk of periprosthetic contracture in such a context, and even of extrusion of the implant if it
is not tolerated by these poorly vascularised tissues;

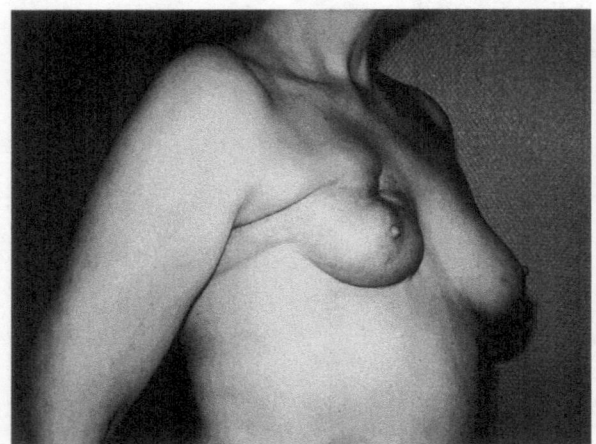
a

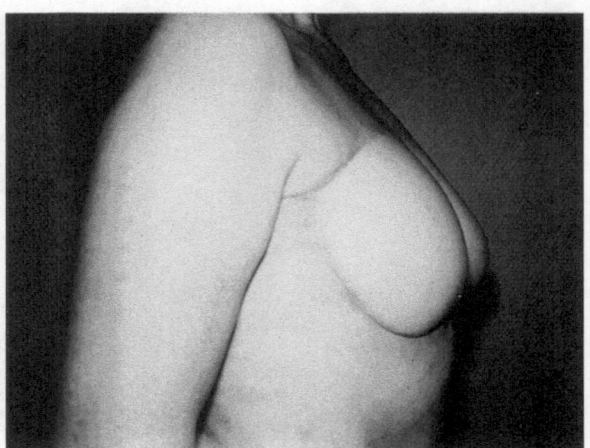
b

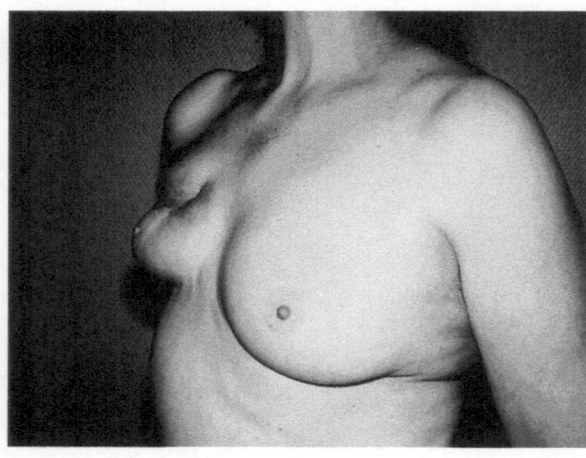
c

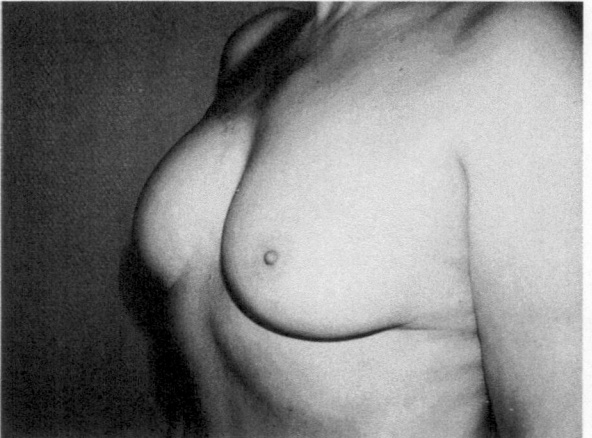
d

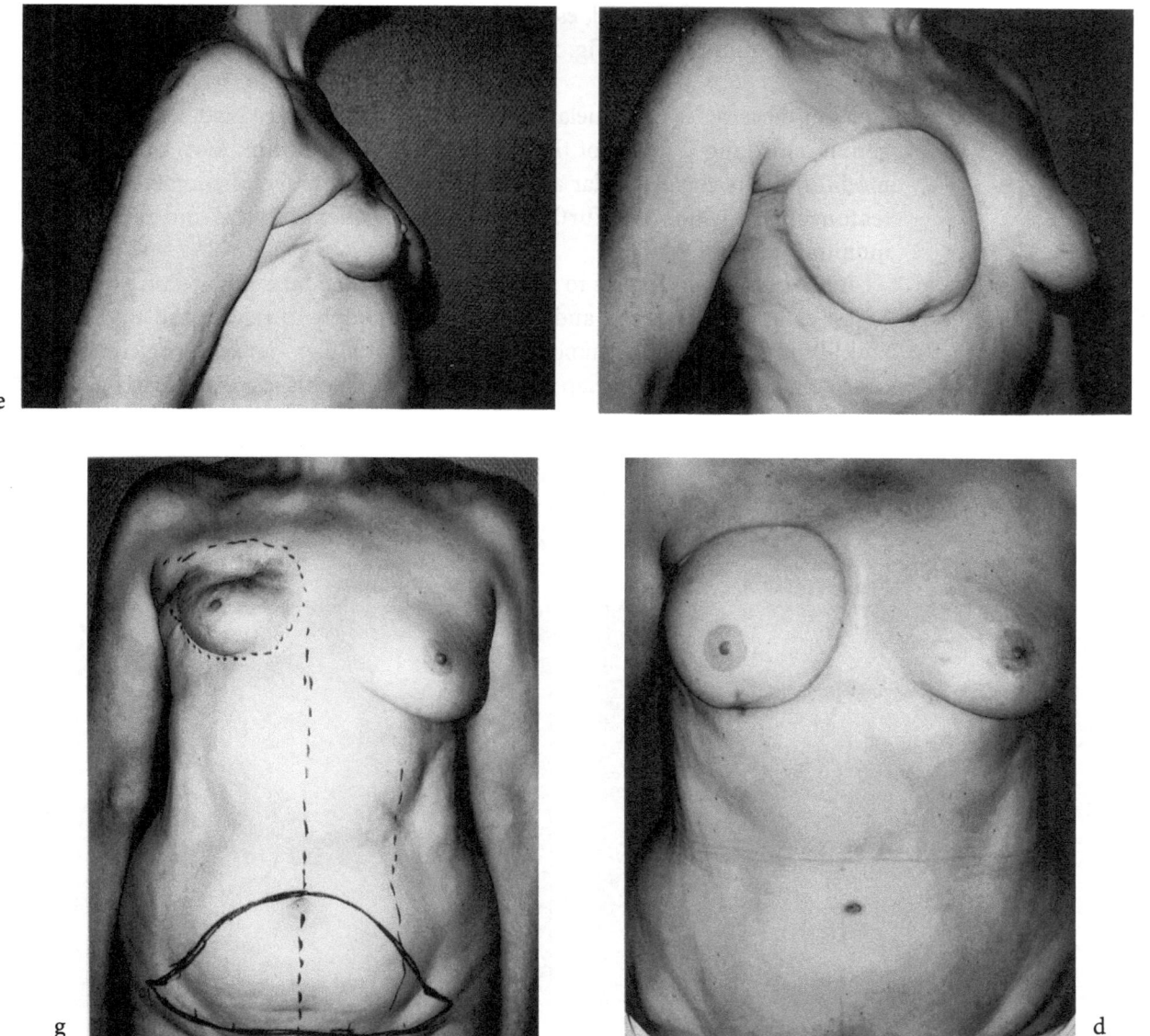

Fig. 246 a-h. "Conservative" treament of right breast. **a, c, e, g** The radiodystrophy and loss of volume are such that only mastectomy with immediate reconstruction can be envisaged; **b, d, f** reconstruction by unipedicled flap of rectus abdominis from opposite side. Note the difference in circumference between the preoperative design and the scar of placement of the flap, due to major expansion at the sides of the loss of substance once the contracted tissue has been removed; **h** appearance at 15 months after 1st stage and 6 months after reconstruction of areola by tattooing and graft from opposite nipple (the scar at the edge of the flap has paled much more slowly than the abdominal scar although there was no tension at this site).

– the breast is deformed, especially by a loss of substance localised to the region of the tumorectomy (fig. 247), a loss of substance fixed by subsequent irradiation.

With these types of sequelae, glandular autoplasties are inadequate and dangerous, since the viability of the irradiated gland is an unknown quantity, and modification of the glandular architecture may lead to the phenomena of cytosteatonecrosis, which will further hinder subsequent clinical and radiological monitoring.

It seems to us preferable to interfere with the glandular architecture of such a breast as little as possible, and rather to seek simply to release the contracture and fill up the loss of substance by provision of a flap, our own preference this time being for a latissimus flap as the loss of substance is less extensive (fig. 248).

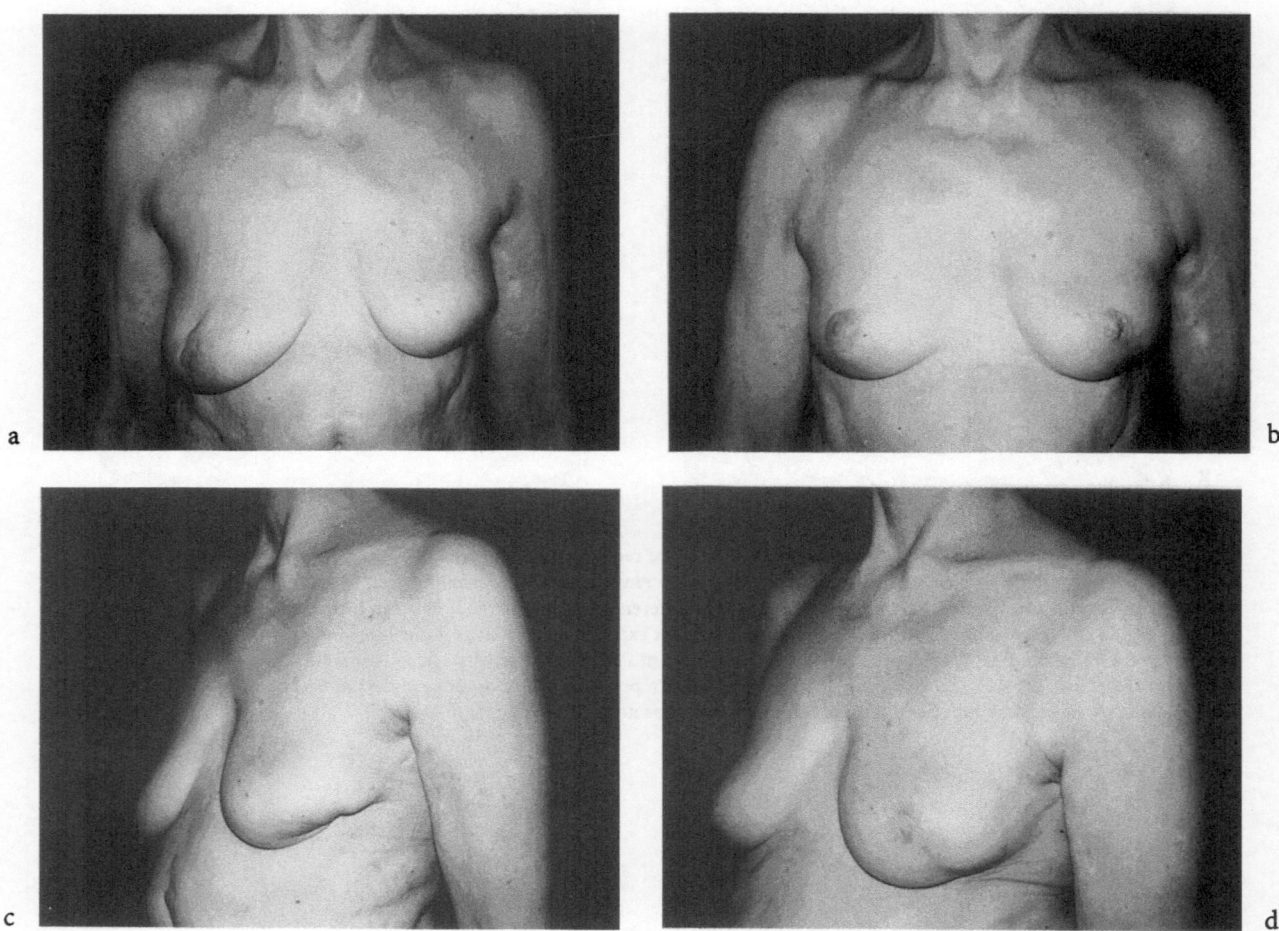

Fig. 247 a-d. Lesion of inferolateral quadrant of left breast treated by tumorectomy and radium therapy. Mammoplasty with superior pedicle, aimed essentially at correction of areolar retraction on left side and reduction of ptosis on the right. Result satisfactory as regards global symmetry of upper quadrants and position of areolae, but residual scar contracture in irradiated zone

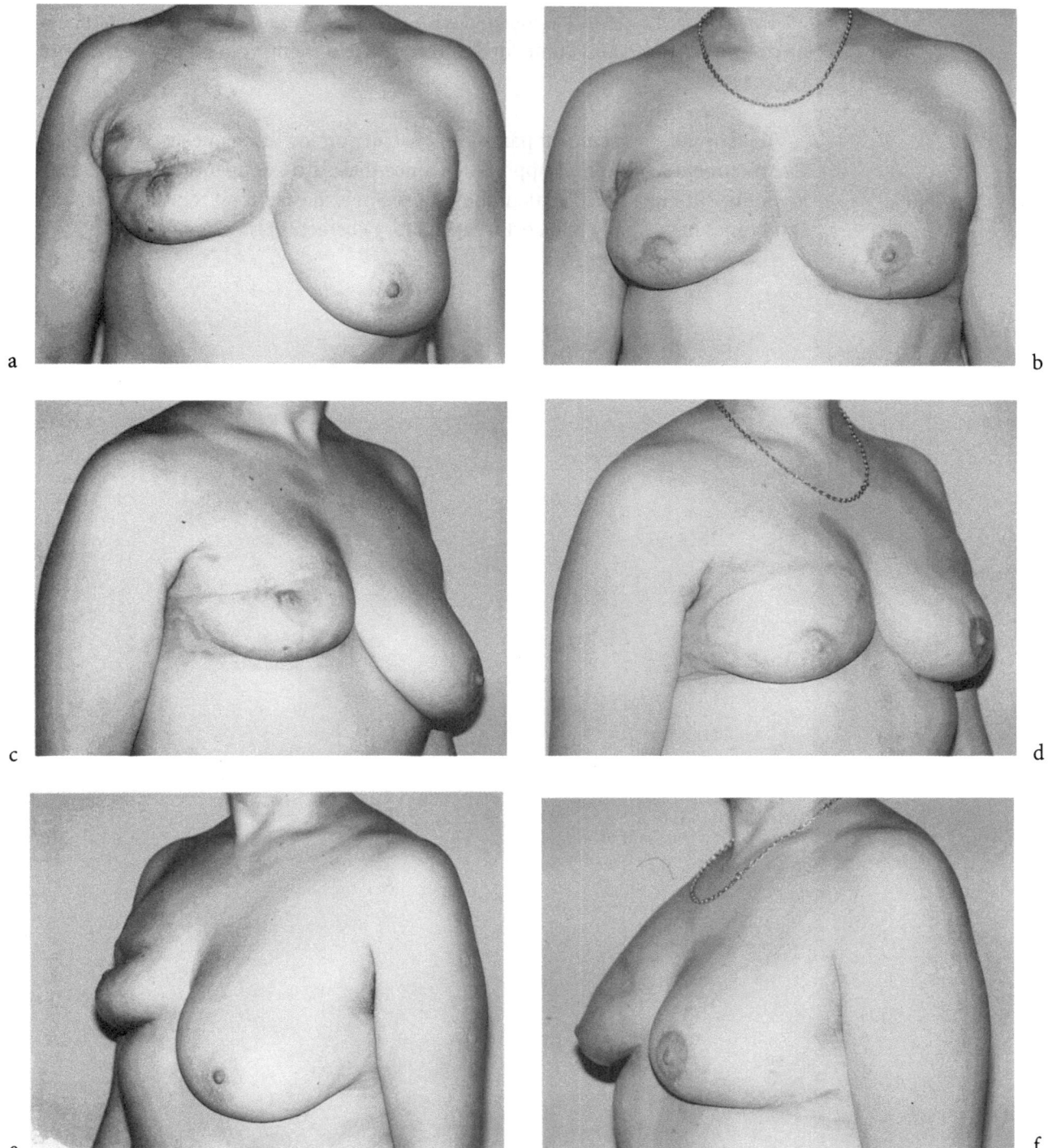

a

b

c

d

e

f

Fig. 248 a-f. Sequelae of wide tumorectomy for lesion of superolateral quadrant followed by irradiation. Correction of tissue contracture by interposition of myocutaneous latissimus flap and mammoplasty of opposite breast to restore symmetry, perfomed 4 months after first stage

Part of the skin island associated with a muscle overlap of variable extent can be de-epithelialised and embedded to restore the missing volume at a precise site (fig. 249).

To sum up, the results of partial reconstruction for the sequelae of conservative treatment are often disappointing, since these are therapeutic problems that are more difficult to resolve than those posed by a mastectomy, to which one may sometimes have finally to resort if satisfactory correction is to be realised.

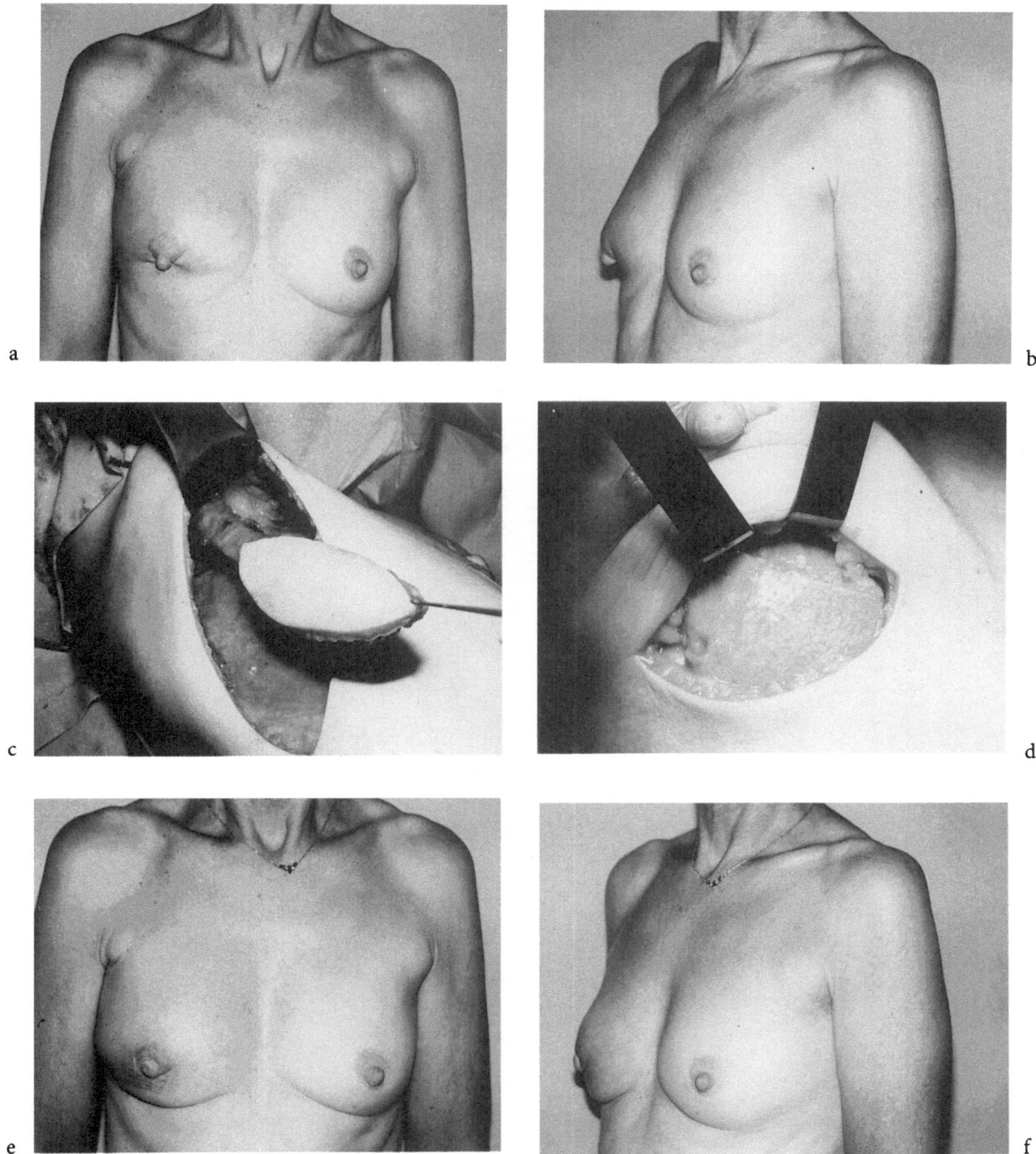

Fig. 249 a-f. Tumorectomy followed by irradiation for lesion situated at junction of inferior quadrants. Loss of substance fixed by irradiation but skin of acceptable quality. Restoration of volume by myocutaneous flap of latissimus dorsi on the anterior part of the muscle, allowing retention in place of intact and innervated posterior part, whose skin island has been entirely de-epithelialised and embedded

Subcutaneous mastectomy

General principles

The principle of subcutaneous mastectomy is simple to separate the skin envelope of the breast from the underlying gland, which is removed with immediate restoration of volume by an implant and of shape by redraping the skin, which is nearly always necessary.

But difficulties begin as soon as one passes from theory to practice. To separate the gland from the skin is a hemorrhagic procedure which takes a great deal of care and precision if an appreciable amount of residual breast gland is not to be left, since it means working at the level of the crests of Duret while avoiding any damage to the skin, and this is frequent at the areola and the nipple.

A compartment is then created behind the pectoral muscles to receive the implant. This pocket, which must be continuous —as in an immediate reconstruction— to prevent dehiscence over the implant and to isolate the subcutaneous plane, is actually retropectoral only in its upper quadrants and a variable extent of the inferomedial quadrant, depending on the shape of the thorax and the implantation of the breast base. In the inferolateral quadrant it is more difficult to dissect as here it consists only of a thin fascia and some fibers of the serratus anterior.

The remaining difficulty consists in the readjustment of container to content, which is almost always necessary except in the case of a small non-ptosed breast. This amounts to the performance of a "mammoplasty of the skin envelope" to recenter the areola at the apex of the reconstructed volume (sometimes by grafting), and reduction of the residual skin.

The quality of the result, which often needs readjustments at a second stage, depends not only on the appearance at the end of the operation, but also involves the factor of a foreign body reaction in contact with the implant, with the risk of periprosthetic contracture, to which are added problems associated with the shape of the skin envelope and its own evolution.

This is a delicate operation, one that may well be considered as the most technically demanding in the plastic surgery of the breast, and one that sometimes gives disappointing results even in the most capable hands; the long-term result is not always as good as might have been expected when contemplating the shape obtained at the end of the procedure.

Operative technique

First stage: subcutaneous mastectomy

The first stage is begun in dorsal decubitus or in very slight head-down tilt to facilitate identification of the inframammary crease, and with the arms beside the body.

The peripheral limits of the mammary gland are marked on the skin.

The approach route must be:

– large enough to allow proper dissection and meticulous hemostasis;

– situated near the areola, as it is here that the glandular cleavage is most tricky, and therefore not to be situated outside the skin excision that may be required at the stage of readjustment of the skin envelope to the prosthesis.

This is why we prefer an inferior hemiareolar incision, to which a vertical subareolar incision is immediately added (fig. 250).

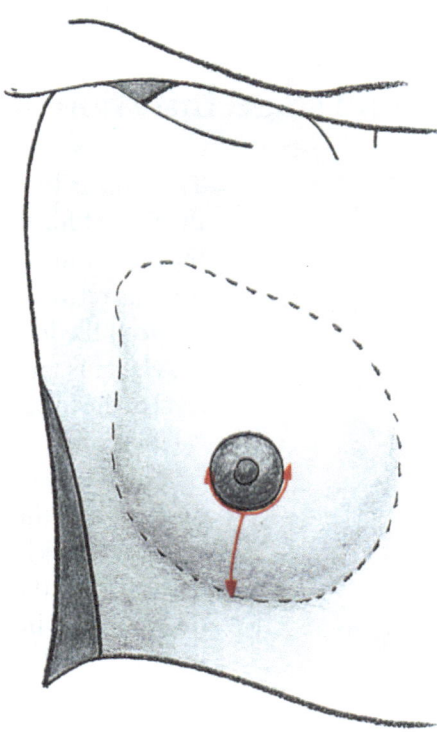

Fig. 250. Tracing the incisions inferior hemiareolar, extended by a subareolar vertical

The skin is incised at first with the scalpel down to the subcutaneous fatty layer and then the dissection is continued with Metzenbaum scissors along the margins of the vertical subarolar incision to free the inferior quadrants first (fig. 251).

With the scissors turned towards the gland, the dissection is made step by step under the entire skin envelope except the immediately retro-areolar region. This glandular freeing, which is effected at the level of the crests of Duret, is difficult and yet must be conducted scrupulously, as there is a constant fear of either leaving too much breast tissue or passing too superficially and risking damaging the superficial circulation. The dissection is easier in thin women, where, though the breast has no true "capsule", the immediately subcutaneous plane is well-differentiated from the glandular plane proper and of a somewhat different color and consistency. It is more awkward in obese women, where the excess of fat infiltrates the tissues and obscures the plane of cleavage.

When the superficial aspect of the gland has been entirely freed, the areola may be dissected. The assistant holds it vertical with the aid of two hooks placed at the edge of the inferior hemiareolar incision, and the deep aspect of the areola is freed with the scalpel very superficially and gradually. This dissection leaves an areola hardly thicker than a full-thickness skin-graft.

The plane of the inframammary crease is then located and freeing of the deep aspect of the gland is made from below upward. The gland is adherent to the underlying infrapectoral plane, where the surgeon must respect what corresponds to the superficial fascia, since preservation of this layer allows continuity of the periprosthetic compartment. The dissection becomes much easier once it crosses the lower border of the pectoralis major, whose perimyisum is preserved.

When the deep and superficial aspects of the gland have been freed, it becomes an easy matter to end the glandular freeing by peripheral section. A stitch identifies the nipple region and another the axillary extension, and the specimen is sent for histologic examination.

Very careful hemostasis is necessary, both at the deep aspect of the skin layer and at the chest wall.

Second stage: insertion of the implant

The table is broken to assist placing the patient in the semi-seated position, and the pocket for the prosthesis is created by transpectoral incision at the middle of the muscle in the direction of its fibers (fig. 225). The difficulty is to preserve a continuous retro- and inframuscular plane, especially below in the region uncovered between the lower border of the pectoralis major medially and the digitations of the serratus anterior laterally. The stripping must be pursued below as far as the level of the inframammary crease, which corresponds to the lower end of the vertical incision.

The hemostasis is checked, with particular attention to the deep aspect of the dissection of the inner attachments of the pectoralis medially and the digitations of the serratus laterally, where there is often bleeding from the perforating vessels derived from the aortic intercostals. A suction drain is placed in the compartment, the implant is inserted and filled and the muscle gap closed.

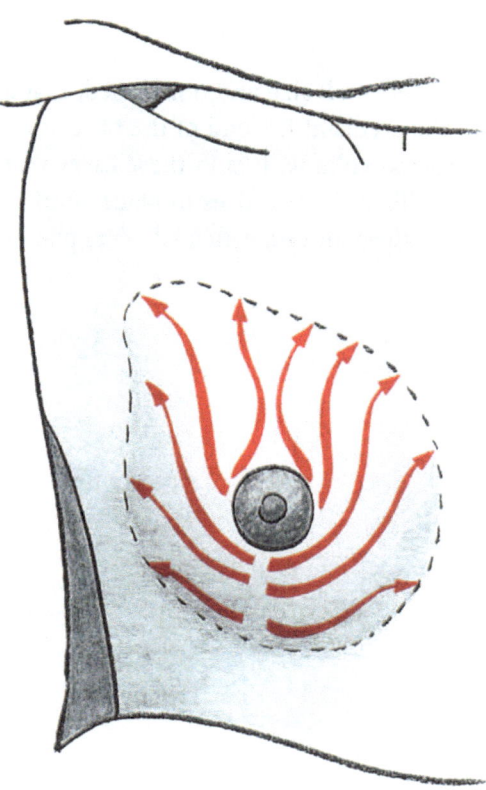

Fig. 251. The dissection begins by superficial freeing of the gland from the subcutaneous layer, first at the lower and then at the upper quadrant, skirting the areola which is dissected last, with the scalpel and in a more superficial plane

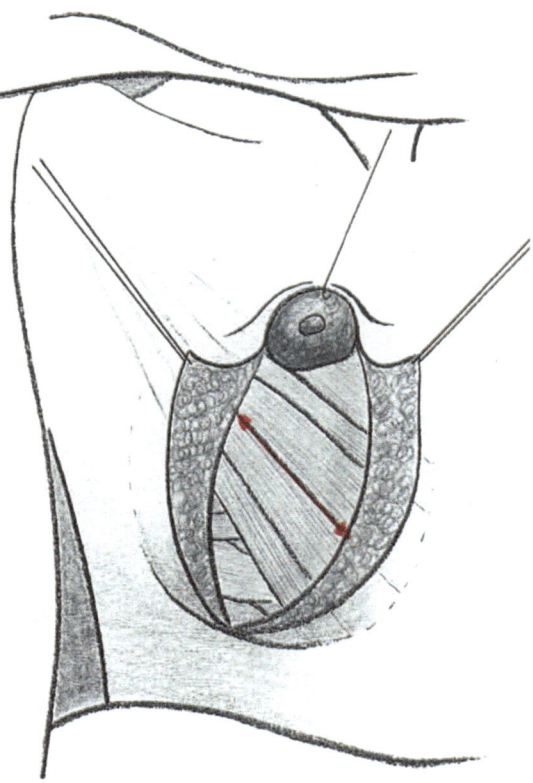

Fig. 251. Transpectoral incision in the direction of the muscle fibers to create the retro- and infrapectoral pocket designed to receive the implant

Third stage: skin plasty

It may sometimes happen, when the breast is of small size and not ptosed, that a skin plasty is unnecessary, the position of the areola at the end of the procedure corrresponding to the apex of the reconstructed volume. It is in these cases that subcutaneous mastectomy gives the best results. It then suffices to place another drain in the zone of stripping, and to close the deep and superficial dermal planes in two layers (fig. 253).

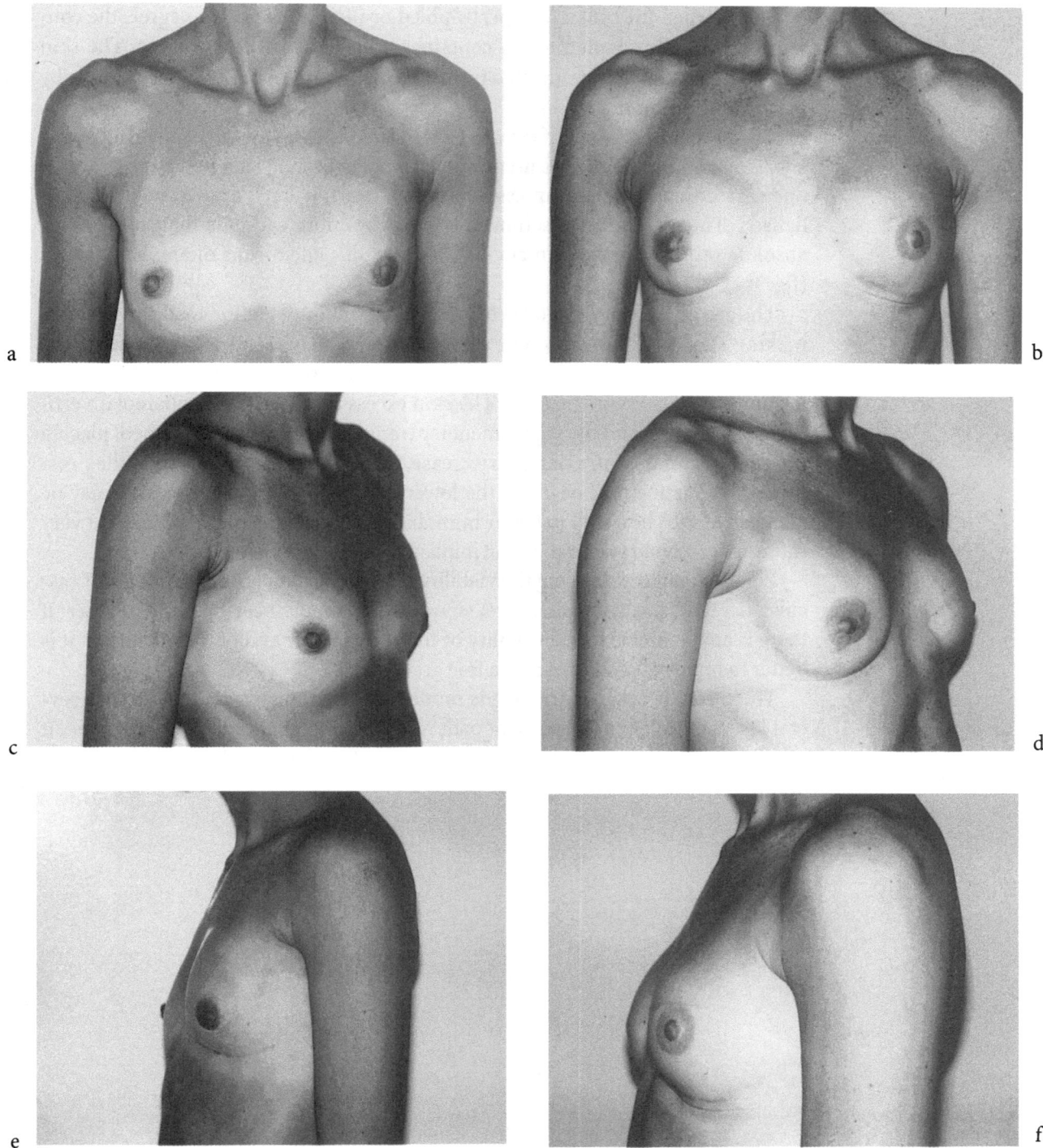

Fig. 253 a-f. Right subcutaneous mastectomy performed at same time as supplementary mastectomy with immediate reconstruction by latissimus flap on left side (previous left tumorectomy for a lesion of the lower quadrants and sacrifice for both carcinologic and reparative reasons of the skin cover of the areola at the inframammary fold).
Right: reconstruction of volume by an implant filled to 140 ml with normal saline
Left: latissimus flap, 13 x 8 cm, implant filled to 130 ml

Often, when the breast is hypertrophied or ptosed in varying degree, the content is no longer adapted to the container, which has become too big. The skin envelope must then be readjusted by means of a "mammoplasty of the skin", ie by performing a skin reduction.

The proper placement of the areola is located with a Dufourmentel ring, using a tracing identical with that used in mammoplasties, the ring being more or less open according to the skin excess. The nipple-bearing flap is drawn and de-epithelialised. This de-epithelialisation must then be more cautious than usual, with absolute respect for the skin circulation, now the sole means of areolar survival (fig. 254).

The areola is closed and tacked down and the skin reduction made on a clamp, making sure that there is good correspondence between the lower end of the clamp and the lower border of the implant, and with uniform and not excessive tension along its limbs (fig. 225). The skin excess is resected, the subareolar vertical tacked dowm, and the supplementary transverse resection performed, placing the scar well in the inframammary crease, ie along the lower margin of the prosthetic compartment. If need be, the lower margin of the transverse scar may be attached to the chest wall to better immobilise it at the level of the crease, but very cautiously to avoid perforating the implant (fig. 256).

Before doing the dressing the viability of the areola is checked. The risk of vascular damage and necrosis is greater when the nipple-bearing flap is longer. If there is any doubt as to the viability of the areola at the end of the operation, it is better to remove it and treat it as a free graft.

The carefully applied dressing is moderately compressive and made with several layers of tulle gras, absorbent pads and hypoallergenic adhesive strapping. It is left untouched until removal of the drains at the 4th or 5th day, when fresh tulle gras is applied.

Postoperative course

This is often a painful procedure, both because of the skin stripping and because the muscle reacts to the insertion of the implant by going into spasm. Analgesics and muscle relaxants are given as required.

The immediate problems consist essentially of the risks of partial or total necrosis of the areola, more rarely skin lesions at the angles of the T (fig. 257). This stresses the importance of the retropectoral position of the implant, and of continuity of the prosthetic compartment, which make it possible to manage this difficult stage with greasy dressings and local attention until complete healing of the skin covering without fear of exposure of the implant.

The remote complications are marked by the morphologic pitfalls of this difficult procedure, not always predictable development of periprosthetic contracture, often asymmetric and then the more troublesome, which modifies the shape of the breast more visibly in the lower quadrants and therefore the position of the inframammary crease; and displacement of the areola in relation to the apex of the reconstructed volume due to unequal distribution of the skin envelope.

A second operative procedure to carry out any necessary adjusments is common, but unfortunately does not always permit correction of all the faults.

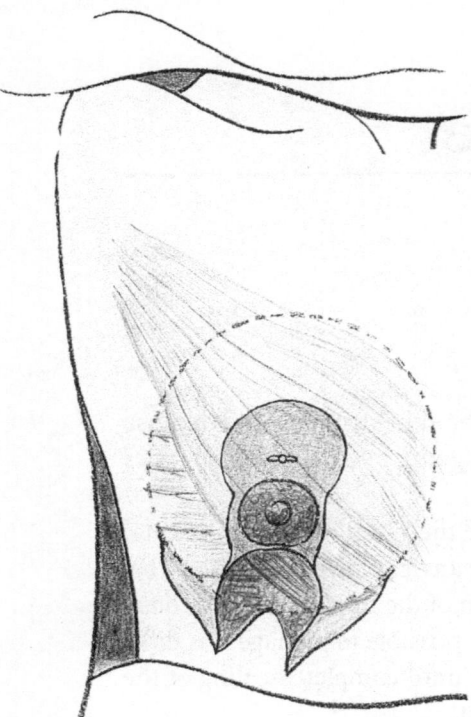

Fig.254. De-epithelialiation of future areolar site centered at apex of volume as reconstructed by implant

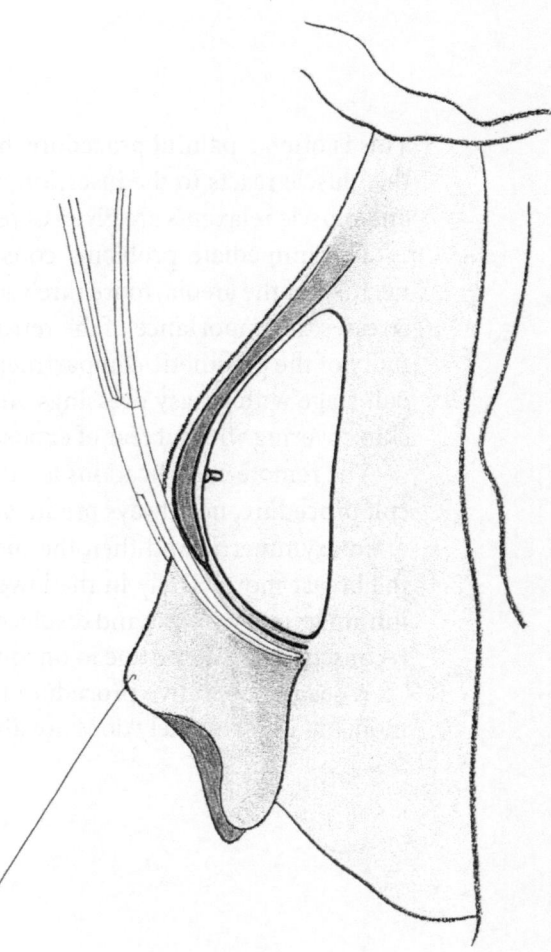

Fig. 255. Skin reduction on clamp, the end of which must correspond to the lower limit of the implant

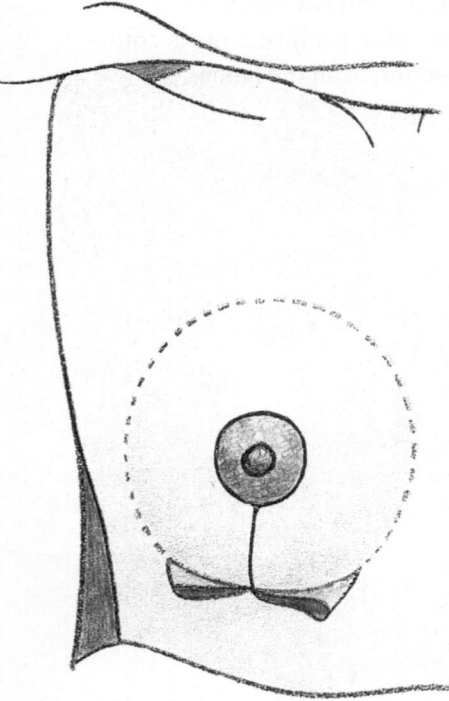

Fig. 256. Supplementary resection placing the inframammary scar in the crease, now indicated by the lower border of the implant

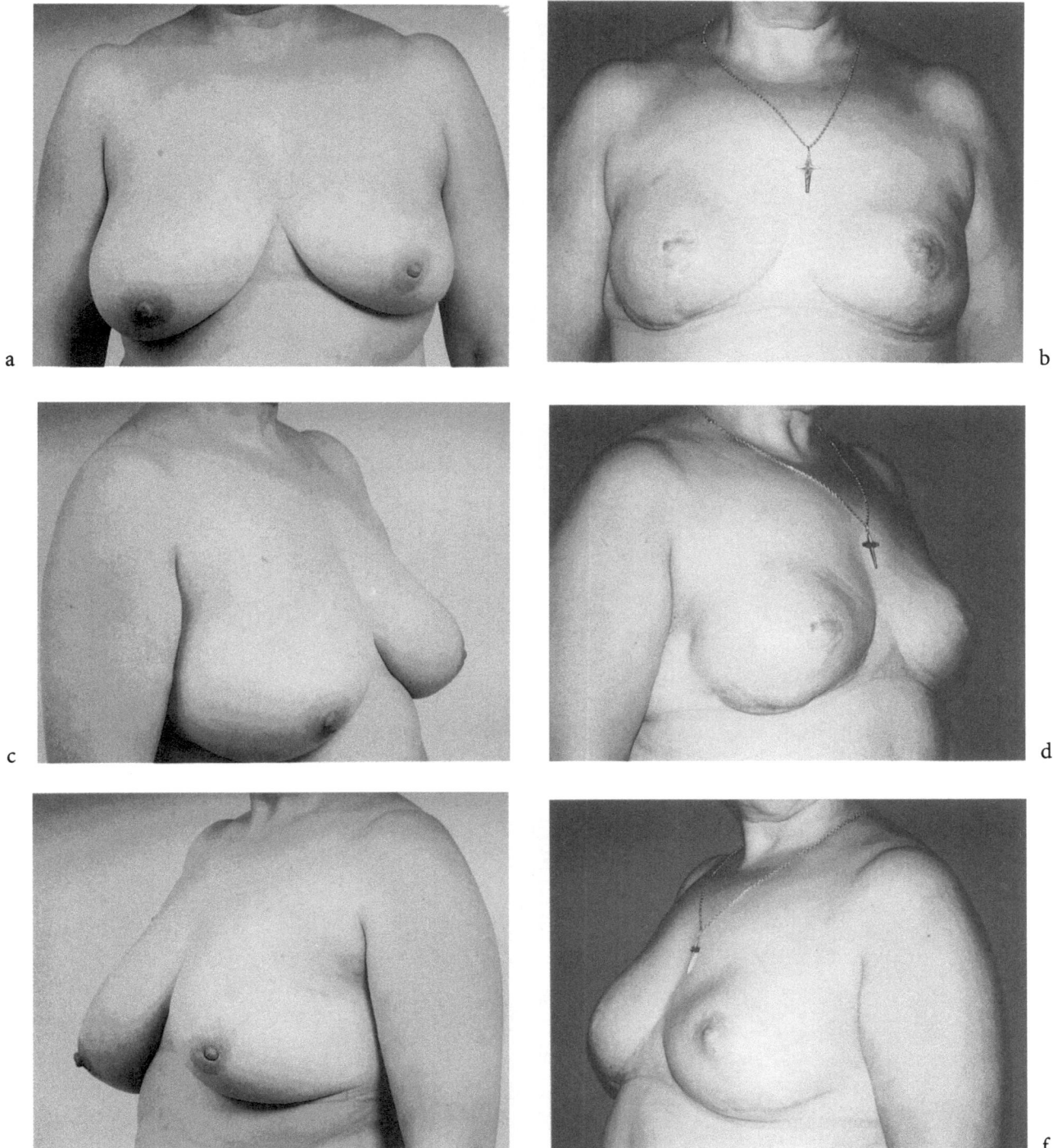

Fig. 257 a-f. Bilateral subcutaneous mastectomy (several previous operations on the left side for high-risk dystrophic lesions). Partial necrosis at angles of T on each side and of right areola, healed after local care but producing depigmentation of right areola. Definitive appearance after change of prosthesis (initial volume 350 ml, definitive volume 480 ml)

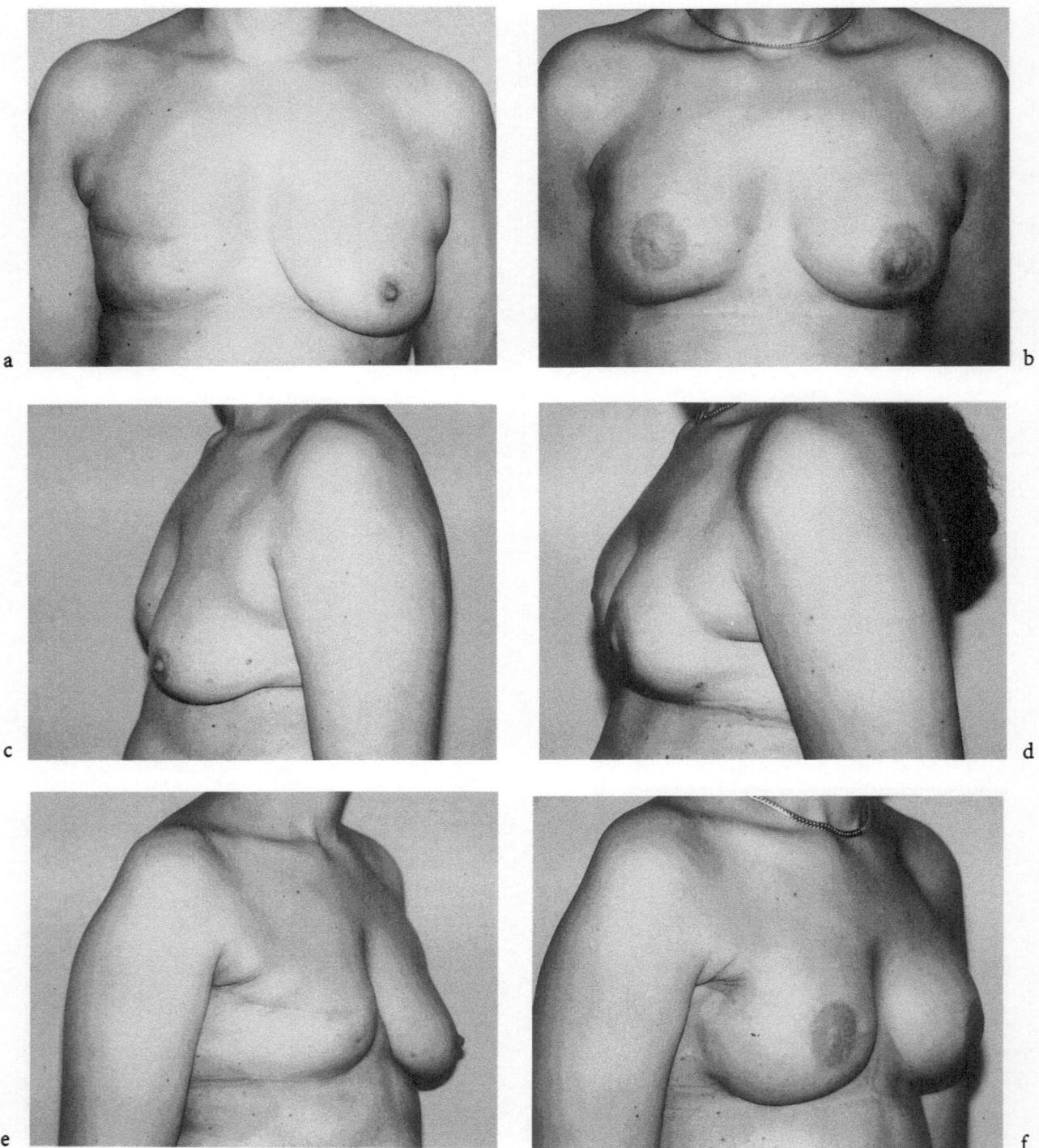

Fig. 258 a-f. Right breast reconstruction and left subcutaneous mastectomy.
Left: before operation
Right: the reconstruction was combined with ablation of the subcutaneous glandular remnant present in the inner quadrants. Reconstruction of volume by smooth inflatable Sebbin LS20 implant of 175 ml filled to 235 ml on each side. Subsequent partial necrosis of areola and loss of nipple contour on left side. Reconstruction of both nipple-areolar plaques by tattooing and ear- lobe grafts

Conclusion

Subcutaneous mastectomy is a difficult procedure as regards both the glandular excision and restoration of shape.

It is much criticised by many because of the inevitable persistence under the skin envelope, which is mammary skin, of a certain amount of gland tissue, at least histologically, if only because of the presence of the crests of Duret. But, if correctly performed, which is admittedly difficult, it leaves no more gland beneath the skin (apart from the areola) than does mastectomy in certain circumstances, when the ellipse of skin incision hardly does more than circumscribe the areola (fig. 258).

The chief criticism that can be leveled against it is really the inconstant quality of the morphologic result, the more difficult to predict when there has been major readjustment of the skin envelope; and since this operation is intended for women in whom the breast carries only a risk of malignant degeneration, a poor cosmetic result is less readily accepted.

References

Lalardrie JP, Morel-Fatio D (1970) Mammectomie totale sous-cutanée suivie de reconstruction immédiate ou secondaire. Mém Acad Chir, 96: 651-662

Extended excisions

Whether due to a wide excision necessitated by a tumoral recurrence after mastectomy or by a problem of radionecrosis, losses of thoracic substance so created need to be covered by a flap because of their size and depth and because the underlying tissues are often of poor nutritional status which would not allow the application of a free graft, the cosmetic outcome of which would naturally be disastrous.

Three types of flaps are perferentially indicated:
– a pedicled omentoplasty,
– a latissimus dorsi flap,
– a rectus abdominis flap.

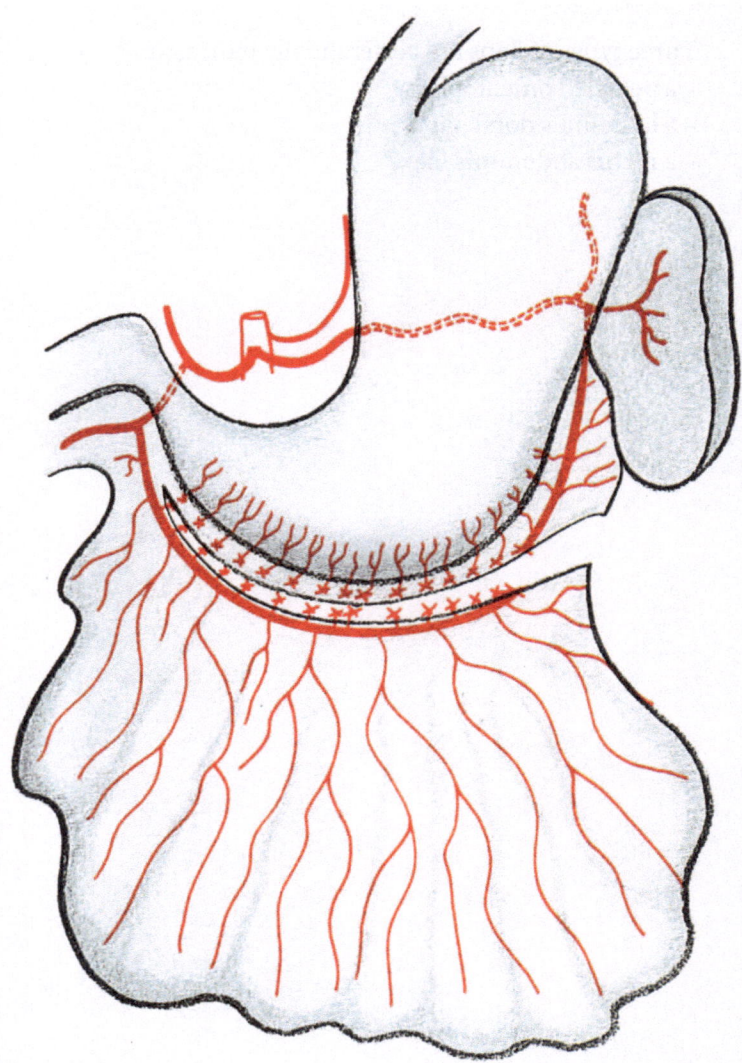

Fig. 259. Isolation of great omentum on right gastroepiploic pedicle

Pedicled omentoplasty

This was described initially by Kiricuta, who first used it extraperitoneally to cover the lesions of thoracic radionecrosis, a technique which remains the one of choice, since the excellent nutritional status of the omentum allows it to adhere to an irradiated substrate without any problems.

The procedure is begun by laparotomy through a midline incision above the umbilicus (if there is the scar of a previous laparomy another technique is advisable if possible, since the omentum is often no longer usable).

The omentum is turned upward, the transverse colon spread horizontally and drawn downward by the assistant, and freeing begins by separating it from the colon, the dissection being very careful in handling the omentum while respecting the mesocolic vessels. It is easier to start this dissection, which is associated with opening of the omental bursa, at the middle and to ʹɔllow it laterally.

When the detachment of the colon from the omentum is completed, freeing of the omentum along the greater curvature of the stomach is performed step by step with ligation at intervals, after identification of the gastroepiploic arch, the short vessels being tied pedicle by pedicle to prevent the formation of a hematoma on either the gastric or the omental side.

The omentum is pedicled on the right gastroepiploic vessels, which are larger than the left gastroepiploic vessels, and its left extremity is freed and sectioned with due care for the splenic vessels (fig. 259).

Once the freeing is completed, its viability is assessed and the omentum is reflected up towards the thoracic region without torsion of its pedicle, while the abdominal cavity is checked and closed. The peritoneal and aponeurotic closure are made so as to leave an opening above just sufficient for passage of the pedicle, and the omentum is brought into the thoracic region by subcutaneous tunneling.

The viability of the omentum is checked (there should be no hesitation in sacrificing its extremity if its viability is dubious) and the irradiated tissues are then excised as widely as possible in relation to the available omental surface, which is often very large (fig. 260).

It is then convenient to anchor the omental margins to the periphery of the loss of substance by a few absorbable sutures to prevent secondary retraction.

Then the omental surface is immediately covered with a thin dermo-epidermal graft, which takes excellently because of the quality of the underlying material. Immediate grafting is preferable for the same reasons: to prevent retraction and drying out of the omentum.

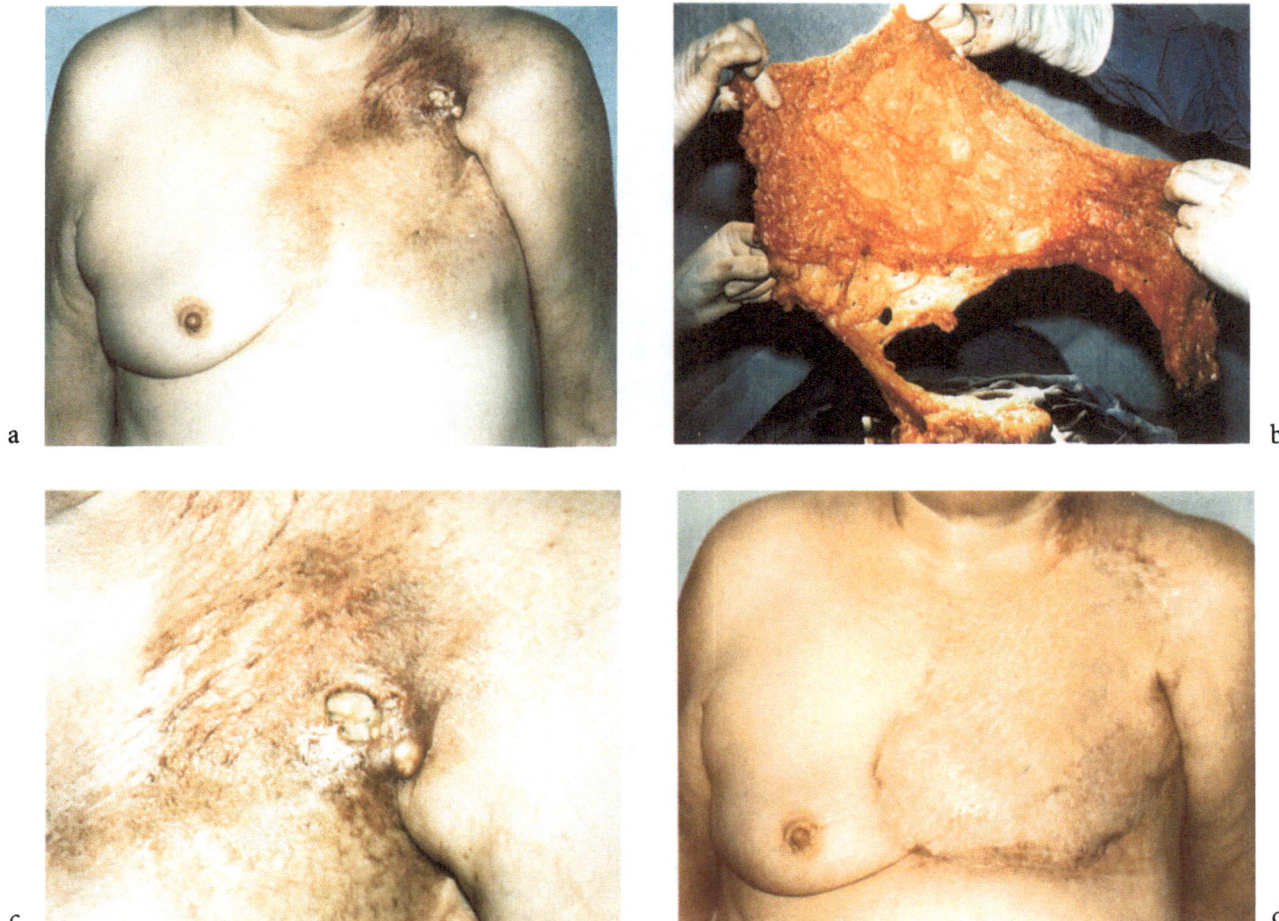

Fig. 260 a-d. 71-year-old patient: Halsted operation + irradiation. Presence of radionecrosis of skin and bone. Excision of necrotic layer, curettage (cautious because of proximity of subclavian vessels to bony lesions) and coverage by pedicled omentoplasty (Drs. Fallouh and Bricout). The left extremity of the omentum, visible at right in **c**, has been sacrificed at the outset as seemingly of poor viability. Coverage of omentum by imediate split-skin graft

Latissimus dorsi flap

Very large skin islands can be obtained with a latissimus dorsi flap, beyond the limits of a cosmetic indication, the size of the skin island no longer being restricted by the need for direct closure of the loss of substance.

The largest and most reliable island is that fashioned astride the anterior border of the muscle, taking the apex of the axillary fossa as the pivotal point of its arc of rotation (fig. 261).

The flap can be raised in dorsal decubitus, the thoracic region being elevated from the plane of the table by a rolled draw-sheet under the scapula.

Unlike pedicled flaps for the cervicofacial region, it is not usually necessary for homolateral use to dissect the island vascular pedicle, but a double pedicle, vascu-

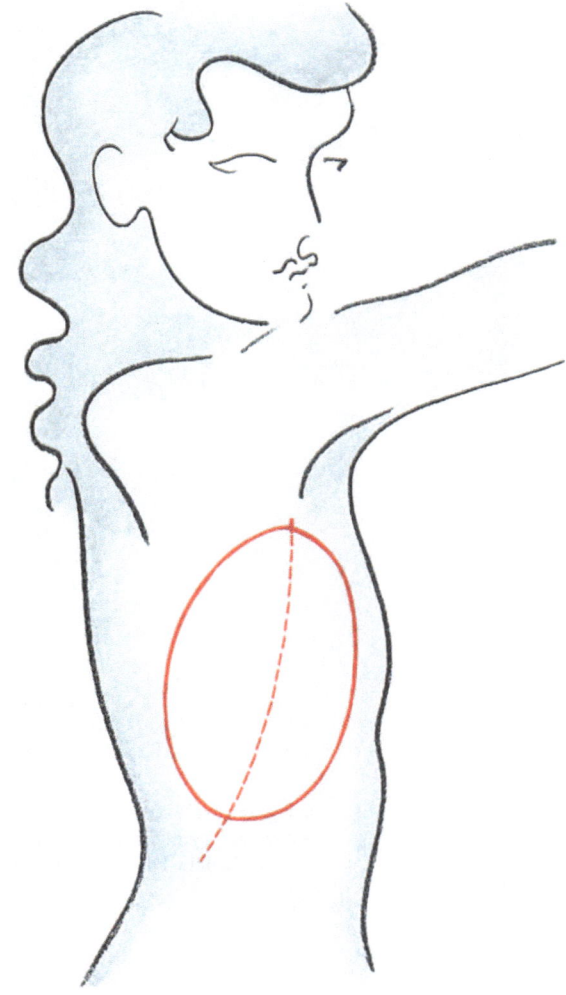

Fig. 261. Raising of a latissimus flap whose skin island straddles the anterior border of the muscle

lar and muscular, can be preserved which provides additional security. In practice, the axilla has often been irradiated, and even with an intact thoracodorsal pedicle the quality of the venous return may be diminished by the adjacent sclerosis. It should also be borne in mind that this flap can be raised on the thoracic branch if the main subscapular pedicle has been damaged. If, at the start of the dissection, a thoracic vessel of abnormally large caliber is discovered, this should be respected until the pedicle has been inspected, since such increased caliber is often a sign of interruption of the subscapular pedicle.

The loss of substance of the donor area is grafted immediately or later, after having reduced the dimensions of the lateral thoracic loss of substance as much as possible by sutures passed at some distance from its margins and taking a firm grip in the deep aspect of the dermis (fig. 262).

A split-skin graft performed secondarily on the granulation tissue which forms after several days under the greasy dressings often takes better than an immediate graft on this foundation, which is too mobile with respiratory movements.

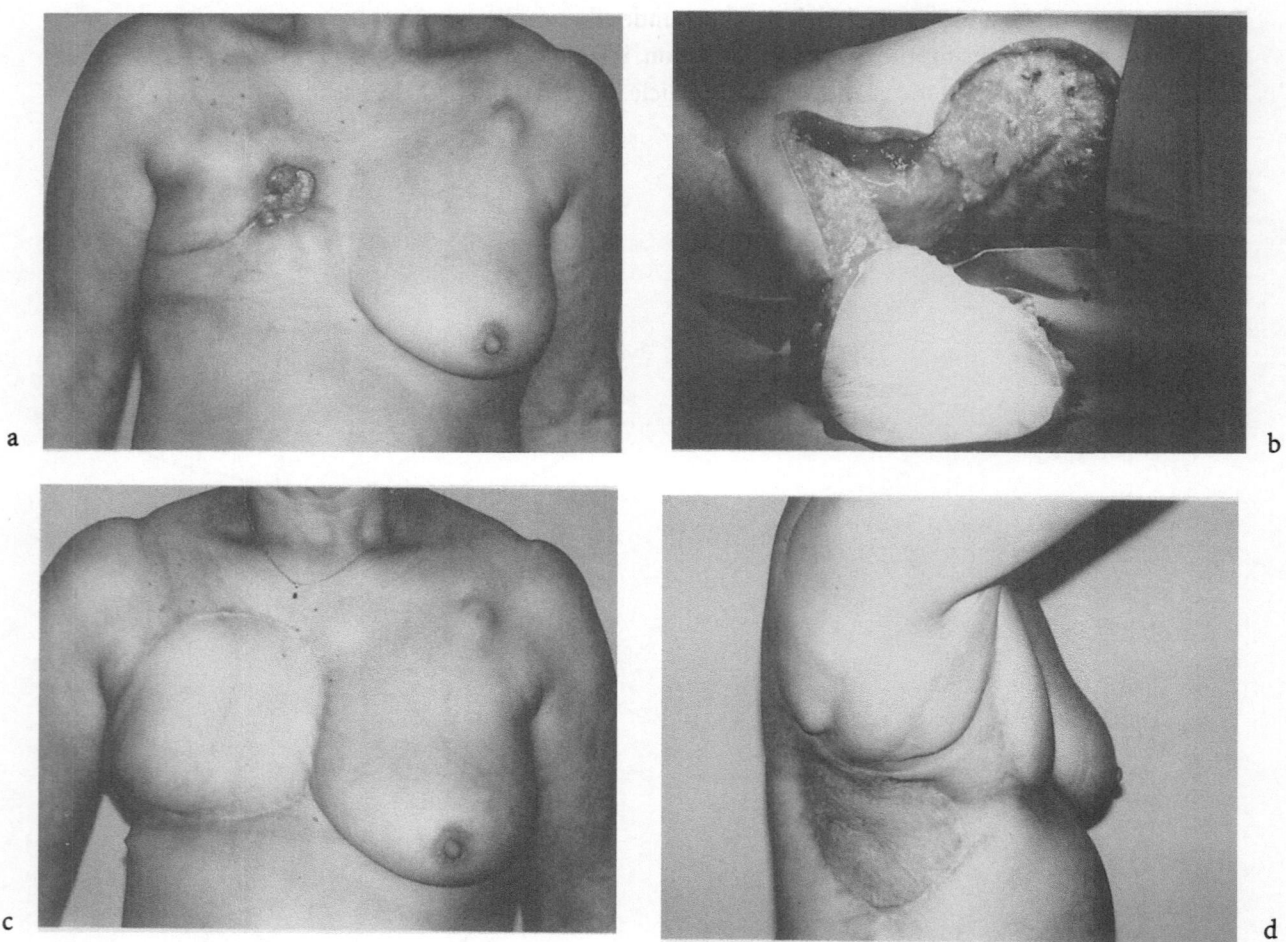

Fig. 262 a-d. Recurrence after mastectomy involving skin and pectoral muscle. Excision down to costal plane, coverage by myocutaneous flap of latissimus dorsi of 17 cm diameter on a muscular and vascular pedicle, raised in dorsal decubitus. Secondary grafting of the donor region at 8 days

The latissimus flap so used allows coverage of very extensive losses of substance created by excision of recurrences after mastectomy, and even of radionecrotic areas if the omentum is not available (fig. 263). If the muscle is of excellent vascularity, its presence and thickness at its deep aspect make it preferable for a

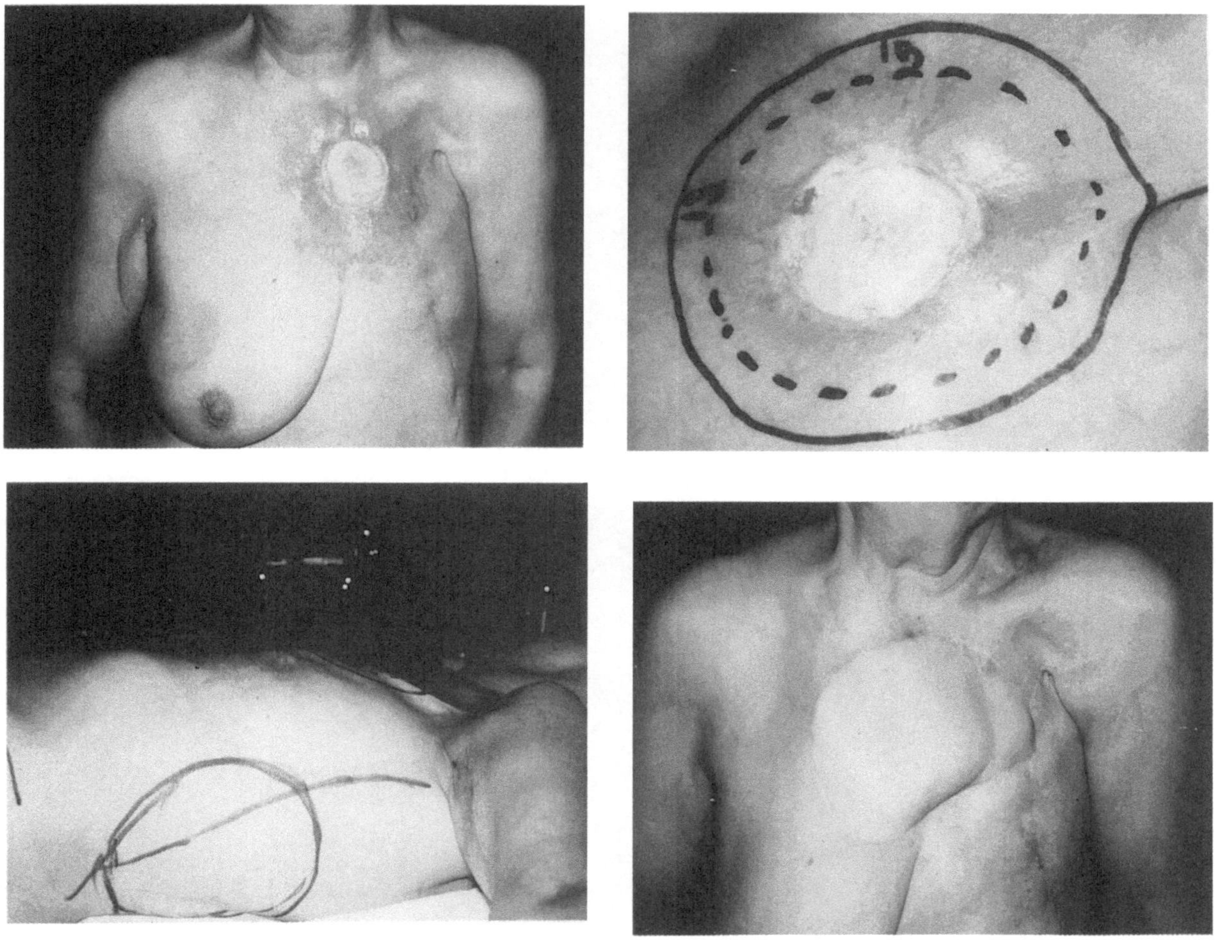

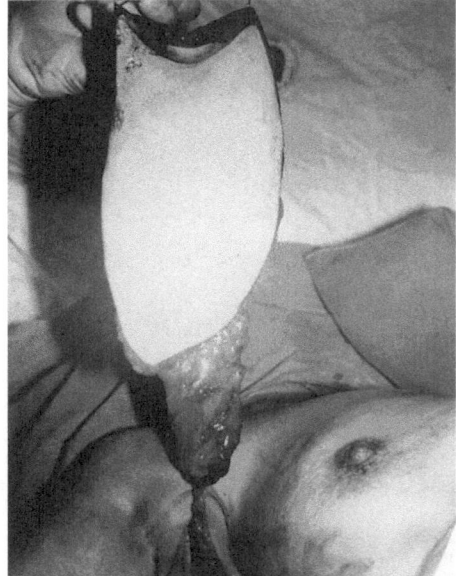

Fig. 263 a-e. 75-year-old patient: Halsted procedure + radiotherapy 15 years previously. Presternal radionecrosis developed after treatment of a local recurrence by (an overdosage of) radium therapy.
Design of a flap of the homolateral latissimus dorsi, but preliminary exploration of the axillary fossa did not reveal the pedicle of the latissimus, injured at the time of nodal clearance. The patient's build allowed coverage of the lesion by a pedicled flap with vascular island of the opposite latissimus, reaching the excisional zone by passage between breast and pectoralis

particular circumstance: when it is intended to perform radium therapy at the site of loss of substance, the guide tubes can be placed by the radiotherapist during the procedure itself (fig. 264).

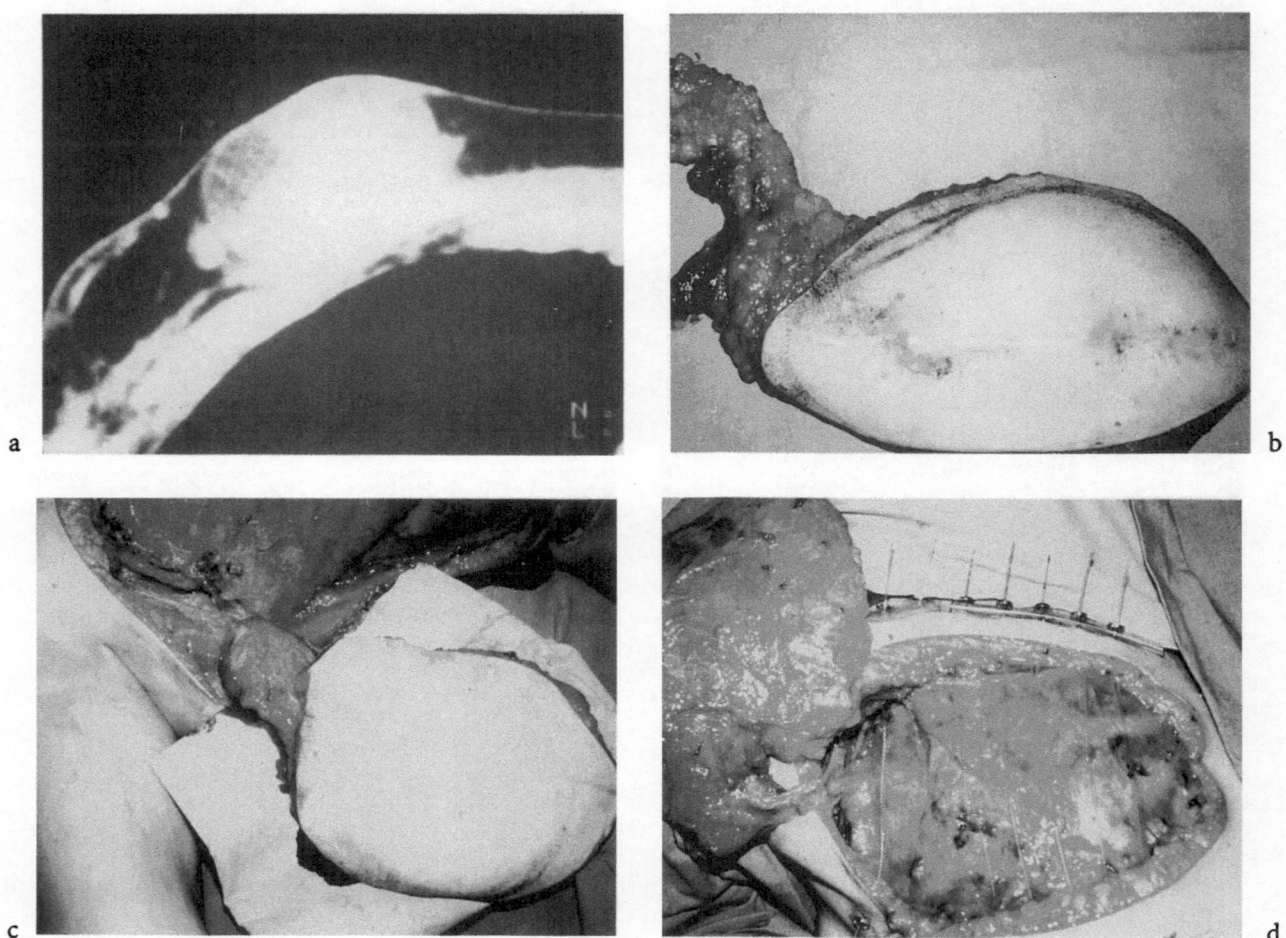

a

b

c

d

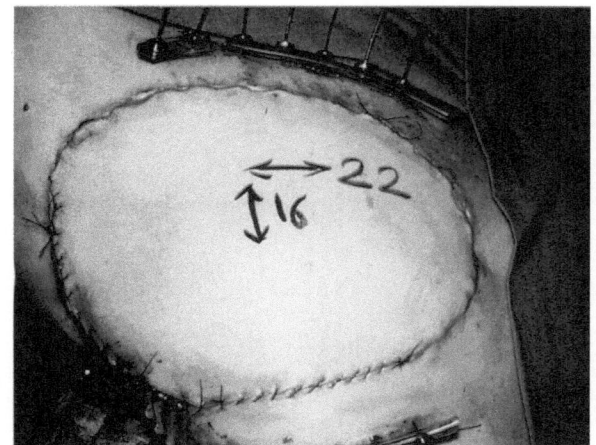

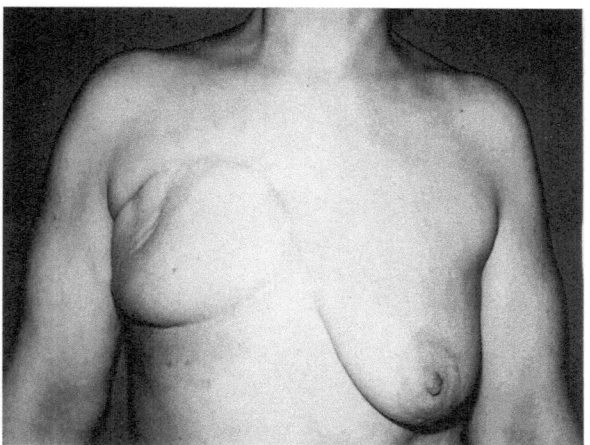

e

f

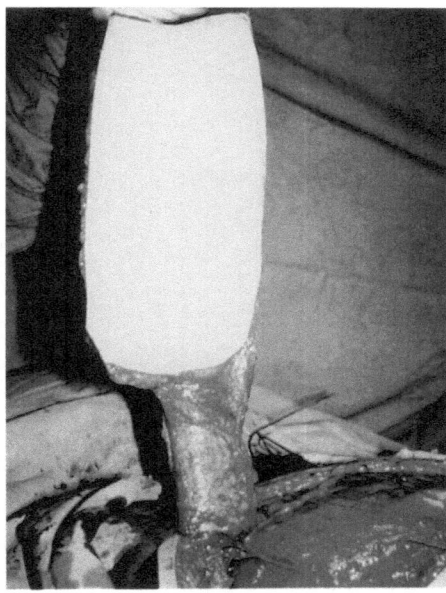

g

Fig. 264 a-g. a Parietal recurrence of comedo-carcinoma; **b** wide excision down to costal plane; **d** placement of guide tubes for radium therapy; **c, g** coverage by homolateral pedicled latissimus flap e radium therapy given at 3rd postoperative day; **f** appearance at 2 years

Rectus abdominis flap

In its bipedicled version (since for the particular indications of wide excision the entire skin island must be preserved without incurring any vascular risks), the rectus flap also allows coverage of extensive losses of thoracic substance, provided always that the patient has sufficient excess of subumbilical tissue (fig. 265).

Compared with the latissimus flap, it has the advantage for an equal surface area of ensuring direct closure of the donor region. On the other hand, its deep aspect consists mainly of fatty tissue and very little muscle.

Therefore it is best reserved for excision of recurrences when radium treatment is not indicated. Nor do we consider it indicated for the coverage of radionecrotic areas, again because of its essentially fatty substrate; in such cases, omental or latissimus flaps are preferable.

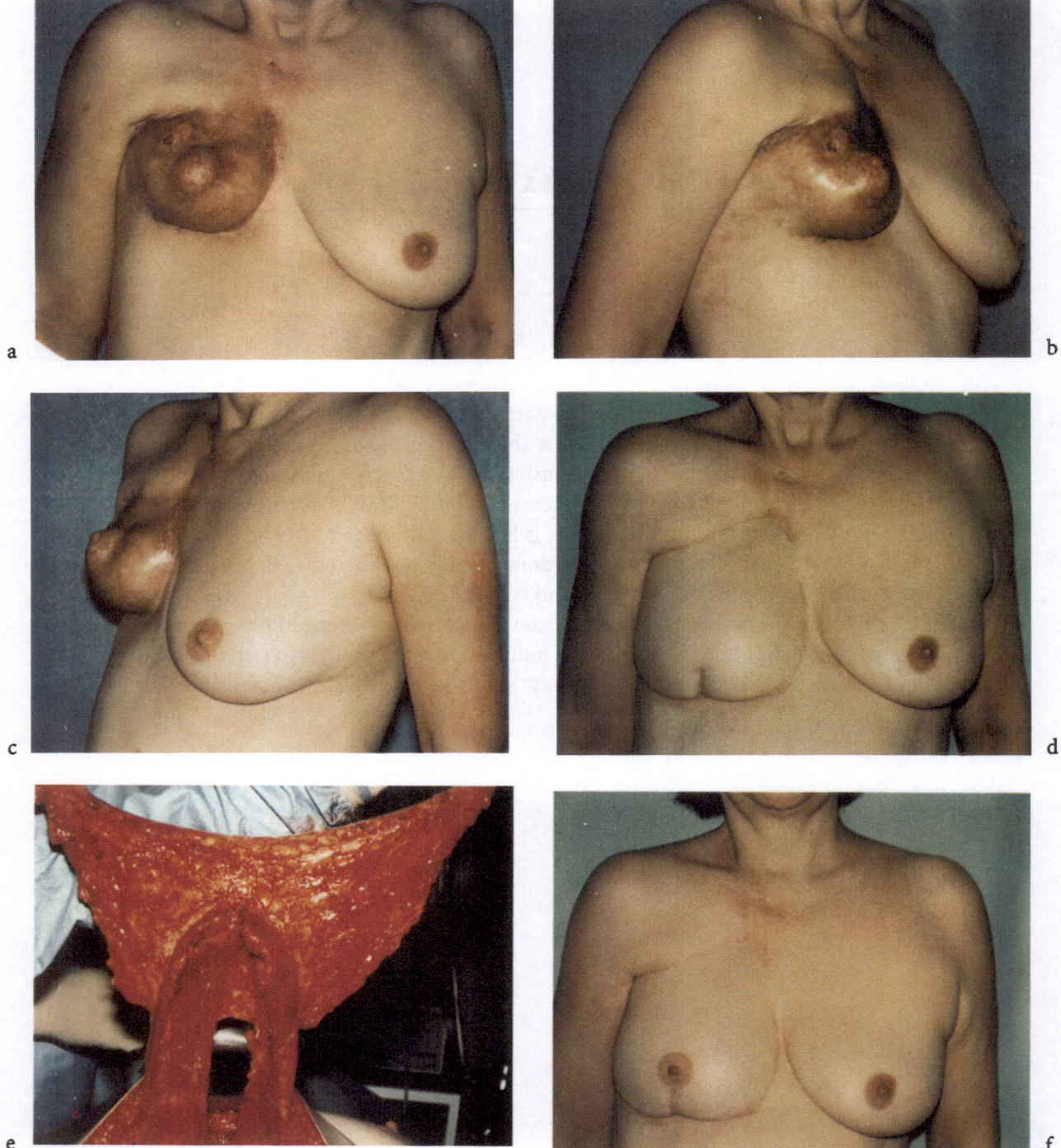

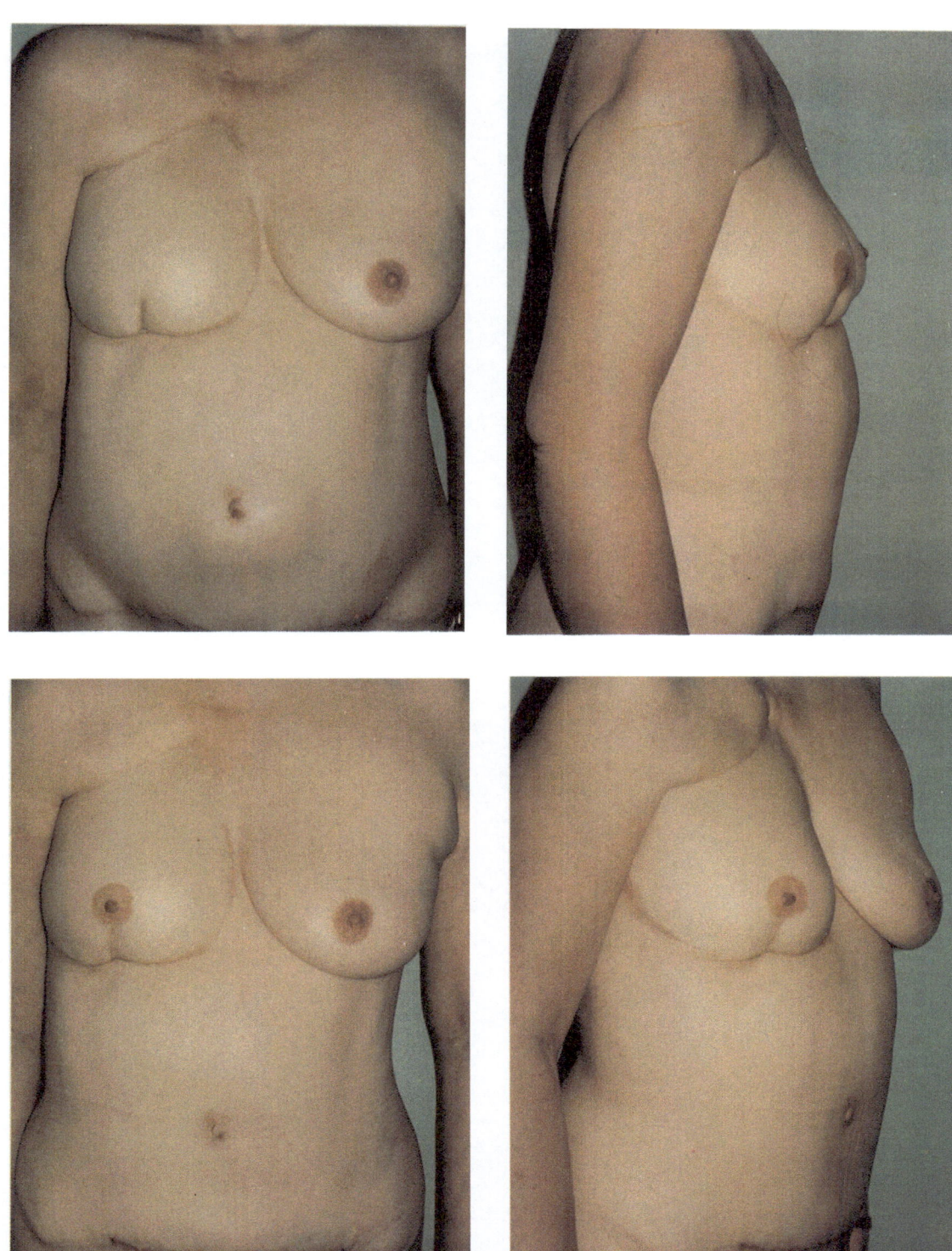

Summary

For ulcerated areas of radionecrosis the preferential method of coverage remains a pedicled omentoplasty, because of its excellent nutritional status, responsible for its cleansing ability and its adhesion to a substrate of poor quality.

Latissimus and rectus flaps share the indications in wide excisions for recurrences, depending on the local and morphologic conditions of the patient.

In these indications, for an equivalent excisional surface area, usally extensive, the donor zone of the latissimus dorsi must be grafted, whereas with a rectus flap direct closure can be made.

The latissimus flap is the only one which, because of the extent of muscle on its deep aspect, allows combined radium treatment.

References

Bricout N, Servant JM (1987) Fermeture de la zone de prélèvement d'un lambeau de grand dorsal. Ann Chir Plast Esth 32/3: 228

Kiricuta (1963) L'emploi du grand épiploon dans la chirurgie du sein cancéreux. Presse Méd 71: 15-17

Index